Patel's Atlas of Transradial Intervention
The Basics and Beyond

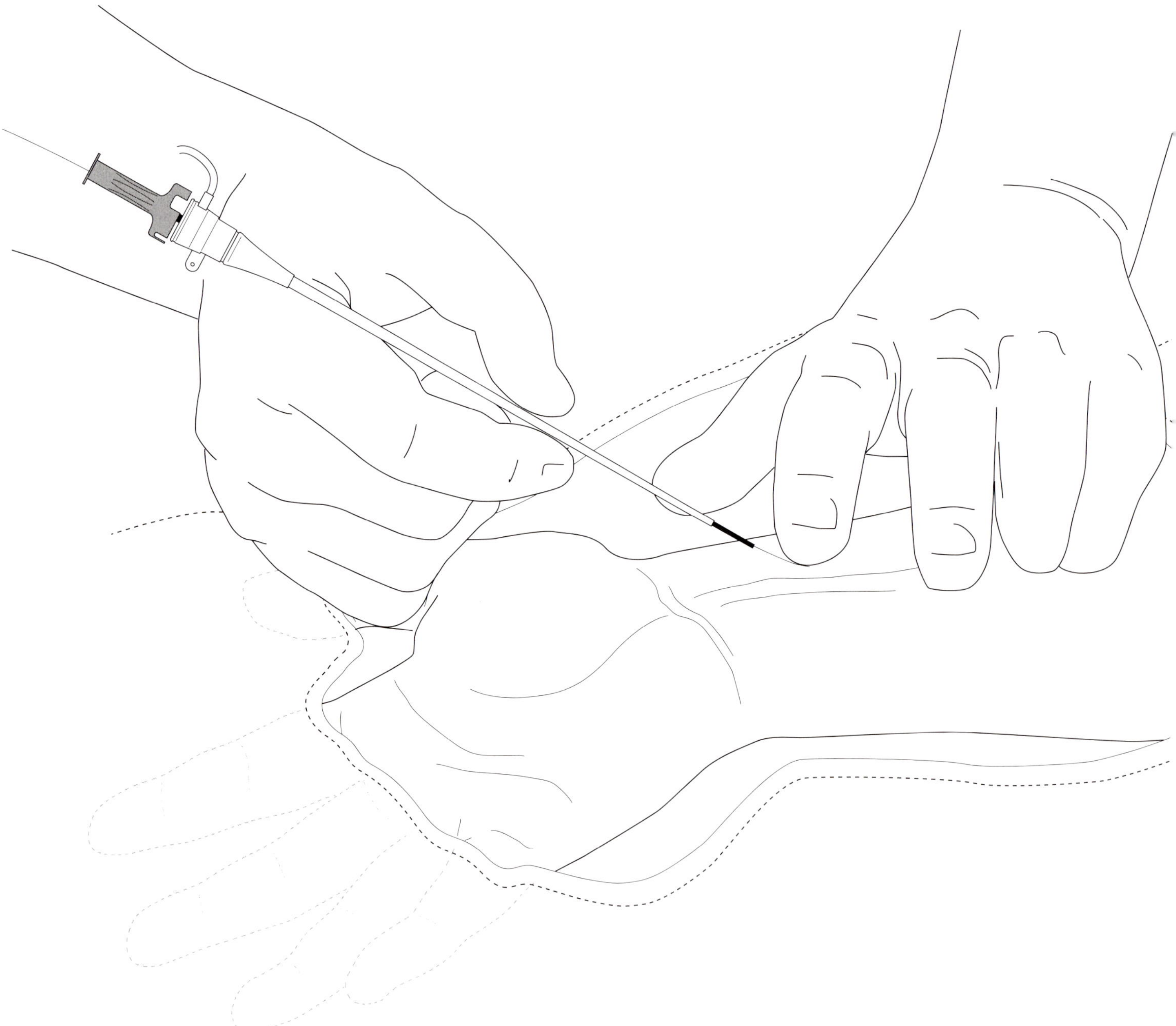

Patel's Atlas of Transradial Intervention
The Basics and Beyond

Editor-in-Chief

Tejas Patel, MD, DM, FACC, FSCAI, FESC
Chairman
Apex Heart Institute
Professor and Head
Department of Cardiology
Smt. N.H.L. Municipal Medical College
Sheth V. S. General Hospital
Ahmedabad, India

Co-Editors

Sanjay Shah, MD, DM
Director
Department of Cardiology
Apex Heart Institute
Assistant Professor of Cardiology
Smt. N.H.L. Municipal Medical College
Sheth V. S. General Hospital
Ahmedabad, India

Samir B. Pancholy
MD, FACP, FACC, FSCAI
Program Director
Cardiology Fellowship
Wright Center for Graduate Medical Education
Associate Professor of Medicine
The Commonwealth Medical College
Scranton, PA, USA

With 29 Contributors

Editorial Assistants
Yash Soni
Chidambaram Iyer

Illustrator
Gopal Limbad

ISBN: 978-1-893446-05-2

First printing March 2012

As the transradial procedure evolves, we can look forward to changes in technique, hardware, and drugs. The authors and publisher have taken extreme care to ensure that this atlas conveys the most accurate, evidence-based information available at the time of publication.

Readers are advised to keep abreast of the latest developments in this elegant, patient-friendly procedure.

Additional information:
www.transradialWORLD.com

Preface

No medical specialty moves faster than contemporary cardiovascular medicine, and no medical specialty depends more on images and graphics than interventional cardiology. Featuring an enhanced and reader-friendly design, this atlas covers basics of the transradial approach (TRA), need-to-know clinical advances, and issues that are becoming increasingly vital to new and experienced radial operators worldwide.

Through the 25 chapters, the reader will find the most complete overview of the TRA, along with a timely focus on evidence-based medicine. Angiographic plates supported by schematic diagrams and concise take-home bullets provide a simple but extremely effective teaching and learning tool. The highly distilled text of the atlas provides a convenient and practical tool to help radial operators master key aspects of TRA. We have especially focused on the most important and common clinical problems that confront radialists on a regular basis. We have also highlighted the availability of different techniques without neglecting the tried-and-true — all while striving to acquaint the reader with the weaknesses and strengths of each of them in balanced fashion.

We express our sincere thanks to the authors and co-authors for their extraordinary dedication and commitment to a rigorous time schedule that allowed publication of this atlas in record time of one year. In a nutshell, this volume is designed to serve as a ready reference for all real world problems as well as a background source for easy perusal during spare moments.

Tejas Patel
Sanjay Shah
Samir Pancholy

Acknowledgment

Our deepest appreciation goes to our cardiology team colleagues who helped us with our challenging cases and shared their thoughtful comments. We express our heartfelt gratitude to Dr. Ian Gilchrist, who not only wrote an excellent chapter but also volunteered to edit the atlas. We owe a lot to the contributors for sparing time and sharing their experiences for this atlas. Very special thanks goes to Dr. Shigeru Saito for mentoring our transradial program. Carol Garzona deserves a very special thanks from us. We also extend our sincere thanks to Chidambaram Iyer, Gopal Limbad, Yash Soni and our publisher, without whom this project would have remained a dream. Thank-yous go to our cath-lab nurses, technicians, secretaries and attendants for doing all the things that make the transradial procedure so easy. We offer our deepest appreciation to our patients, who unconditionally stood by us. We offer our apologies and gratitude to our wives Sonali, Komal and Dipti, who put up with our moods as we assembled a first-of-its-kind book.

List of Contributors

Olivier F. Bertrand, MD, PhD, FSCAI
Interventional Cardiologist
Quebec Heart-Lung Institute
Associate Professor
Faculty of Medicine, Laval University
Quebec City, Canada

Ronald P. Caputo, MD, FACC, FSCAI
Director of Cardiac Services
St. Joseph's Hospital
Associate Clinical Professor of Medicine
SUNY Health Science Center
Syracuse, NY, USA

John Coppola, MD, FACC, FSCAI
Clinical Assistant Professor
NYU Langone Medical Center
New York, NY, USA

Keith Fonseca, MBBS
Medical Officer
Apex Heart Institute
Ahmedabad, India

Biren Gandhi, MBBS
Medical Officer
Apex Heart Institute
Ahmedabad, India

Ian C. Gilchrist
MD, FACC, FAHA, FSCAI, FCCM
Professor of Medicine
Pennsylvania State University
Heart And Vascular Institute
Hershey, PA, USA

Rajiv Gulati, MD, PhD, FACC, FSCAI
Consultant
Division of Cardiovascular Diseases
Assistant Professor of Medicine
College of Medicine
Mayo Clinic
Rochester, MN, USA

Sasko Kedev, MD, PhD, FESC, FACC
Director
University Clinic of Cardiology,
"Ss. Cyril and Methodius" University
President
Macedonian Society of Cardiology
Skopje, Macedonia

Mitchell W. Krucoff
MD, FACC, FAHA, FSCAI, FAPSIC
Professor Medicine/Cardiology
Duke University Medical Center
Director
CV Devices Unit
Duke Clinical Research Institute
Durham, NC, USA

Tak W. Kwan, MD, FACC, FACP, FSCAI
Associate Clinical Professor of Medicine
Albert Einstein College of Medicine
Adjunct Clinical Associate Professor of Medicine
NYU School of Medicine
Senior Associate Director
Cardiac Catheterization Laboratory and Interventional Cardiology
Beth Israel Medical Center
New York, NY, USA

Yves Louvard, MD, FSCAI
ICPS
Hopital privé Jacques Cartier
Massy, France

Josef Ludwig, MD, PhD
University Clinic
Erlangen, Germany

Tift Mann, MD, FACC, FSCAI
Wake Heart and Vascular Associates
Raleigh, NC, USA

Samir B. Pancholy
MD, FACP, FACC, FSCAI
Program Director
Cardiology Fellowship
Wright Center for Graduate Medical Education
Associate Professor of Medicine
The Commonwealth Medical College
Scranton, PA, USA

Tejan B. Patel, MD, FACC, FSCAI
Director
Interventional Cardiology
Unity Health System
Rochester, NY, USA

Tejas Patel
MD, DM, FACC, FSCAI, FESC
Chairman
Apex Heart Institute
Professor and Head
Department of Cardiology
Smt. NHL Municipal Medical College
Sheth VS General Hospital
Ahmedabad, India

Chistopher Pyne, MD, FACC, FSCAI
Department of Interventional Cardiology
Lahey Clinic Medical Center
Burlington, Massachusetts, USA

Ramon Quesada
MD, FACP, FACC, FSCAI
Medical Director
Interventional Cardiology, Cardiac Research & Outcomes
Baptist Cardiac & Vascular Institute
Clinical Associate Professor of Medicine
Herbert Wertheim College of Medicine at Florida International University
Miami, FL, USA

Rajnikant Radadiya, MD
Medical Intensivist
Apex Heart Institute
Ahmedabad, India

Alok Ranjan, MD, DNB, MRCP, DM
Senior Consultant
Interventional Cardiology
Wockhardt Hospital
Surat, India

Sunil V. Rao, MD FACC FSCAI
Associate Professor of Medicine
Duke University Medical Center
Director
Cardiac Catheterization Laboratories
VA Medical Center
Durham, NC, USA

Charanjit S. Rihal, MD, MBA
Professor of Medicine
Chair of the Division of Cardiovascular Diseases
Mayo Clinic
Rochester, MN, USA

Kintur Sanghvi, MD, FACC, FSCAI
Director of Transradial Program
Interventional Cardiology & Endovascular Medicine
Deborah Heart and Lung Institute
Browns Mills, NJ, USA

Leena Shah, MD
Medical Intensivist
Apex Heart Institute
Ahmedabad, India

Pinak B. Shah, MD, FACC, FSCAI
Director
Interventional Cardiology Training Program
Brigham and Women's Hospital
Assistant Professor of Medicine
Harvard Medical School
Boston, MA, USA

Sanjay Shah, MD, DM
Director
Department of Cardiology
Apex Heart Institute
Assistant Professor of Cardiology
Smt. N.H.L. Municipal Medical College
Sheth V. S. General Hospital
Ahmedabad, India

Kimberly A. Skelding MD, FACC, FAHA, FSCAI
Associate, Interventional Cardiology
Geisinger Medical Center
Director of Cardiovascular Genomics and Cardiovascular Research
Geisinger Health System
Director of Women's Heart and Vascular Health Program
Danville, PA, USA

Jennifer A. Tremmel, MD, MS
Assistant Professor of Medicine
Stanford University Medical Center
San Francisco, CA, USA

Chirayu Vyas, MD, DM
Interventional Cardiologist
Apex Heart Institute
Visiting Interventional Cardiologist
Sheth V. S. General Hospital
Ahmedabad, India

Contents

Foreword

Ian C. Gilchrist, MD, FACC, FAHA, FSCAI, FCCM

Andreas Gruentzig is quoted as having said, "If I have an enemy, I will teach him angioplasty." The modern corollary for the interventional cardiology may be that if I am a friend, I will teach him transradial techniques. Since the introduction of modern percutaneous transradial cardiac catheterization and, subsequently, angioplasty in the late 1980s and early 1990s, no other addition to the invasive cardiologist's toolbox has promised to reduce overnight the operator's vascular complication rate to nearly-zero and endear the patients to the extent transradial techniques have. Despite outcomes that might otherwise be considered a patient-care breakthrough, worldwide dissemination has been slow — even reminiscent of Darwin's finches evolving diverse approaches in geographic isolation. Textbooks that detail transradial approaches have been rare and, in many countries (not the least being the United States), educational resources have been few and far between.

After 20 years, a definitive guide for transradial can now be found in The Atlas of Transradial Interventions: The Basics and Beyond. This is the successor to Dr. Tejas Patel's basic atlas, first published in 2007. It has grown from the extensive local experience of Dr. Patel and his colleagues from Ahmedabad, India, to a now-international volume that combines the best of many practices around the world in a highly readable text. The results of many Darwinian radial experiences have been cultivated in this latest atlas and summarized in one text. Emblematic of the personal and open exchange of ideas found in the radial community, many of the authors have been featured at one time or another at Dr. Patel's TRICO courses in Ahmedabad. TRICO has grown to one of the largest of such teaching courses in the world, convening radialists from around the world, and ultimately has enriched this Atlas.

The Atlas, while expanded, has retained the visual focus and clarity of the initial volume. Interventional cardiologists are visually oriented, and this style is ideal for rapidly transferring information to the reader. The subject matter is escalated through the initial chapters, starting from the basics of access and patient preparation into techniques to succeed in interventional procedures. The later, coronary-based chapters explore essentially all the complex patient subsets and touch on the advanced non-balloon techniques that can be done transradially. It beautifully demonstrates that transradial can be the default strategy for most coronary procedures and shows the reader how to succeed.

After the spectrum of transradial coronary procedures are discussed, the Atlas leads the reader beyond the heart into non-cardiac circulation. Peripheral vascular, reno-vascular and neurovascular techniques are shown again in a format that relies on illustration and pictures, with support from focused text. Many different situations are shown and solutions demonstrated. While no guide can cover every possible situation, the understanding and the thought processes demonstrated in the illustrations leaves the reader with knowledge that can feed further exploration and imagination.

The Atlas finishes with several didactic chapters. More words, fewer pictures and illustrations than the earlier chapters, these later chapters are well-written discussions of the state of transradial, the data supporting its use and the logistics of establishing a transradial program. These later chapters compliment the pictorial approach to the individual components of transradial techniques that predominate the procedural part of the Atlas. They wonderfully summarize how the techniques demonstrated in the earlier chapters come together in the bigger picture of practice.

Transradial techniques are gaining traction after 20 years of development by a diverse group of dedicated cardiologists. Patients are talking about it, regulators and insurance payers are talking about it, clinical studies are driving evidence of its effectiveness, and now even cardiologists in the United States are understanding the importance of learning these techniques. A few traditional textbooks on transradial are available, but no guidebooks exist. Patel's Atlas is the guidebook every transradial operator needs. Whether recently trained or a long-term operator, all expertise levels can learn from the diverse, illustrative techniques and ideas contained herein. It can be read quickly in an evening, but contains many years of culminated experience from trial and error to share and even provide seeds for novel applications not yet considered by the authors. This is the guidebook to transradial techniques that should compliment all operators' experiences and remain a resource for transradial catheterization.

Ian C. Gilchrist, MD, FACC, FAHA, FSCAI, FCCM
Professor of Medicine
Pennsylvania State University
Heart and Vascular Institute
Hershey, Pennsylvania, USA

Jeffrey J. Popma, MD

Over the 4 years since Patel's Atlas of Transradial Intervention: The Basics was published, interventional cardiology has evolved dramatically. I have to admit, I didn't see such profound changes coming so quickly. As the interventional landscape develops, I'm reminded of an old proverb: "The more things change, the more they stay the same." I think the 2012 paraphrase would be "Things have to change to stay the same."

Interventionalists need to evolve to maintain a central position in medical decision-making. We're now under increased scrutiny for our decisions, held accountable by our patients and colleagues, payers responsible for hospital and professional reimbursement, and governmental agencies that oversee responsible and ethical medical practice. The value of our decisions is no longer based solely on our clinical acumen and experience, but increasingly on our adherence to an expanding number of published societal practice guidelines[1] culminating in "appropriateness criteria."[2,3]

"Compliance to guidelines" and "attainment of performance measures" are key phrases for those responsible for quality and public reporting. I actually think this is good for interventionalists, because it makes us think about what we're doing. If we disagree, we're obligated to present an evidence-based rationale for what we do for our patients. In short, standardization and acceptance of the new techniques and therapies based on patient outcomes is a laudable goal.

Since Atlas of Transradial Intervention: The Basics was published, an explosive number of clinical studies have emphasized the important role of bleeding and access-site complications, particularly in patients with acute coronary syndromes undergoing percutaneous coronary intervention (PCI).4-7 We all seek ways to reduce procedural complications in our clinical practices and, based on the results of recent randomized clinical trials and registries,[4-7] the evidence has dramatically shifted in favor or transradial access to improve patient outcomes.

Crucially, the 2011 ACCF-AHA-SCAI guidelines state, "the use of radial access can be useful to decrease access site complications (Class IIa, Level of Evidence A)."1 This seems like profound vindication to those who have historically advocated that transradial catheterization is actually better for our patients. It's also the mandate for interventionalists to begin to embrace transradial access to improve patient outcomes.

I'd like to think the Atlas of Transradial Intervention: The Basics in some way contributed to transradial catheterization's use in the United States increasing from 1% in 2006 to 6% in 2010 — although, still, less than 1 in 10 U.S. PCI patients undergoes transradial access.

I know the many reasons that interventionists shy away from radial access: unfamiliarity with the technique; resistance from cath lab staff; concerns over excess contrast, radiation, and time on the table; and the general feeling that complex procedures are compromised by radial access. But I am hopeful that the recent ACCF-AHA-SCAI recommendations will nudge more interventionalists to embrace radial transradial access.[1]

The new Atlas of Transradial Intervention: The Basics and Beyond is welcome as use of transradial access further increases. So many aspects of the atlas make it a wildly effective teaching source. The side-by-side angiograms and illustrations are unique to interventional textbooks, and the easy-to-read outline format simulates the expert formal presentation of the authors at their international teaching symposium.

The Atlas of Transradial Intervention: The Basics and Beyond dramatically expands on previous edition, with 9 new chapters and additional perspectives of international experts in transradial intervention. The thorough and thoughtful approach to the major issues of transradial catheterization addressed by the this volume have made it the definitive teaching source for transradial intervention.

For the novice radialist, the basics of patient selection (chapter 1), puncture technique (chapter 2), post-procedural management (chapter 3), complications (chapter 4) and establishing a transradial program (chapter 23) are presented clearly and concisely, to aid physicians and catheterization laboratory staff in the fundamentals of the radial approach. Initial procedures that focus on the basics with low-risk patients are the surest way to gain confidence with this technique. Mastering the fundamental maneuvers in straightforward cases renders the complex cases less problematic.

As the radial experience increases, so does the recognition of the challenges in patients with complex anatomy. An understanding of the anatomic variations of the radial and brachial arteries (chapter 5), navigation of the subclavian, innominate, and aorta (chapter 6), left radial radial (chapter 19), right heart catheterization (chapter 20), ulnar artery catheterization (chapter 24), and cannulation of the coronary ostia (chapter 7) will improve the procedural success rates with the transradial approach.

Many new techniques for specific anatomic subsets have been added to this edition, including transradial access for saphenous vein graft lesions (chapter 8), bifurcations lesions (chapter 9), left main coronary artery disease (chapter 10), chronic total occlusion (chapter 11) and acute myocardial infarctions (chapter 12). These sections are particularly valuable for the advanced interventionalist.

One of the most valuable aspects of this Edition is the dramatically expanded attention to peripheral vascular intervention, including internal carotid stenosis (chapter 13), vertibrobasilar disease (chapter 14), subclavian and innominate lesions (chapter 15), renal artery stenosis (chapter 16), iliac artery lesions (chapter 17), and mesenteric, celiac and superficial femoral artery lesions (chapter 18).

The Atlas of Transradial Intervention: The Basics and Beyond is a must-have for all interventional cardiologists. It will be on my shelf for ready access, and we'll use it as our teaching guide for our interventional fellows.

Whether you're a beginner considering becoming a radialist or an experienced radialist who wishes to fine-tune skills, you'll find this atlas an important part of your interventional library. This is our chance to evolve.

Jeffrey J. Popma, MD
Director, Interventional Cardiology Clinical Services
Beth Israel Deaconess Medical Center
Associate Professor of Medicine
Harvard University
Boston, Massachusetts, USA

References

1. Levine GN, Bates ER, Blankenship JC, et al. 2011 ACCF/AHA/SCAI Guideline for Percutaneous Coronary Intervention: a report of the American College of Cardiology Foundation/American Heart Association Task Force on Practice Guidelines and the Society for Cardiovascular Angiography and Interventions. Circulation. [Consensus Development Conference]. 2011;124:e574-651.
2. Patel MR, Dehmer GJ, Hirshfeld JW, et al. ACCF/SCAI/STS/AATS/AHA/ASNC/HFSA/SCCT 2012 appropriate use criteria for coronary revascularization focused update: A report of the American College of Cardiology Foundation Appropriate Use Criteria Task Force, Society for Cardiovascular Angiography and Interventions, Society of Thoracic Surgeons, American Association for Thoracic Surgery, American Heart Association, American Society of Nuclear Cardiology, and the Society of Cardiovascular Computed Tomography. J Am Coll Cardiol. 2012; DOI:10.1016/j.jacc.2011.12.001. Available at content.onlinejacc.org.
3. Patel MR, Dehmer GJ, Hirshfeld JW, et al. ACCF/SCAI/STS/AATS/AHA/ASNC 2009 appropriateness criteria for coronary revascularization: A report by the American College of Cardiology Foundation Appropriateness Criteria Task Force, Society for Cardiovascular Angiography and Interventions, Society of Thoracic Surgeons, American Association for Thoracic Surgery, American Heart Association, and the American Society of Nuclear Cardiology. J Am Coll Cardiol. 2009;53:530-553.
4. Jolly SS, Amlani S, Hamon M, et al. Radial versus femoral access for coronary angiography or intervention and the impact on major bleeding and ischemic events: a systematic review and meta-analysis of randomized trials. Am Heart J. 2009;157:132-140.
5. Jolly SS, Yusuf S, Cairns J, et al. Radial versus femoral access for coronary angiography and intervention in patients with acute coronary syndromes (RIVAL): a randomised, parallel group, multicentre trial. Lancet. 2011;377:1409-1420.
6. Vavalle JP, Rao SV. The association between the transradial approach for percutaneous coronary interventions and bleeding. J Invasive Cardiol. 2009;21:21A-24A.
7. Rao SV, Cohen MG, Kandzari DE, et al. The transradial approach to percutaneous coronary intervention: historical perspective, current concepts, and future directions. J Am Coll Cardiol. 2010;55:2187-2195.

"That which we persist in doing becomes easier, not that the task itself has become easier, but that our ability to perform it has improved."

Ralph Waldo Emerson (1803–1882)

Patient Selection, Cath Lab Setup and Patient Preparation

1

Tejas Patel, Sanjay Shah and Samir Pancholy

An experienced radialist can complete virtually every coronary angiogram and intervention through the radial route. However, when an interventionalist is first establishing a radial program, it is important that the first 200 cases be chosen carefully. Being selective in the beginning will build the understanding and confidence needed to convert oneself into a seasoned radialist.

In this chapter, the essential patient selection criteria for inclusion and exclusion for the beginning radialist are listed. These initial standards for patient selection have been used successfully to start transradial programs.

The Modified Allen's Test, the Inverse Allen's Test and alternative tests are discussed in detail. Although many expert radialists no longer perform these tests, the new radial operator will build confidence by incorporating them into the procedure.

The Ideal Patient for New Radialists

- Hemodynamically and clinically stable
- Strong radial pulse
- Simple coronary anatomy
- Relatively young (< 70 years old)

Exclusion Criteria for New Radialists

- Absence of radial artery pulse
- Absence of functional collaterals between the radial and the ulnar arteries, as judged by the Modified Allen's Test or alternative tests
- Clinically unstable, e.g., acute coronary syndromes
- Complex or problematic anatomy, e.g., bypass grafts, unprotected left main stenosis, chronic total occlusions and peripheral vascular lesions
- Elderly (> 70 years old), especially with hypertension (often have dilation and/or distortion of the aortic arch that impedes entry into the ascending aorta)
- Arteriovenous shunt for renal dialysis on the procedure forearm
- Raynaud's phenomenon
- Any procedure requiring > 8 Fr catheter

Modified Allen's Test

The Modified Allen's Test is a measure of functional collaterals between the radial and ulnar arteries through the deep and superficial palmer arches. It should be performed on both forearms before the procedure.

1. Palpate the radial and the ulnar arteries. Obliterate both pulses with the thumbs and fingers of both hands.
2. Ask the patient to clench the fist repeatedly until the palm blanches white.
3. Ask the patient to open the palm.
4. Release only the ulnar pulse and count the time to reappearance of normal palm color.

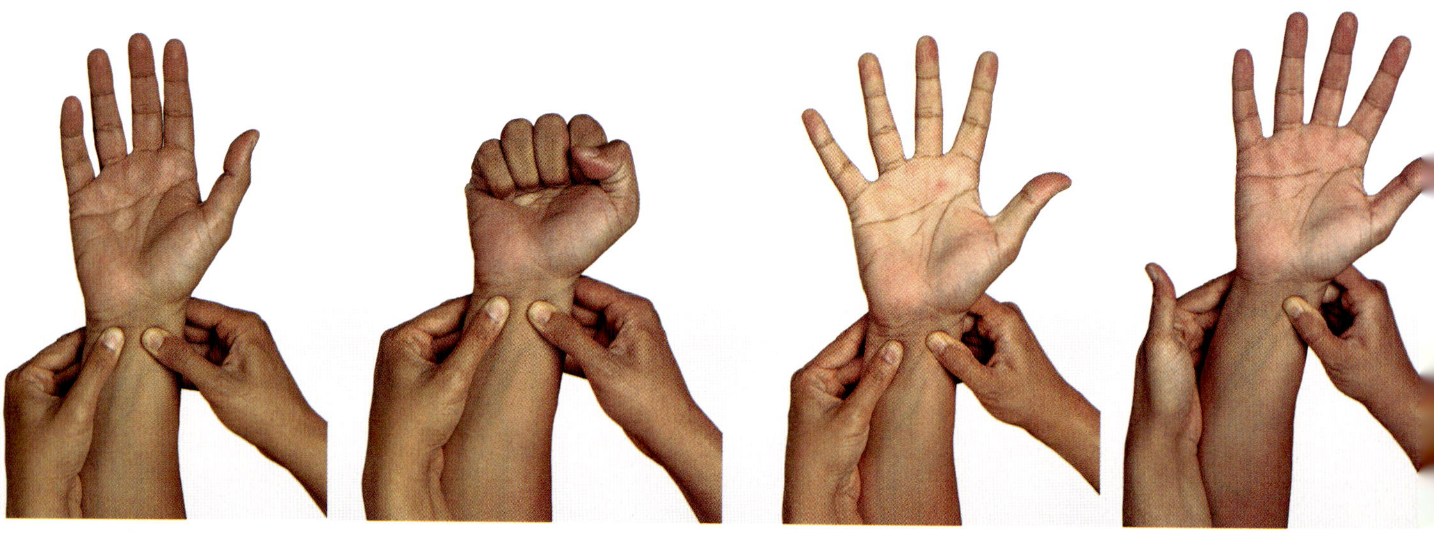

1 2 3 4

Interpretation of the Modified Allen's Test

1. **Normal (positive) Modified Allen's Test**

   Normal palm color returns within 7 seconds.

2. **Abnormal (negative) Modified Allen's Test**

   a. Borderline abnormal

   Delayed return of palm color, in 8 to 15 seconds.

   b. Absolutely abnormal

   No return of palm color until more than 15 seconds.

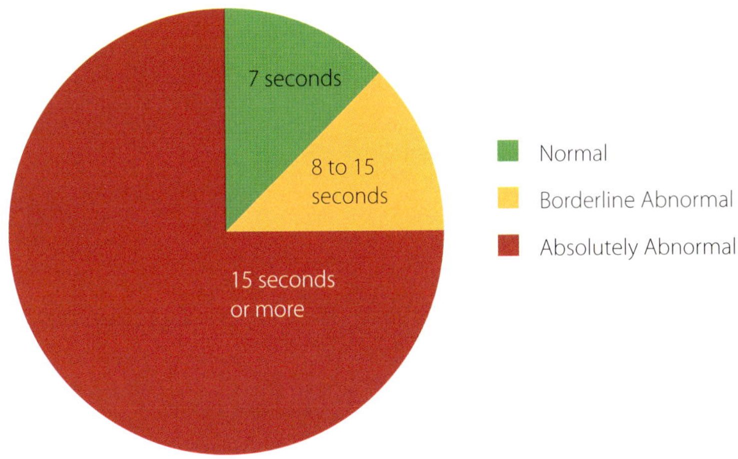

Inverse Allen's Test

This test is performed to determine the patency of the radial artery. It is useful in repeat procedures with the same radial artery. The steps in this test are similar to those in the Modified Allen's Test, except the radial pulse is released instead of the ulnar pulse. The interpretation is the same as in the Modified Allen's test.

If the Inverse Allen's Test is abnormal, the radial artery is not suitable for the procedure. Therefore, both the Modified Allen's Test and the Inverse Allen's Test should be normal before the patient is selected for a transradial procedure.

Alternative Tests

Perform alternative tests if the Modified Allen's Test is abnormal (negative). These tests require finger plethysmography and is also known as the Barbeau's Test.

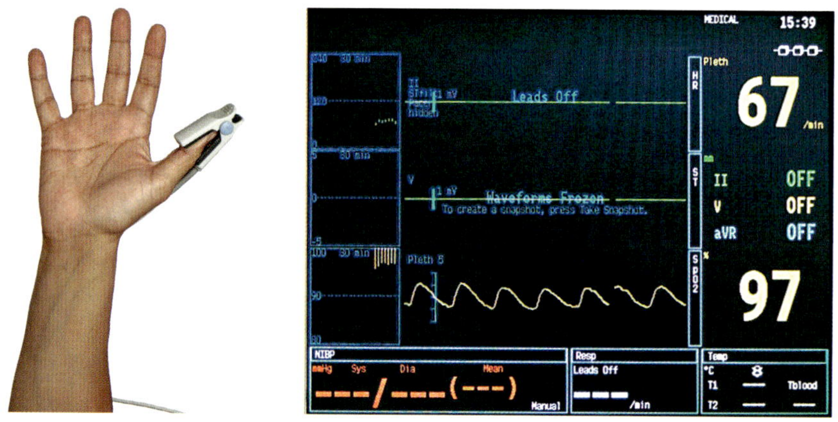

Clip the sensor to the thumb of the patient and confirm a normal (sharp) tracing and pulse oximeter reading.

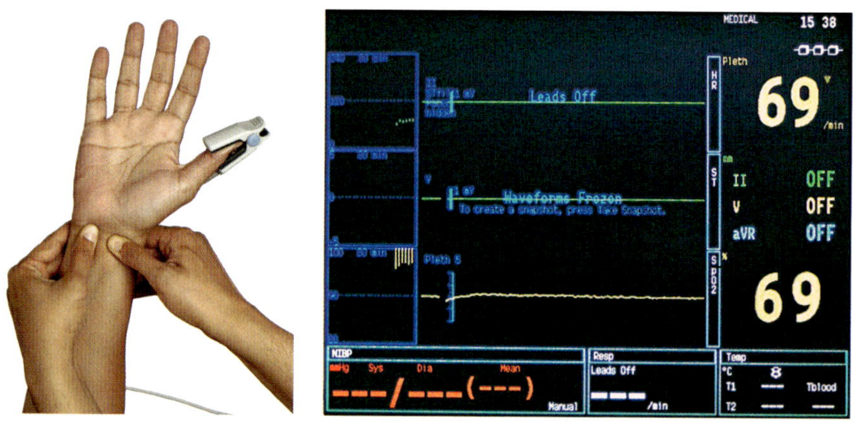

Compress the radial and the ulnar arteries as described in the Modified Allen's Test. The plethysmographic signal will be replaced by a flat line.

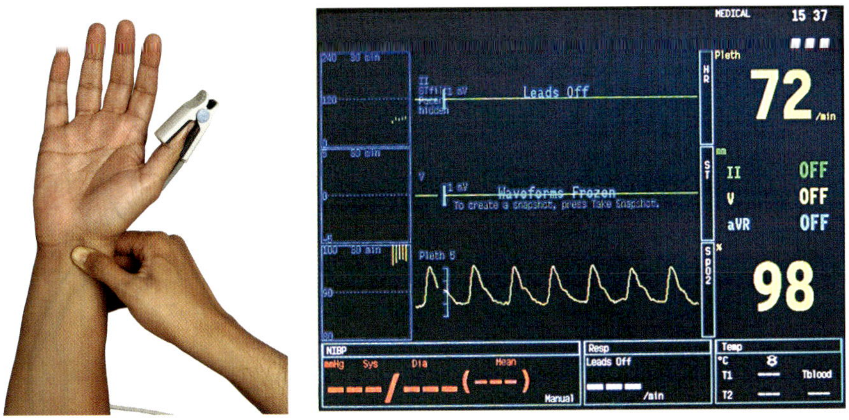

Release the pressure over the ulnar artery and watch for the tracing and pulse oximetry reading. Immediate return of a normal pulsatile waveform suggests a normal (positive) test, indicating the presence of collaterals.

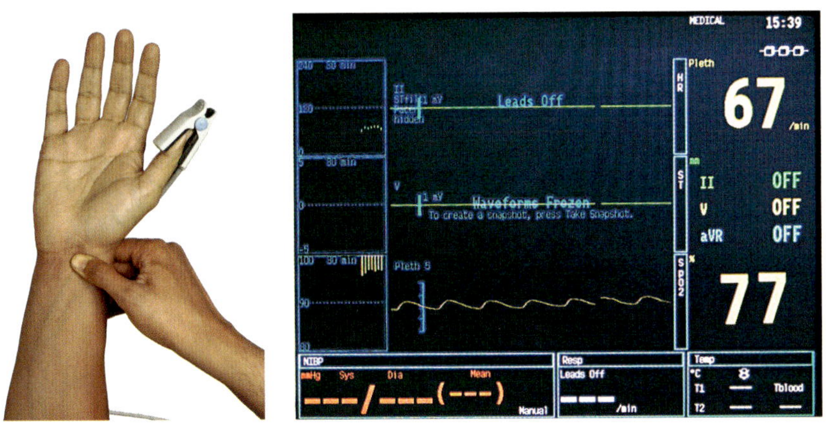

If the tracing does not return immediately, wait an extra minute. If a normal tracing and the SpO_2 normalize slowly, it indicates recruiting collaterals. A repeat Modified Allen's Test on the same forearm will show a rapid return of the normal tracing. This indicates the collaterals are functional and the radial artery can be used for the procedure.

If the tracing persistently flattens, this indicates there are no collaterals between the radial and ulnar arteries. In this case, the radial artery is not suitable for the beginning radialist.

Cath Lab Setup and Patient Preparation

With a few minor modifications, the same laboratory setup and patient preparation used for the femoral approach can be used for the radial approach.

An arm board is one helpful modification. Several have been described in the literature. Most laboratories use relatively simple modifications that allow external rotation of the arm and support for wrist flexion during the procedure.

Excessive sedation can defeat the "walk in, walk out" benefit of the radial approach; in fact, these procedures can be done successfully without sedation. Showing the patient a short video of the procedure and explaining what can be expected may alleviate much of the anxiety and obviate the need for systemic sedation.

Beginning radialists should prep the groin area for their first 200 procedures in case there is a need to switch to the femoral approach. Patients should be told there is a small chance the femoral artery may be needed to complete the procedure.

The hardware, anticoagulants and spasmolytic cocktails used vary depending upon the operator and the laboratory. All transradial intervention equipment discussed throughout the book is suggested, commonly used and based on experience with over 32,000 cases.

Equipment and Hardware

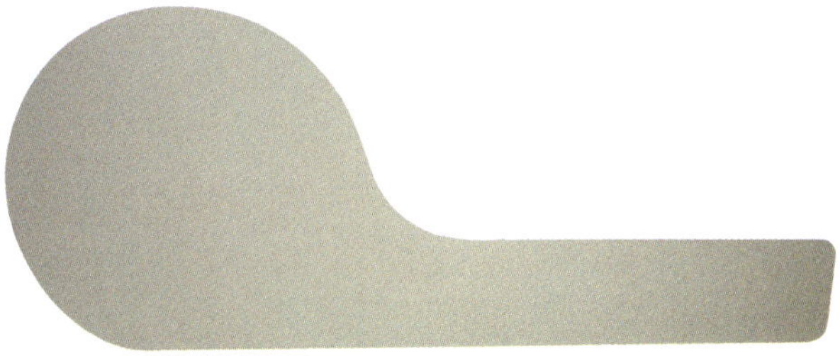

The patient rests the procedure arm on the support. It is 45 inches (114 cm) long, 18 inches (46 cm) at its widest, and 6 inches (15 cm) at its narrowest.

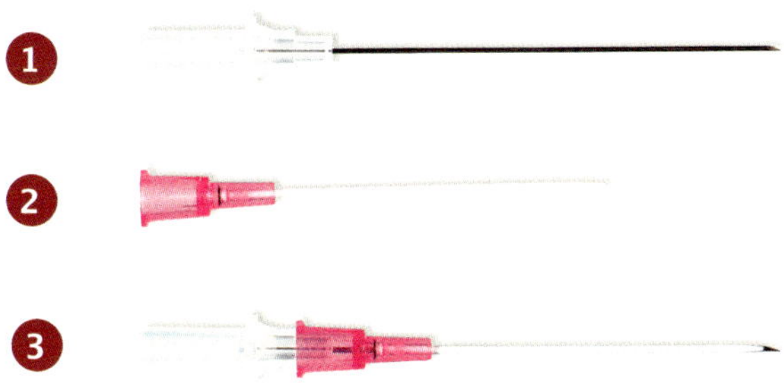

1. Needle
2. Plastic cannula
3. 45 mm 20G needle with plastic cannula*

*Note: A 20G, one-piece, metal needle can be used instead.

Straight-tip hydrophilic 0.025-inch guidewire.

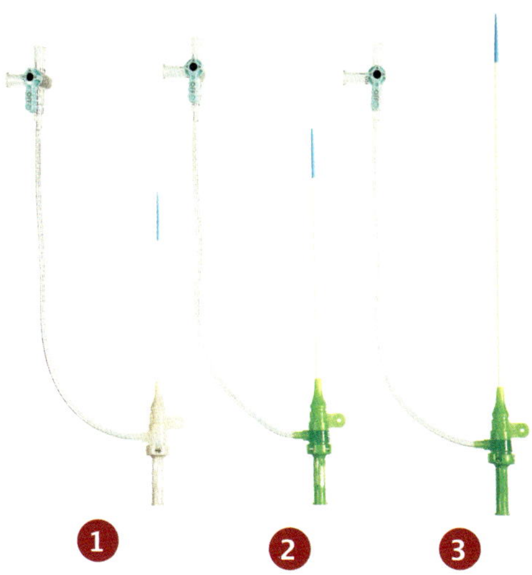

Introducer sheaths

5 Fr for diagnostic; 6 Fr for interventions

1. Short: 5 Fr, 70 mm
2. Medium: 6 Fr, 100 mm
3. Long: 6 Fr, 160 mm

If necessary, the introducer sheath can be downsized to 4 Fr. For interventions, 5 Fr to 7 Fr can be used. Reserve the 8 Fr introducer sheath only for very special situations.

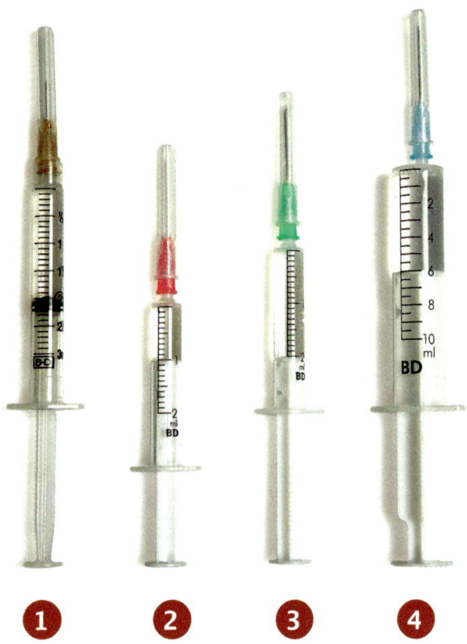

1. 2% Xylocaine
2. Intravenous heparin: 5,000 IU for diagnostic study; 100 IU/kg for interventions; use 70 IU/kg if abciximab is planned
3. Intra-arterial spasmolytic cocktail: injectable nitroglycerine (NTG) 200 mcg
4. Intra-arterial spasmolytic cocktail: injectable verapamil 5 mg or diltiazem 5 mg. Choice of spasmolytic cocktail is left at the discretion of an operator.

Preparation of The Forearm

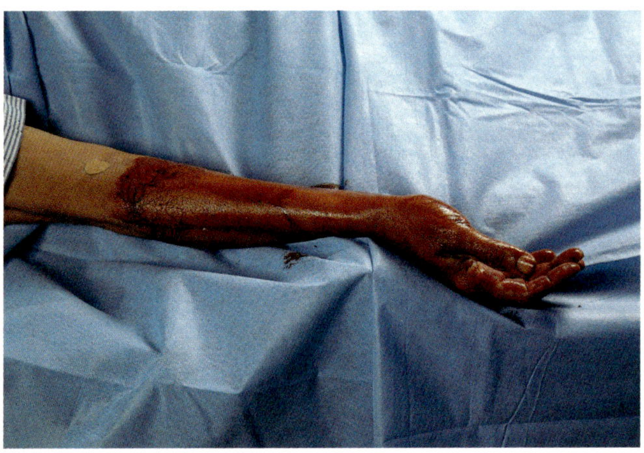

Shave the forearm up to the mid-part. Paint and drape both the flexor and extensor surfaces. The forearm should be supinated and hyperextended at the wrist joint for puncture. Position the arm parallel to the table.

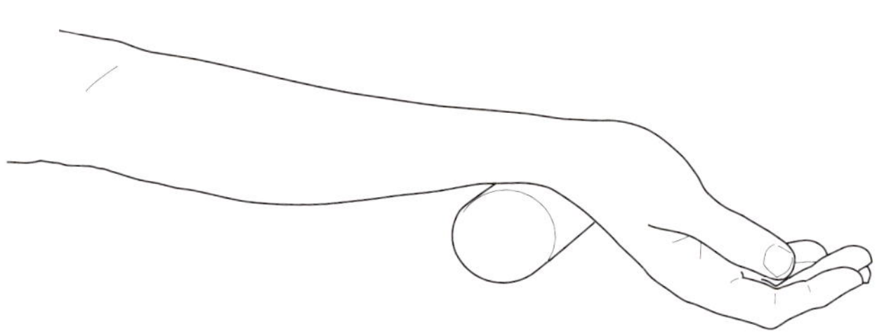

Hyperextension at the wrist joint can be achieved by putting a saline bag or similar soft, rounded object under the wrist.

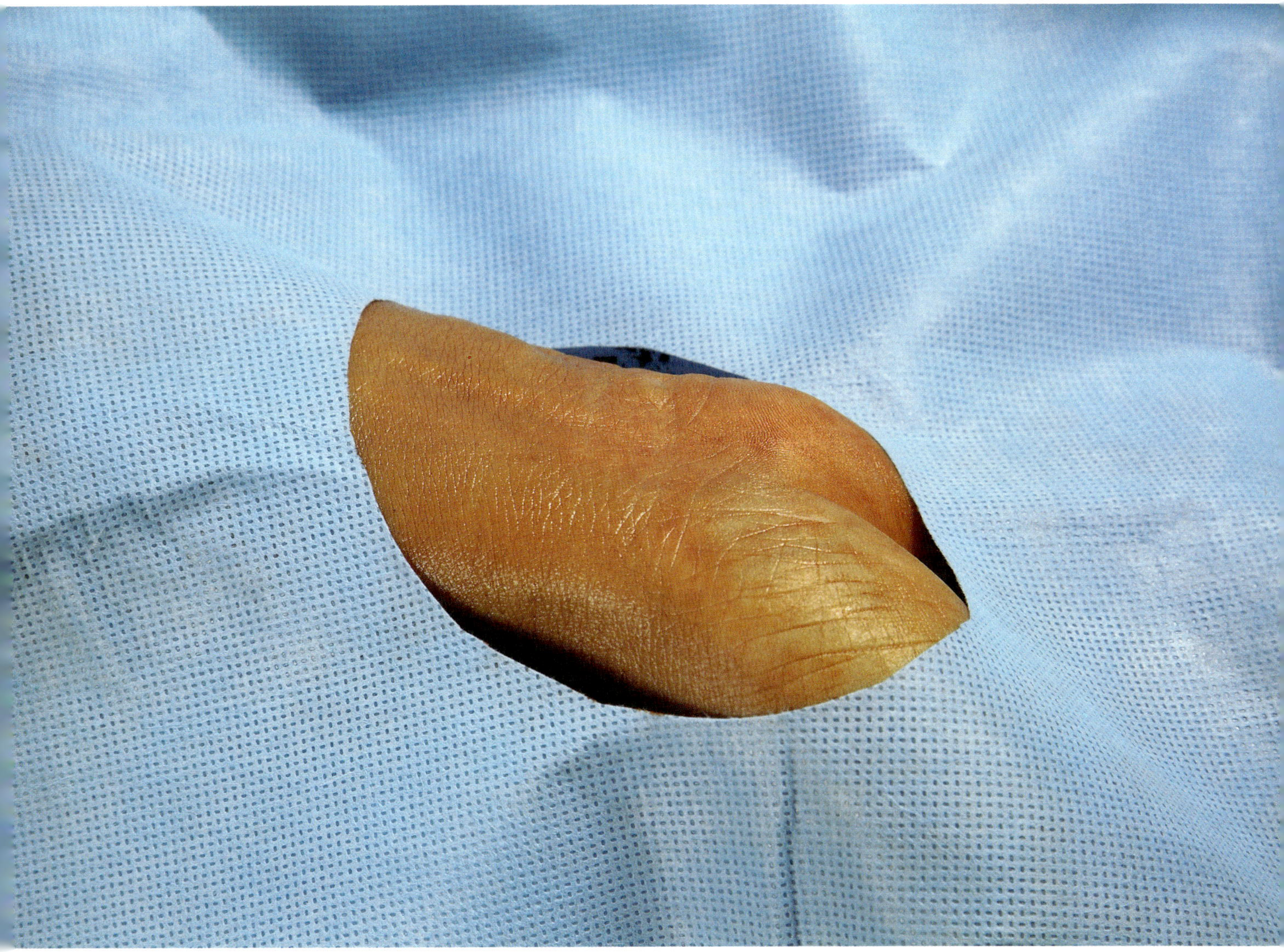

The forearm is ready for puncture.

Recommended Reading

1. Barbeau G, Arsenault F, Dugas L, et al. Evaluation of the ulnopalmar arterial arches with pulse oximetry and plethysmography: comparison with the Allen's test in 1010 patients. Am Heart J. 2004; 147 (3): 489-93.
2. Behan M, Haworth P, Colley P, et al. Decreasing operators' radiation exposure during coronary procedures : the transradial radiation protection board. Catheter Cardiovasc Interv. 2010: 76 (1): 79-84.
3. Chen C, Lin C, Lin T, et al. A simple and effective regimen for prevention of radial artery spasm during coronary catheterization. Cardiology. 2006; 105: 43-47.
4. Cohen M, Alfonso C. Starting a transradial vascular access program in the cardiac catheterization laboratory. J Invasive Cardiol. 2009; 21 (8 Suppl A): 11A-17A.
5. Coppola J, Patel T, Kwan T et. al. Nitroglycerin, nitroprusside, or both, in preventing radial artery spasm during transradial artery catheterization. J Invasive Cardiol. 2006; 18 (4): 155-58.
6. Ghuran A, Dixon G, Holmberg S, et al. Transradial coronary intervention without pre-screening for a dual palmar blood supply. Int J Cardiol. 2007; 121 (3): 320-22.
7. Gilchrist I. Is the Allen's test accurate for patients considered for transradial coronary angiography? J Am Coll Cardiol. 2006; 48 (6): 1287.
8. Greenwood M, Della-Siega A, Fretz E, et al. Vascular communications of the hand in patients being considered for transradial coronary angiography: is the Allen's test accurate? J Am Coll Cardiol. 2005; 46 (11): 2013-17.
9. Hildick-Smith D. Use of the Allen's test and transradial catheterization. J Am Coll Cardiol. 2006; 48 (6): 1287.
10. Kiemeneij F, Fraser D, Slagboom T, et al. Hydrophilic coating aids radial sheath withdrawal and reduces patient discomfort following transradial coronary intervention: a randomized double-blind comparison of coated and uncoated sheaths. Catheter Cardiovasc Interv. 2003; 59 (2): 161-64.
11. Kiemeneij F, Vajifdar B, Eccleshall S, et al. Evaluation of a spasmolytic cocktail to prevent radial artery spasm during coronary procedures. Catheter Cardiovasc Interv. 2003; 58 (3): 281-84.
12. Pancholy S, Coppola J, Patel T. Subcutaneous administration of nitroglycerin to facilitate radial artery cannulation. Catheter Cardiovasc Interv. 2006; 68 (3): 389-91.
13. Rathore S, Stables R, Pauriah M, et al. Impact of length and hydrophilic coating of the introducer sheath on radial artery spasm during transradial coronary intervention: a randomized study. JACC Cardiovasc Interv. 2010; 3 (5): 475-83.
14. Varenne O, Jégou A, Cohen R, et al. Prevention of arterial spasm during percutaneous coronary interventions through radial artery: the SPASM study. Catheter Cardiovasc Interv 2006; 68 (2): 231-35.
15. Yokoyama N, Takeshita S, Ochiai M, et al. Direct assessment of palmar circulation before transradial coronary intervention by color Doppler ultrasonography. Am J Cardiol. 2000; 86 (2): 218-21.

The Puncture Technique

Sanjay Shah, Alok Ranjan and Tejas Patel

2

"Well begun is half done."

Taking a little extra care at the time of puncture will pay off later. The radial puncture is a critical part of the transradial procedure and it takes some time to master, even for the experienced interventionalist.

This chapter will describe how to successfully perform the puncture. There are several puncture techniques, but this particular, simplified approach is very helpful for the beginning radialist. Once access is mastered, the successful radialist may eventually evolve personalized methods.

In rare situations, a high puncture site is useful. This will be explained along with the standard site for radial access.

The Ideal Site for Puncture

The ideal site for puncture is 2 cm to 3 cm proximal to the flexor crease of the wrist.

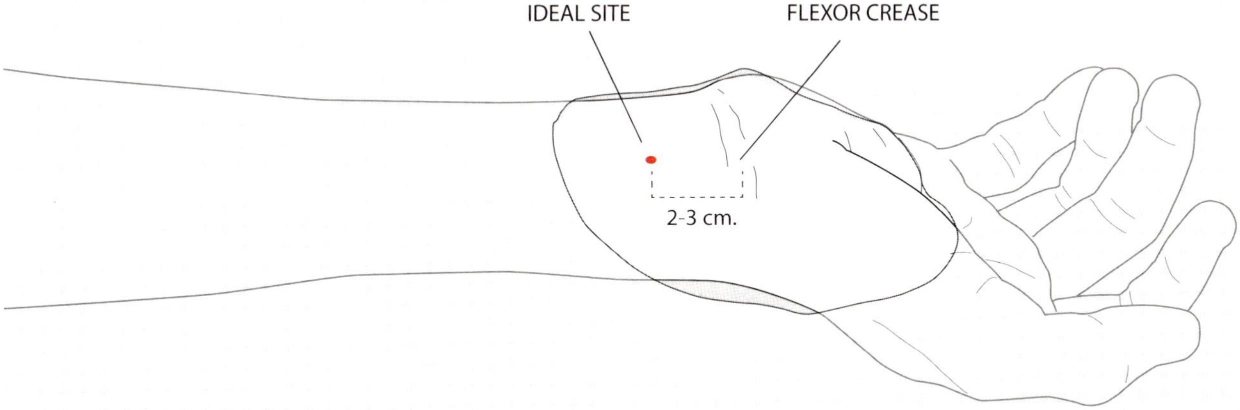

If the puncture is too distal, hemostasis may be difficult due to proximity to the wrist joint, where even minor movement may change the compression pressure over the radial puncture site. In addition, a distal puncture may also lead to perforation of the reticular ligament of the wrist.

If the puncture is attempted too proximally, it may be difficult to palpate the radial artery beneath the forearm muscles. After the procedure is completed, a proximal radial artery puncture may also be difficult to compress, and risk of hematoma formation may be increased. Finally, the proximal segments of the radial artery are probably best preserved for re-puncture or repeat procedures at a later date.

Local Anesthesia

❶ Inject a small amount (1 ml) of 2% lidocaine HCl at the planned site of puncture. Larger amounts may obliterate the pulse and cause difficulty in the puncture.

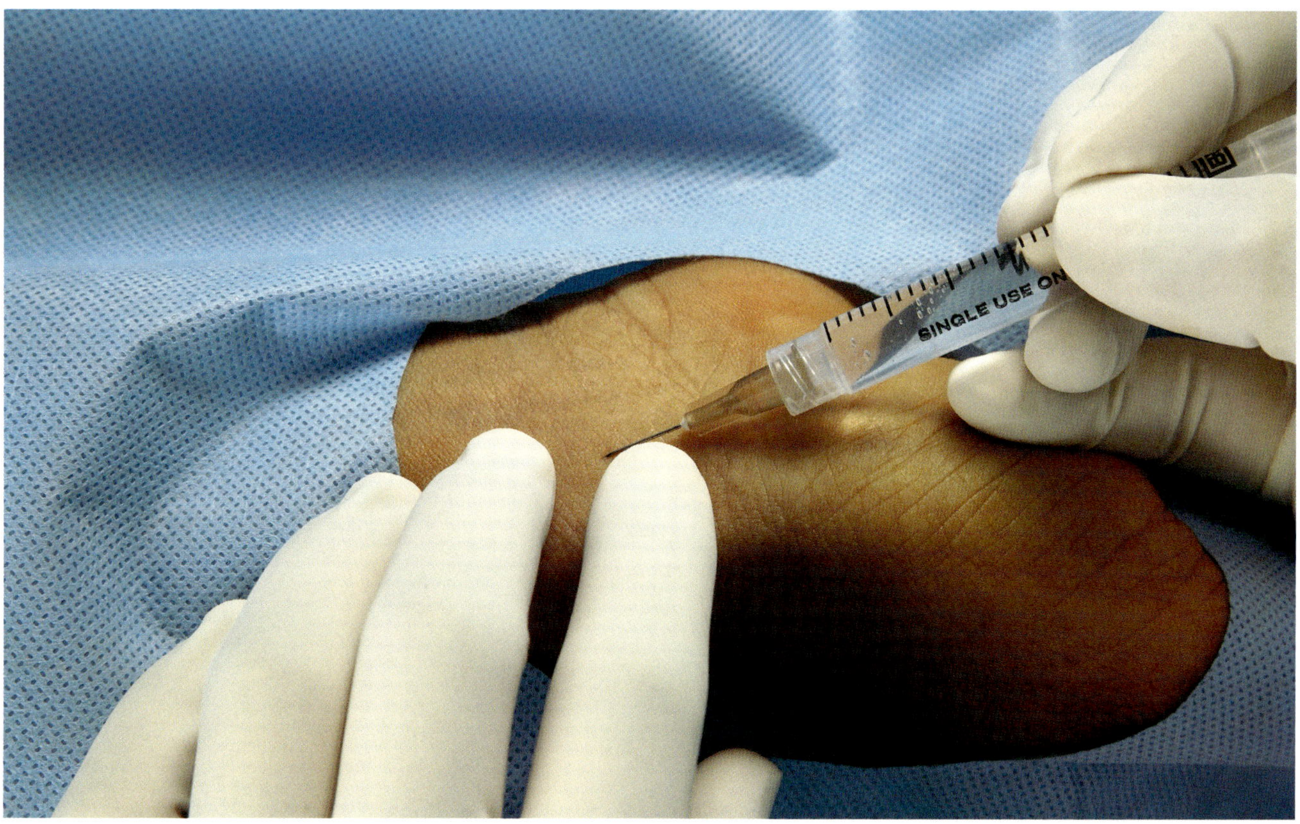

Radial Puncture

❶ The radial artery is fixed with the index and middle fingers of the operator's left hand. Puncture the radial artery using a needle with plastic cannula, with the bevel pointing upward. The angle between the needle and the forearm should be about 30°–45°.

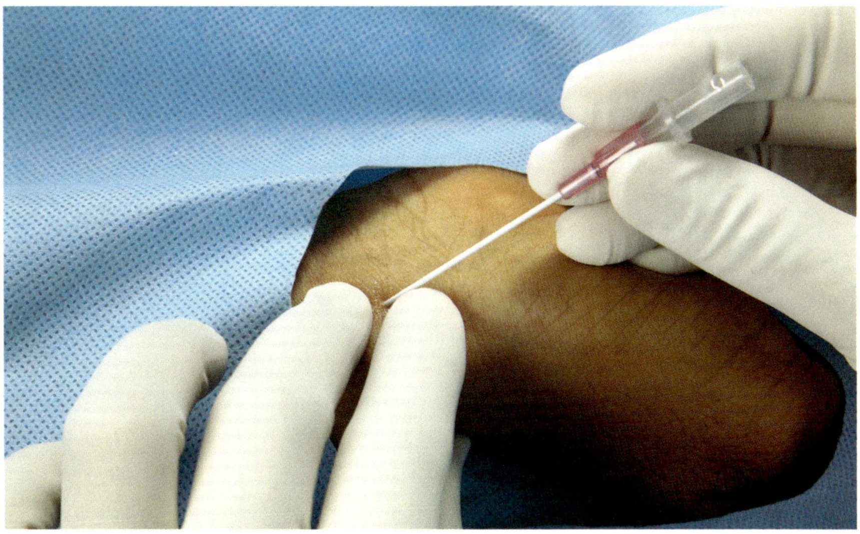

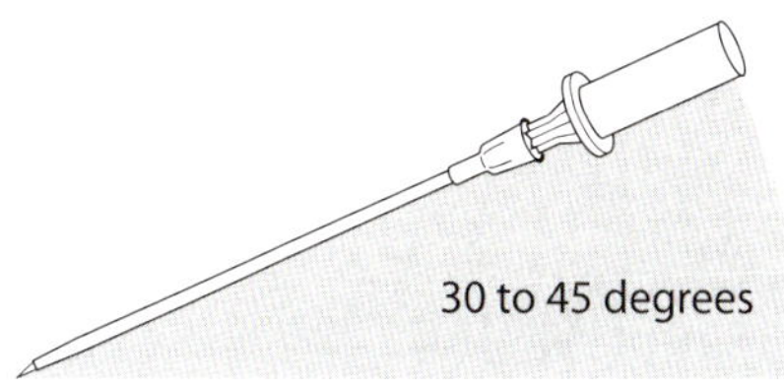

❷ Push the needle along the line of the arterial pulsations and watch for the backflow of blood in the hub of the needle. Backflow indicates a successful puncture of the radial artery.

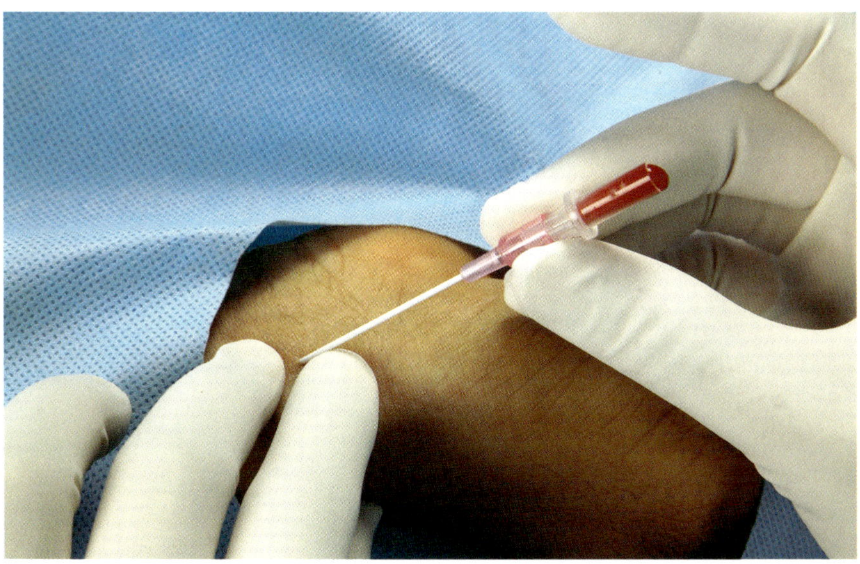

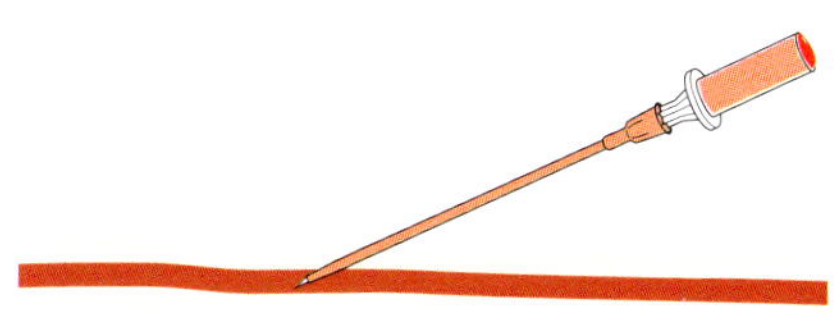

❸ Push the needle forward to counter-puncture the radial artery through the posterior wall. Counter-puncture of the artery is recommended for beginners because it is difficult to reliably perform a usable anterior puncture with this type of access device. (Note: Anterior-only puncture is more feasible with a one-piece metal needle.)

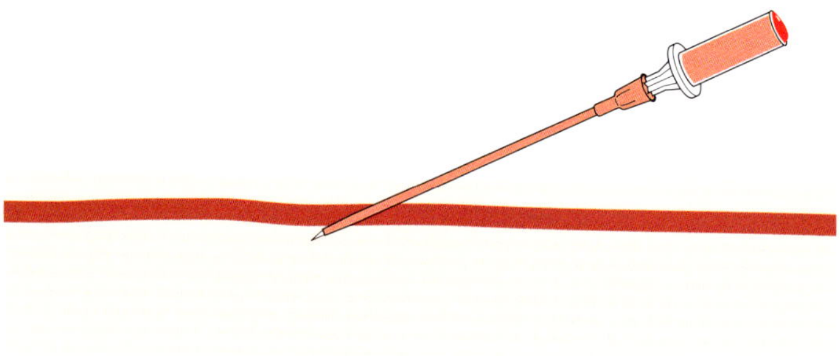

❹ Remove the needle and leave the plastic cannula. Reduce the angle between the plastic cannula and skin to 10°–20°. Slowly pull back the plastic cannula and watch for a free backflow of blood. Free flow of blood indicates intraluminal position of the plastic cannula. This shallower angle leaves the cannula more coaxial to the radial artery, and facilitates the passage of a 0.025-inch straight-tip, hydrophilic or metallic guidewire. This ability to coaxially align the cannula with the radial artery is a distinct advantage of this counter-puncture technique.

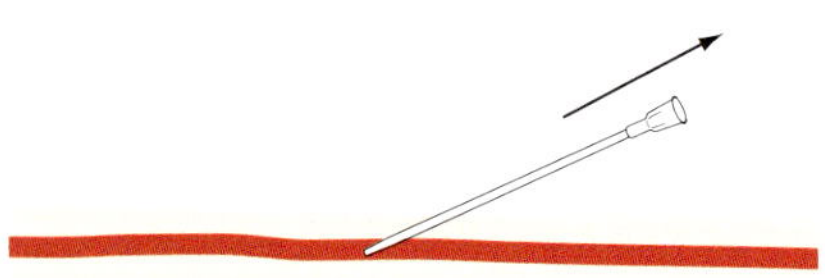

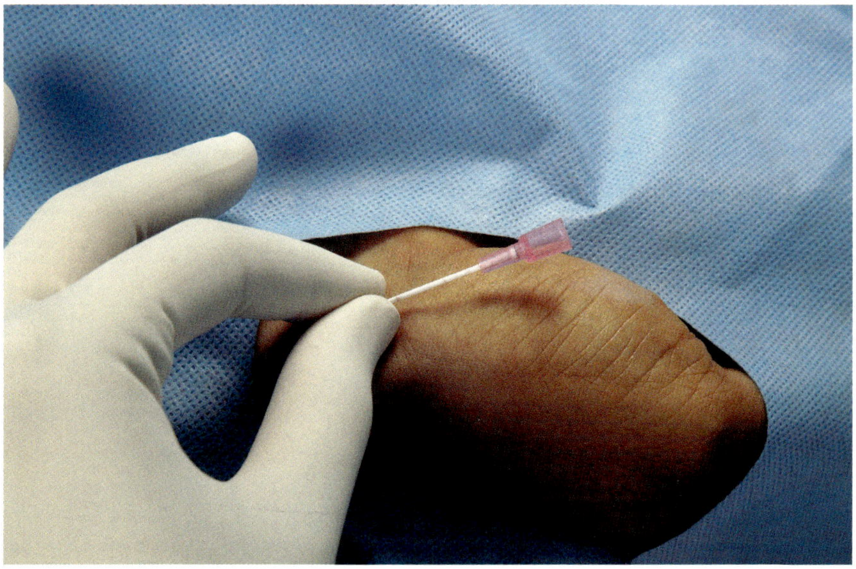

Guidewire Insertion

❶ Insert the 0.025-inch, straight-tip, hydrophilic or metallic guidewire into the radial artery through the plastic cannula.

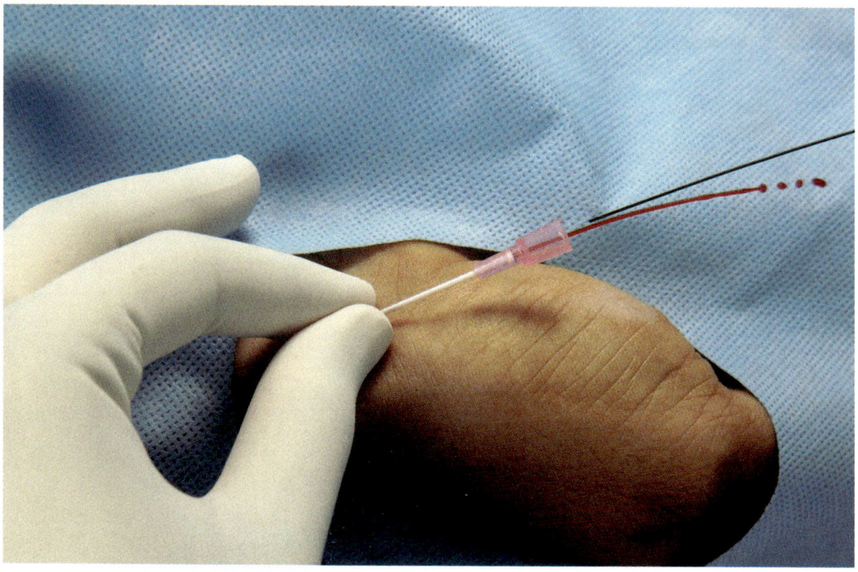

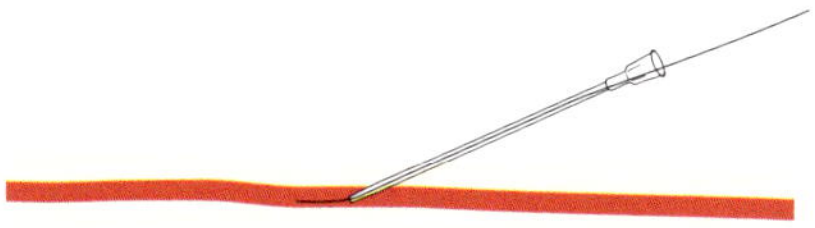

❷ Once the guidewire is well within the artery, remove the plastic cannula and leave the guidewire.

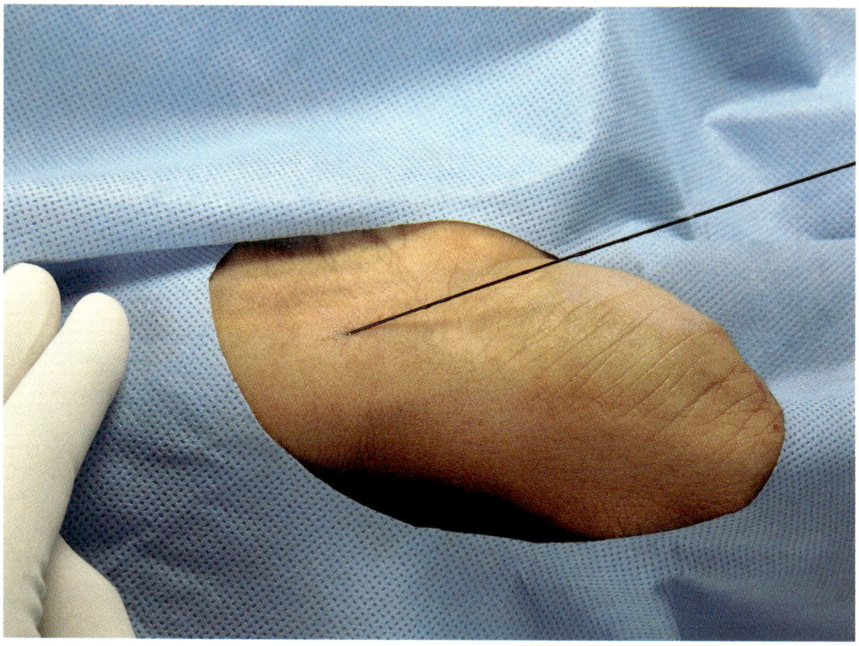

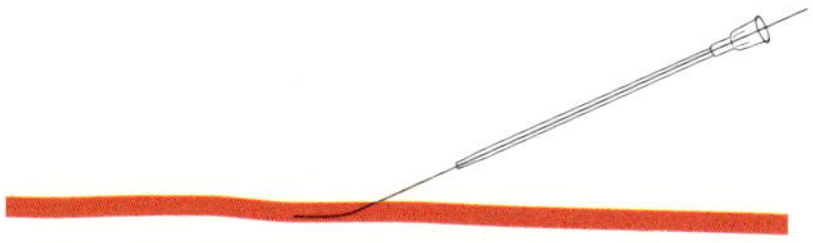

Sheath Insertion

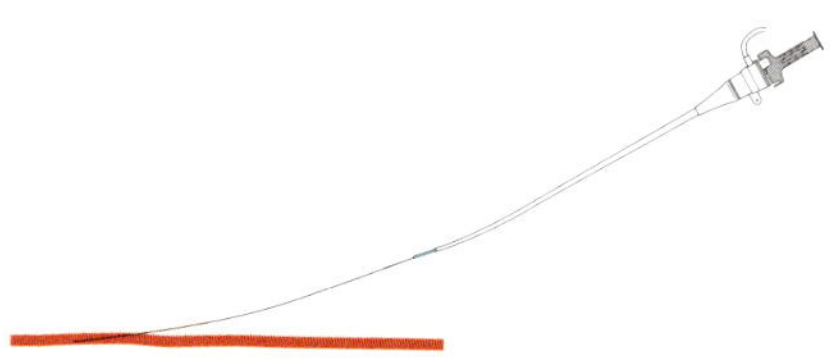

❶ Insert the sheath over the guidewire. In case of difficulty, the skin can be nicked with a #11 scalpel to facilitate insertion. A corkscrew motion may also help overcome minor resistance when inserting the sheath.

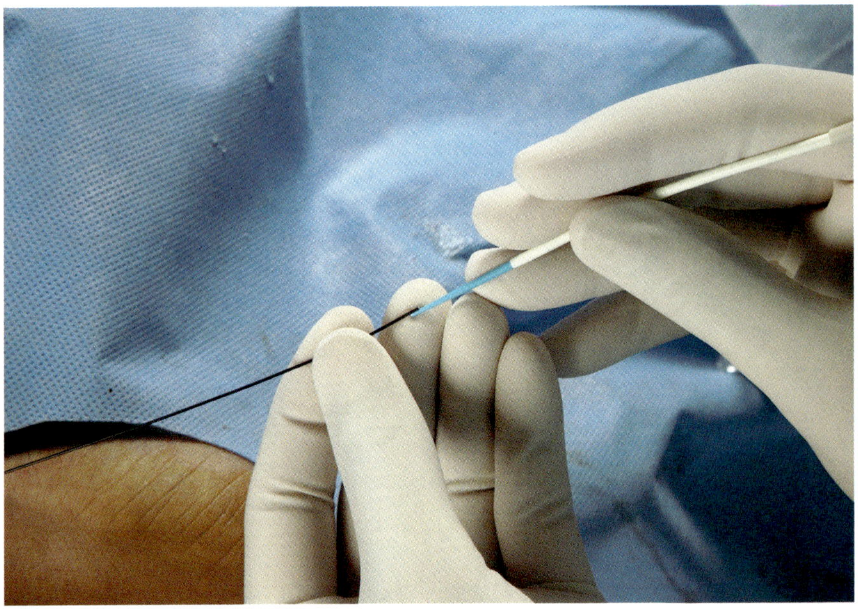

❷ Remove the sheath's dilator and the guidewire.

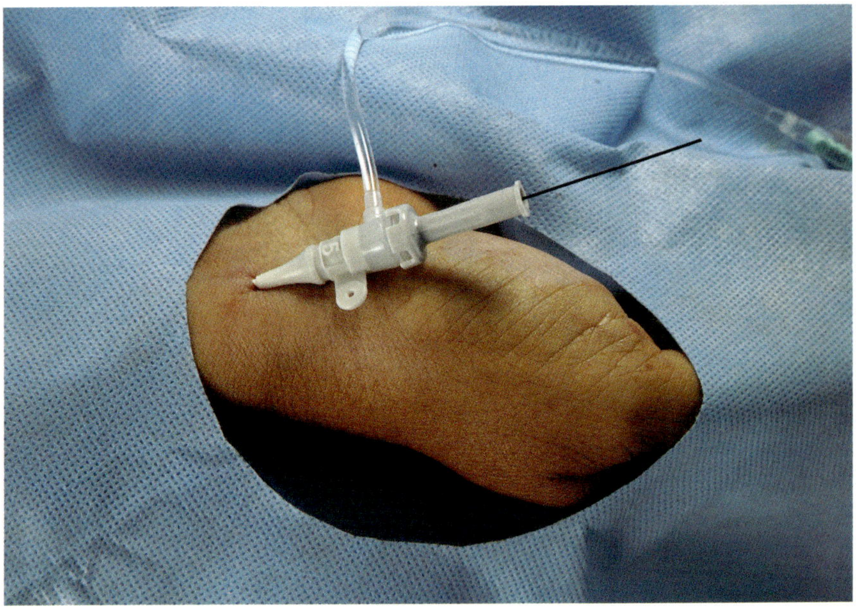

8 The sheath is in place.

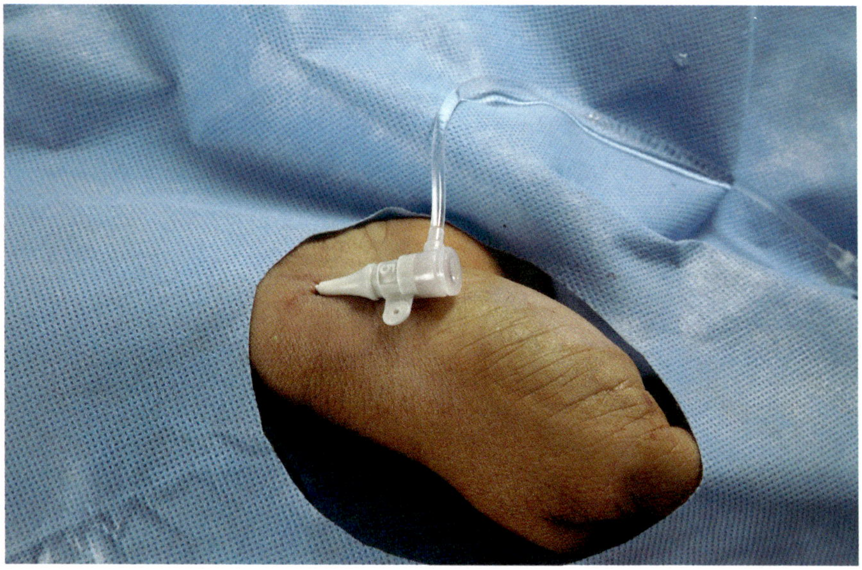

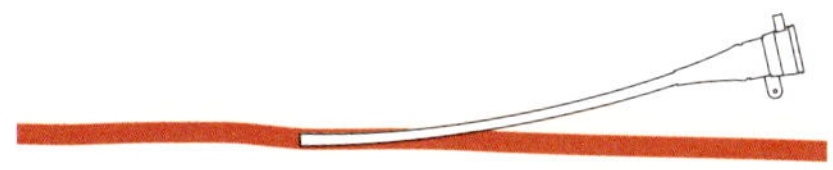

Spasmolytic Cocktail Administration

1 Warn the patient that there may be a slight burning sensation with administration of the cocktail. Aspirate blood into the syringe before injecting the spasmolytic cocktail through the sidearm of the sheath. (Mixing blood with the spasmolytic

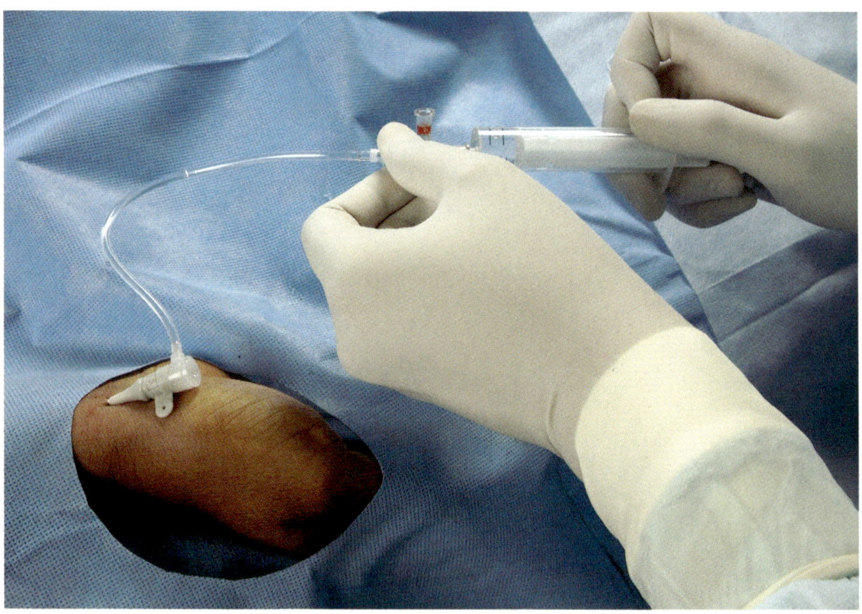

cocktail buffers the pH of the mixture closer to that of blood and attenuates the burning sensation.) Heparin should be administered intravenously.

❷ The puncture is complete and the patient is ready for the procedure.

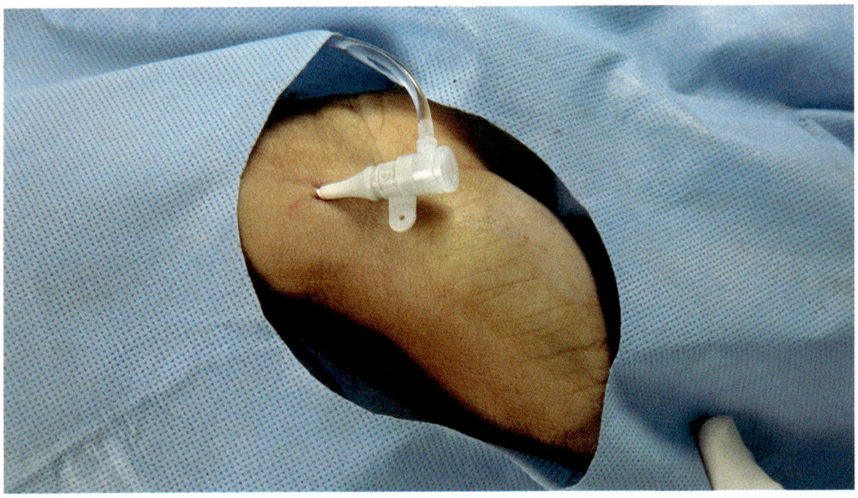

High Puncture of the Radial Artery

Although the ideal site for puncture is 2 cm to 3 cm proximal to the flexor crease of the wrist, the radial artery can be punctured right up to the mid-forearm, as long as the radial pulsation can still be felt and the artery can be localized.

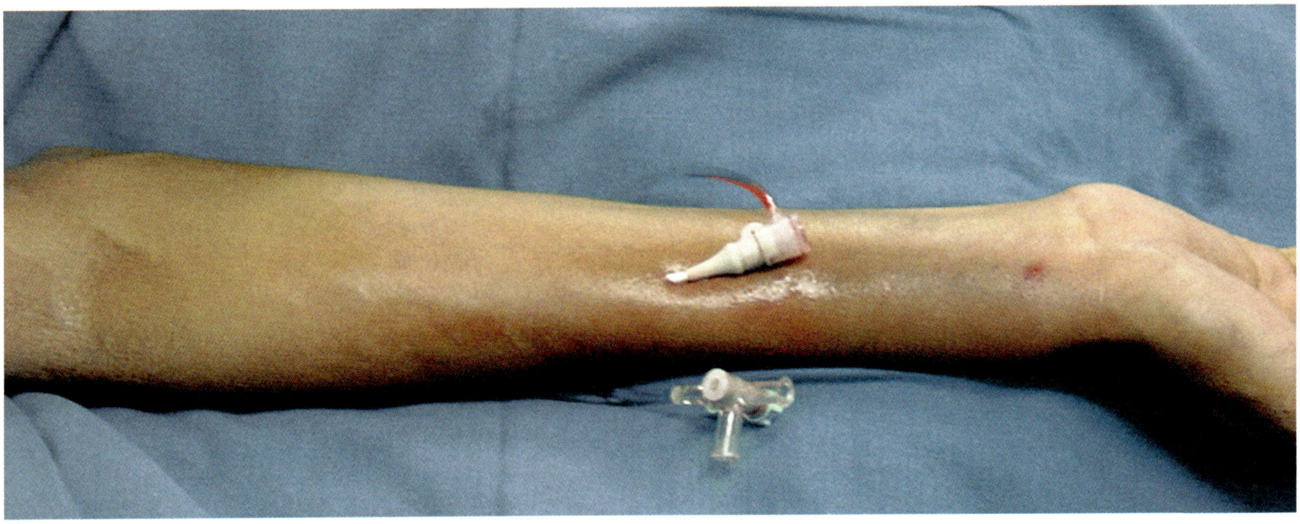

Angiogram showing a high radial puncture.

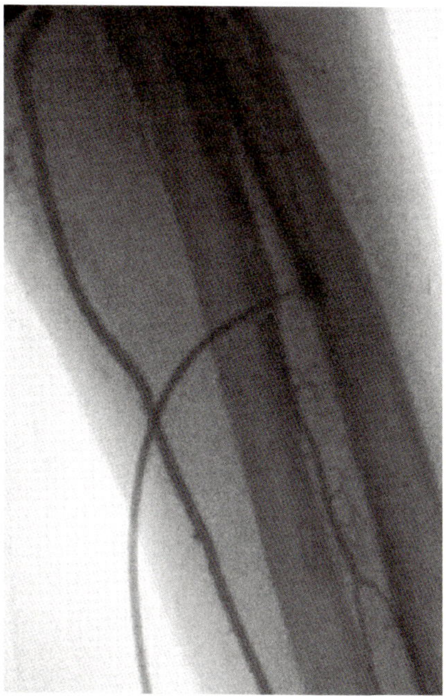

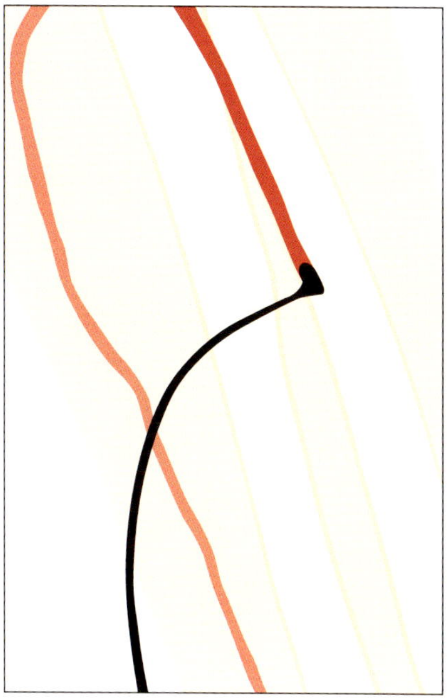

Very Lateral Puncture

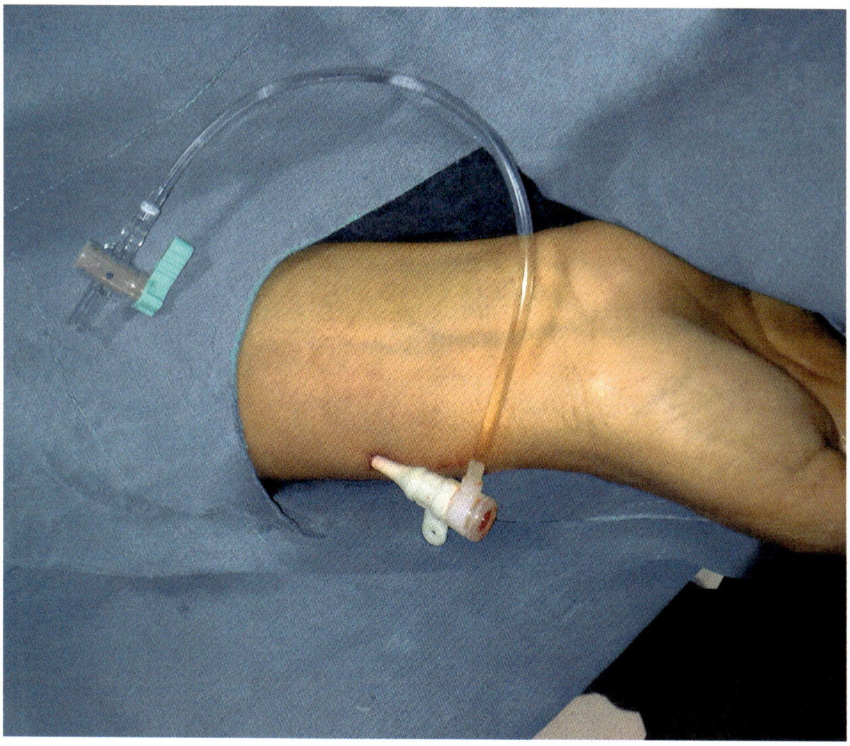

Important Concepts

- Take enough time to locate and fix the radial artery before the puncture.
- The first stick is usually the best stick because repeated sticks can induce spasm.
- Do not worry about having to counter-puncture the radial artery; it is not a problem. The radial artery lies superficially and, because of bone support beneath, it is easily compressible. As a result, there is little chance of hematoma.
- Do not hesitate to perform a high puncture when necessary. High puncture is used for infradiaphragmatic lesions, sometimes for repeat transradial puncture and, rarely, in patients with very low radial loops.

Recommended Reading

1. Babunashvili A, Dundua D. Recanalization and reuse of early occluded radial artery within 6 days after previous transradial diagnostic procedure. Catheter Cardiovasc Interv. 2011; 77 (4): 530-36.
2. Campeau L. Entry sites for coronary angiography and therapeutic interventions: from the proximal to the distal radial artery. Can J Cardiol. 2001; 17 (3): 319-25.
3. Caputo R, Simons A, Giambartolomei A, et al. Safety and efficacy of repeat transradial access for cardiac catheterization procedures. Catheter Cardiovasc Interv. 2001; 54 (2): 188-90.
4. Fujii T, Masuda N, Toda E, et al. Analysis of right radial artery for transradial catheterization by quantitative angiography - anatomical consideration of optimal radial puncture point. J Invasive Cardiol. 2010; 22 (8): 372-76.
5. Ludwig J, Achenbach S, Flachskampf F. Transradial approach: a modified puncture technique for arterial access. EuroIntery. 2010; 6 (2): 280-82.
6. Pancholy S, Coppola J, Patel T. Subcutaneous administration of nitroglycerin to facilitate radial artery cannulation. Catheter Cardiovasc Interv. 2006; 68 (3): 389-91.
7. Pancholy S. Transradial access in an occluded radial artery : new technique. J Invasive Cardiol. 2007; 19 (12): 541-44.
8. Patel T, Shah S, Sanghavi K, Pancholy S. Reaccessing an occluded radial artery: a 'proximal entry' technique. J Interv Cardiol 2011; 24 (4): 378-81.

Post-Procedure Management

Tejas Patel, Sanjay Shah, Keith Fonseca, Biren Gandhi and Samir Pancholy

3

It is noted that with experience, nurses, technicians and attendants become very relaxed about patient care because transradial post-procedure management is comparatively stress-free.

With femoral patients, the staff spends long hours attending to patients — adjusting their beds, making sure they do not move or cross their legs, and helping them with bedpans. There is the constant worry about bleeding and groin complications. Transradial patients can recover with less reliance on staff care and little risk of a sudden life-threatening bleed, resulting in a more relaxed work environment for the staff.

In this chapter, techniques for hemostasis with a closure device and manual compression will be described.

Sheath Removal and Hemostasis

Remove the sheath in the cath lab immediately after the procedure. But, before doing so, the patient should be warned that there may be some slight discomfort in the forearm while the sheath is removed. Inject an additional dose of spasmolytic cocktail if there are any concerns about vasospasm.

Sheath Removal and Hemostasis After Diagnostic Procedures

❶ Before removing the sheath, use the left hand to apply gentle pressure on the radial artery, proximal to the puncture site.

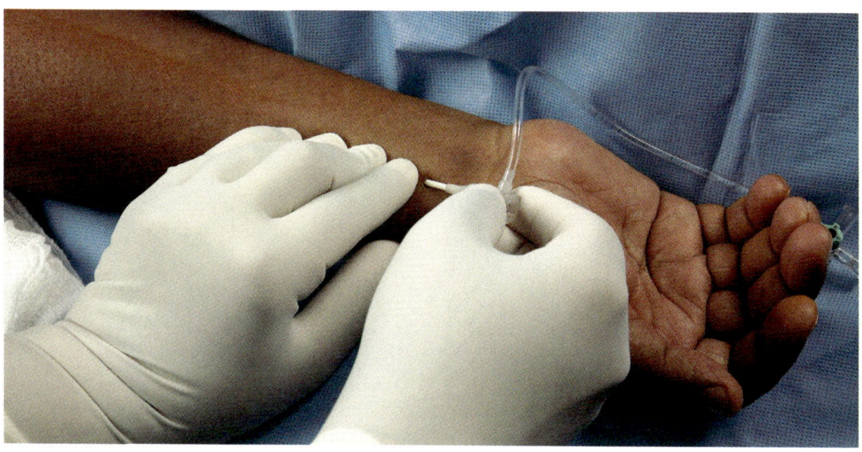

❷ Remove the sheath in the usual fashion.

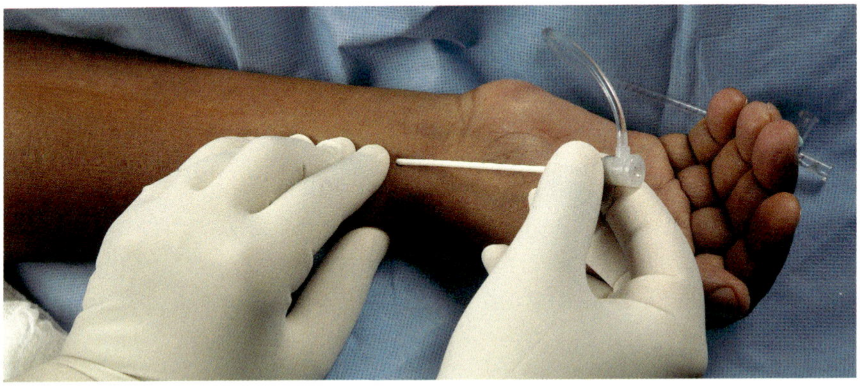

❸ Allow a slight back-bleed from the puncture site, then compress the radial artery.

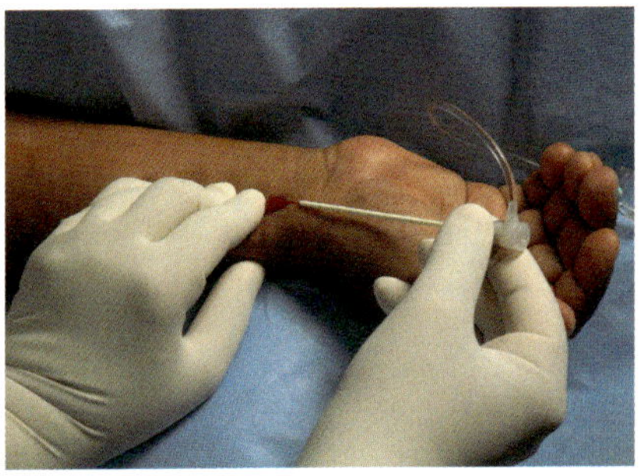

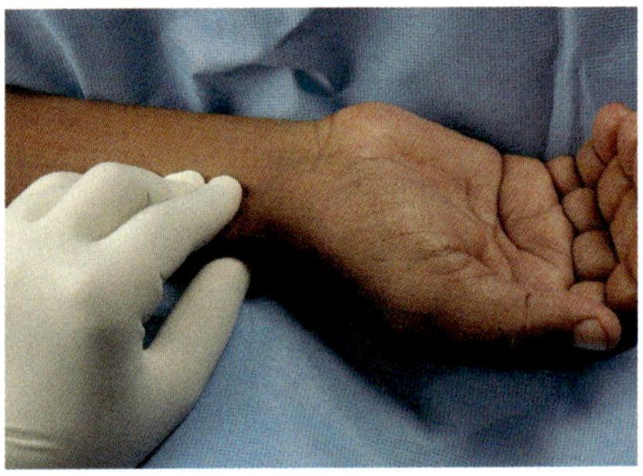

❹ Once hemostasis has been achieved, apply several gauze pads over the puncture site. Place an adhesive tape in a crisscross fashion over the gauze so it applies compression to the radial artery, but not the ulnar artery. Using several gauze pads over the radial puncture site helps keep the ulnar side free of undue pressure, preventing venous stasis. The bandage should be kept in place for 4 to 6 hours.

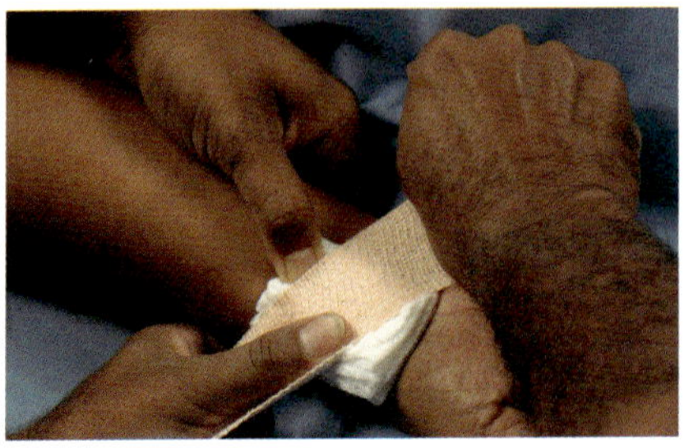

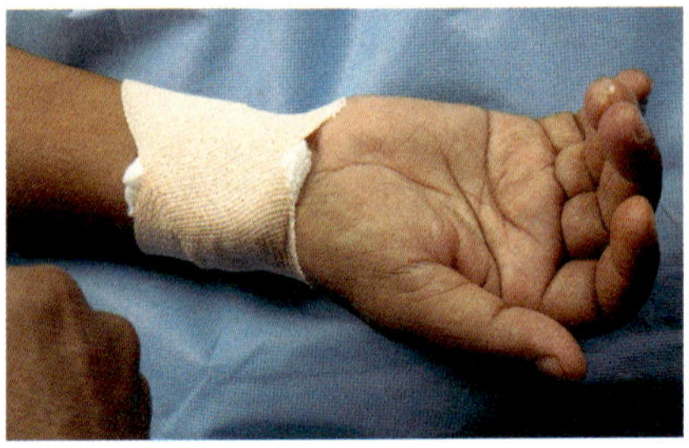

Attributes to Prevent Radial Artery Occlusion

Procedural attributes

- Sheath-to-artery ratio of > 1 is associated with an increased risk of RA occlusion.
- Therefore, use the lowest profile equipment to successfully complete the procedure.
- Systemic anticoagulation with heparin (50 U/kg up to 5,000 U) or equivalent antithrombin agent, either IV or IA, minimizes the incidence of RA occlusion.

Post-procedural attributes

- Maintaining RA patency during hemostatic compression after transradial catheterization is associated with a lower incidence of RA occlusion.
- Hemostasis with frequent monitoring of RA flow, with the goal to maintain RA patency throughout the hemostatic compression duration (termed "patent hemostasis"), combined with adequate intraprocedural anticoagulation is considered best practice.

Definition of patency

RA patency is defined as the presence of plethysmographic signal with ulnar artery occlusion and the amplitude of that plethysmographic signal should be at least 33% of the amplitude noted at baseline.

WEAK (< 33%) UNDULATION OF PLETHYSMOGRAM SHOULD NOT BE ACCEPTED AS EVIDENCE OF PATENCY.

Definition of Radial Artery Occlusion

Plethysmographic technique

Absence of plethysmographic waveform with manual occlusive compression of the ulnar artery. This finding is very accurate in detecting radial artery occlusion, although it assumes the presence of a normal baseline, as determined by the Reverse Barbeau's Test.

Duplex-Doppler evaluation

Absence of antegrade flow in the radial artery distal to the radial puncture site, as evidenced by reversal of the flow signal in the radial artery where it crosses over and dives into the palm, using pulse-Doppler technique.

Presence of echogenic material in the presumed lumen is not adequate evidence. Total absence of flow is not expected due to high prevalence of palmar macrocollateral circuits.

Audible Doppler signal is frequently preserved in the radial artery proximal and distal to the occluded segment and, hence, the presence of an audible Doppler signal is not of value in evaluating radial artery patency

Radial pulse and radial artery occlusion

The presence of radial artery pulsation is not a sign of radial artery patency.

Decrease in pulsation volume or a gap in radial pulsation around the entry site is frequently seen in radial artery occlusion.

Stepwise approach to patent hemostasis

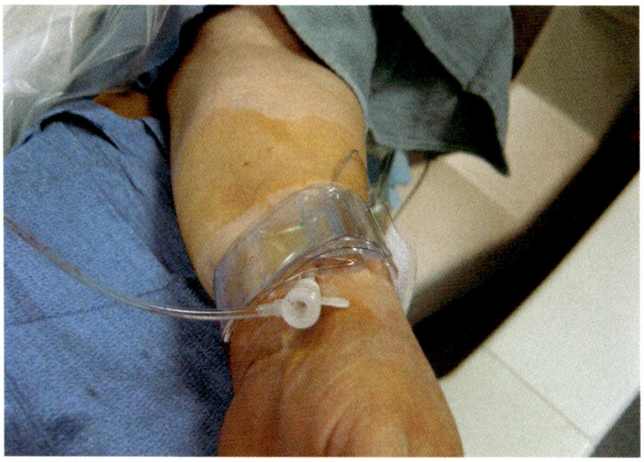

❶ Apply hemostatic compression at the entry site with sheath in place.

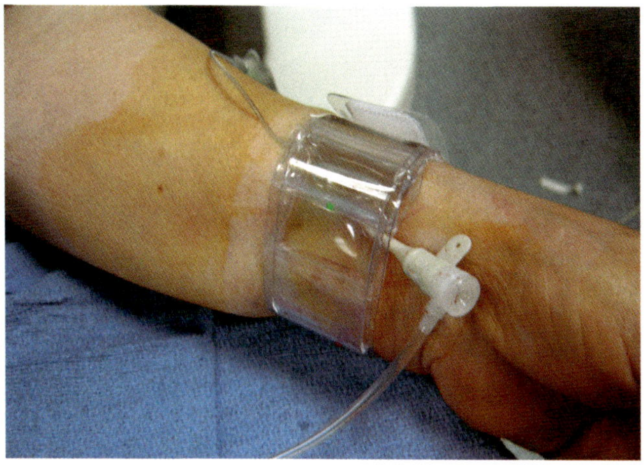

❷ Pull the sheath partially. Open the stopcock and let it bleed freely for 3-4 cardiac cycles (to purge any thrombus in the radial lumen).

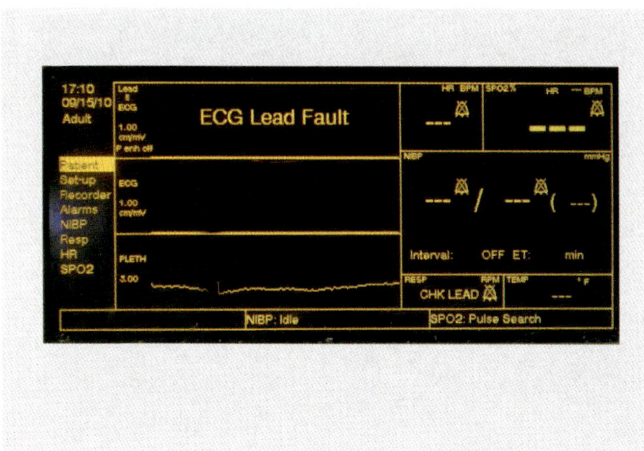

❸ Apply the plethysmographic sensor on the index finger and monitor signal. Inflate the TR band. Sheath is usually occlusive.

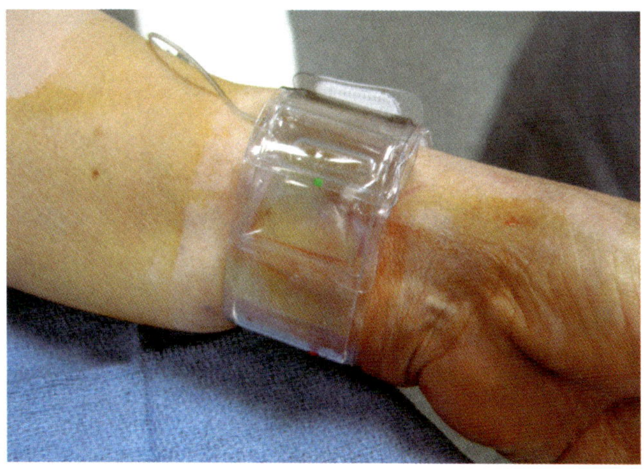

❹ Remove the sheath. Inflate the TR band and remove with sheath with the back-bleed valve open, letting it bleed while coming out.

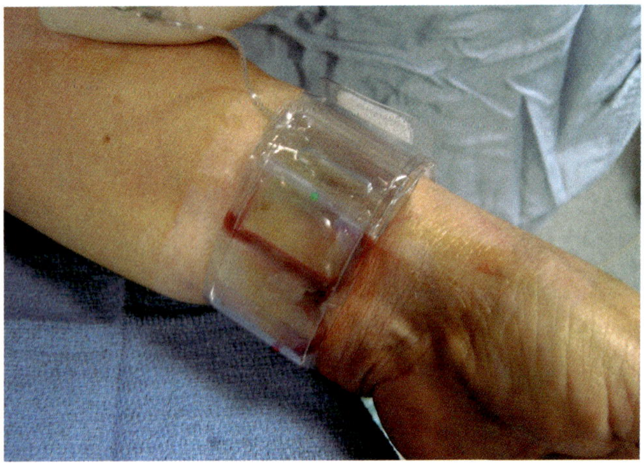

❺ Decrease the pressure at the site by loosening/deflating the band until some pulsatile bleeding is seen.

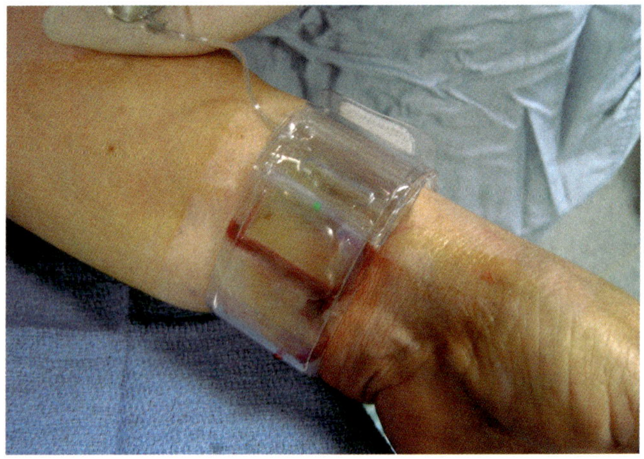

❻ Increase the pressure at the site just enough to eliminate this bleeding (i.e., inflate the band slightly).

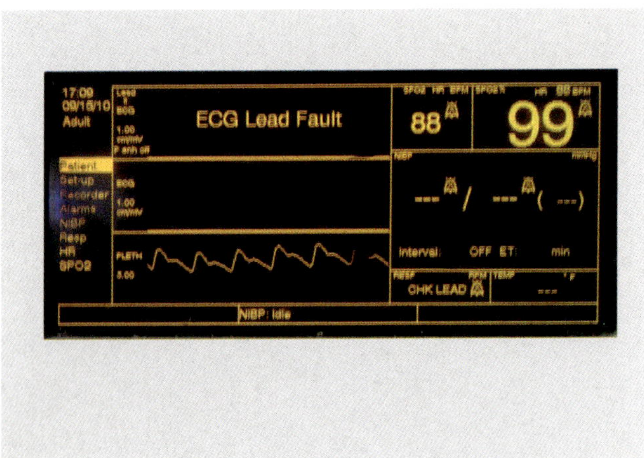

❼ Perform a Reverse Barbeau's Test by compressing the ulnar artery and observe the plethysmographic signal. If the radial artery is patent, there should still be a pulsatile signal.

Tips

- While performing Reverse Barbeau's Test, occlude the ulnar artery at Guyon's canal between the pisiform and hamate bones at the level of the wrist.
- Avoid compression at the forearm level, as the resultant increase in pressure in the enclosed forearm compartment may lead to inadvertent pressure on the radial artery.

Frequency of monitoring

- RA flow should be monitored every 15 minutes after initial hemostatic pressure application.
- If radial flow is evident by plethysmography, the status should be re-evaluated in 15 minutes.
- If radial flow is interrupted, hemostatic pressure should be decreased, unless bleeding occurs.

Duration of compression

- Manual hemostatic compression should be performed until hemostasis is evident, the duration of which is determined by repeated assessment on an individual basis.
- When hemostatic compression is performed using a dedicated device, approximately 2 hours may be required. Longer compression duration is associated with a higher risk of RA occlusion. Much shorter compression times may be needed in non-anticoagulated patients.

Removal of hemostatic device

- Devices must be removed very carefully to avoid tenting of the skin that may have adhered to the band.
- Application of a thin film of lubricant (e.g., antibiotic ointment or saline) to the point of pressure usually eliminates this problem.

- If an adherent device is pulled and causes tenting of the skin, recurrent bleeding may occur, necessitating reapplication of the hemostatic device.

- After the hemostatic device is removed and the site is dry, re-evaluate RA patency using a Reverse Barbeau's Test.

- Apply sterile dressing to the site without applying any pressure.

Converting non-patent hemostasis to patent hemostasis

- Reduce pressure at the access site.

- Apply pressure on the ulnar artery to interrupt ulnar artery flow. This increases the flow volume in the radial artery and improves patency with frequent re-establishment of flow.

- Ask the patient to open and close the fist with the ulnar artery compressed. This maneuver may also re-establish radial artery flow by reducing the palmar vascular resistance, leaving the radial as the only choice for forward flow.

Recommended Reading

1. Badheka A, Cohen M. Bivalirudin and transradial access - the end of the bleeding era for catheterization procedures? J Invasive Cardiol. 2011; 23 (3): 105-106.
2. Brueck M, Bandorski D, Kramer W, et al. A randomized comparison of transradial versus transfemoral approach for coronary angiography and angioplasty. JACC Cardiovasc Interv. 2009; 2 (11): 1047-54.
3. Cubero J, Lombardo J, Pedrosa C, et al. Radial compression guided by mean artery pressure versus standard compression with a pneumatic device (RACOMAP). Catheter Cardiovasc Interv. 2009; 73 (4): 467-72.
4. Gilchrist I. Laissez-faire hemostasis and transradial injuries. Catheter Cardiovasc Interv. 2009; 73 (4): 473-74.
5. Kiemeneij F, Fraser D, Slagboom T, et al. Hydrophilic coating aids radial sheath withdrawal and reduces patient discomfort following transradial coronary intervention: A randomized double-blind comparison of coated and uncoated sheaths. Catheter Cardiovasc Interv. 2003; 59 (2): 161-64.
6. Kim J, Yoon J, Yoo B, et al. The effect of a eutectic mixture of local anesthetic cream on wrist pain during transradial coronary procedures. J Invasive Cardiol. 2007; 19 (1): 6-9.
7. Mamas M, D'Souza S, Hendry C, et al. Use of the sheathless guide catheter during routine transradial percutaneous coronary intervention: a feasibility study. Catheter Cardiovasc Interv. 2010; 75 (4): 596-602.
8. Pancholy S. Impact of two different hemostatic devices on radial artery outcomes after transradial catheterization. J Invasive Cardiol. 2009; 21 (3): 101-104.
9. Pancholy S, Coppola J, Patel T, et al. Roke-Thomas M. Prevention of radial artery occlusion-patent hemostasis evaluation trial (PROPHET study): a randomized comparison of traditional versus patency documented hemostasis after transradial catheterization. Catheter Cardiovasc Interv. 2008; 72 (3): 335-40.
10. Pancholy S. Comparison of the effect of intra-arterial versus intravenous heparin on radial artery occlusion after transradial catheterization. Am J Cardiol. 2009; 104 (8): 1083-85.
11. Pancholy S. Transradial access in an occluded radial artery: new technique. J Invasive Cardiol. 2007; 19 (12): 541-44.
12. Patel T, Shah S, Sanghavi K, Pancholy S. Reaccessing an occluded radial artery: a 'proximal entry' technique. J Interv Cardiol. 2011; 24 (4): 378-81.
13. Politi L, Aprile A, Paganelli C, et al. Randomized clinical trial on short-time compression with kaolin-filled pad: a new strategy to avoid early bleeding and subacute radial artery occlusion after percutaneous coronary intervention. J Interv Cardiol. 2011; 24 (1): 65-72.
14. Rathore S, Stables R, Pauriah M, et al. A randomized comparison of TR band and radistop hemostatic compression devices after transradial coronary intervention. Catheter Cardiovasc Interv. 2010; 76 (5): 660-67.
15. Takeshita S, Saito S. Transradial coronary intervention using a novel 5-Fr sheathless guiding catheter. Catheter Cardiovasc Interv. 2009; 74 (6): 862-65.

Complications and Management

Sanjay Shah, Tejas Patel, Kimberly Skelding and Chirayu Vyas

4

The data from several randomized studies comparing the transfemoral and transradial approach have shown major vascular complication rates of between 1.5% and 6.5% for the femoral approach and near zero for the radial approach. (See Recommended Reading at the end of this chapter.)

However, no medical procedure is free of complications. In this chapter, the relatively rare and minor local complications that have been seen while performing over 32,000 cases will be discussed. Management technique of these same complications will also be reviewed.

Minor Local Complications

❶ Radial artery spasm and pain were present in 5.6% and 3% of patients (respectively) of more than 32,000 procedures. Only 0.5% patients experienced severe spasm.

❷ Infraclavicular hematoma due to perforation of a small branch of the axillary artery was present in only 1 of more than 32,000 procedures.

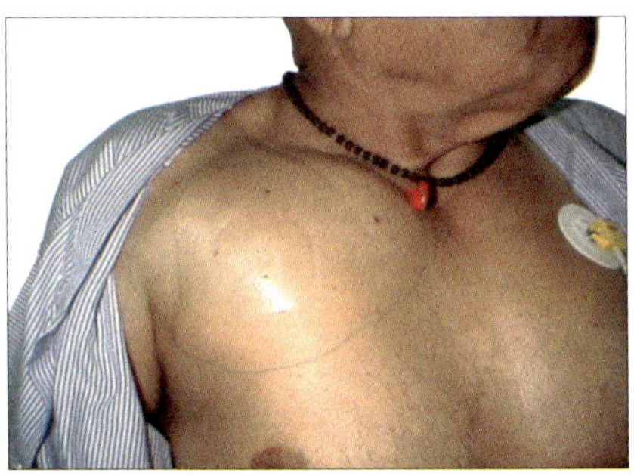

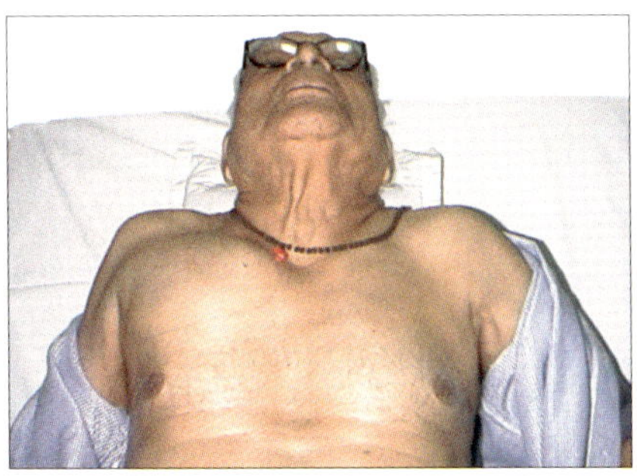

❸ Depigmented scar at the puncture site due to excessive compression by the hemostatic device was present in 7 of over 32,000 procedures.

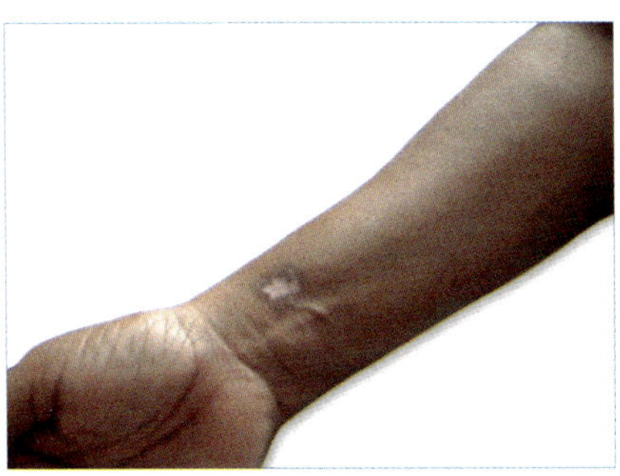

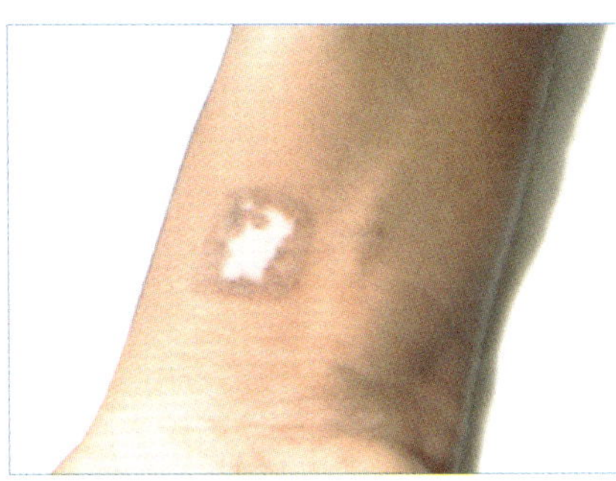

❹ Small pseudoaneurysm at the radial artery puncture site was present in 10 of more than 32,000 procedures. If manual compression fails to resolve the issue, minor surgery may be required.

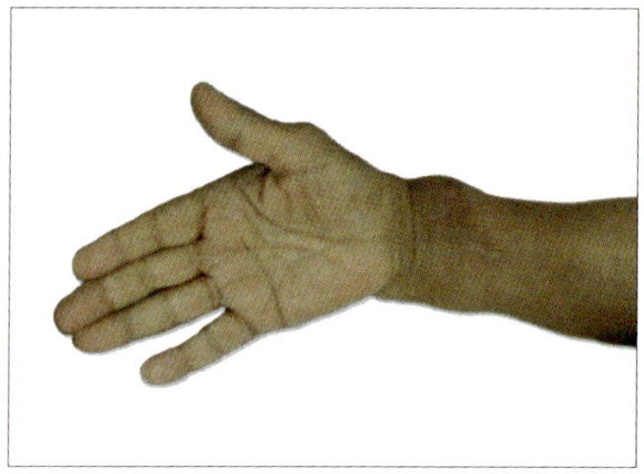

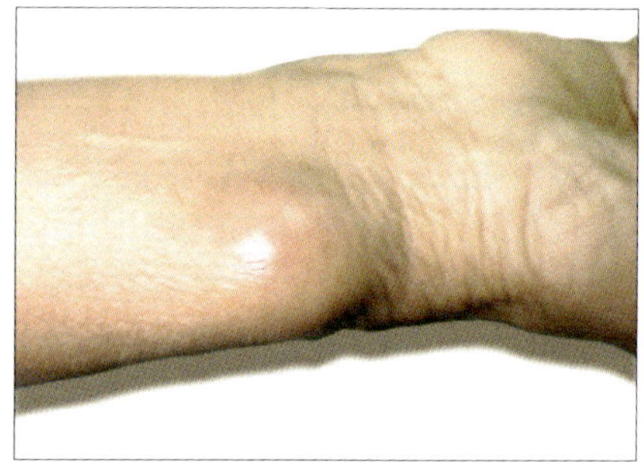

Perforations

Perforations in the radial-brachial region were present in 30 of more than 32,000 procedures.

❶ Radial artery perforation leading to extravasation of contrast material into the surrounding tissue.

❷ Brachial artery perforation.

Management of perforations in this region is discussed in Chapter 5.

Rare Minor Complications

- Asymptomatic radial-artery occlusion (2.5% in series)
- Forearm discomfort that usually disappears within several days (0.2% of cases)

Potential Minor Complications

The following minor complications are mentioned in the literature, but are so rare they have not been seen after performing over 32,000 transradial procedures:

- Nerve injury leading to causalgia

1

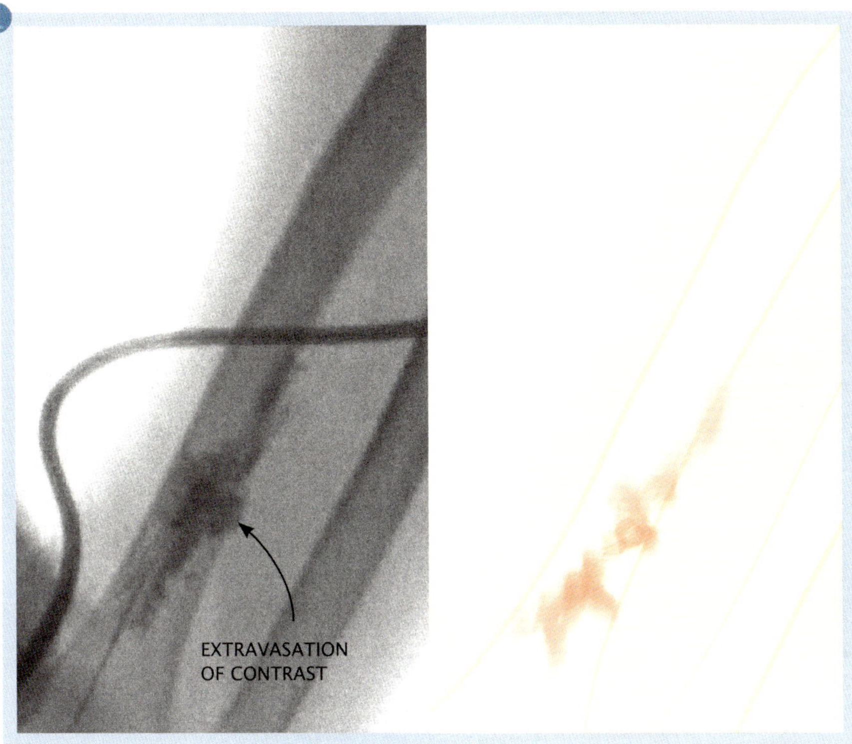

2

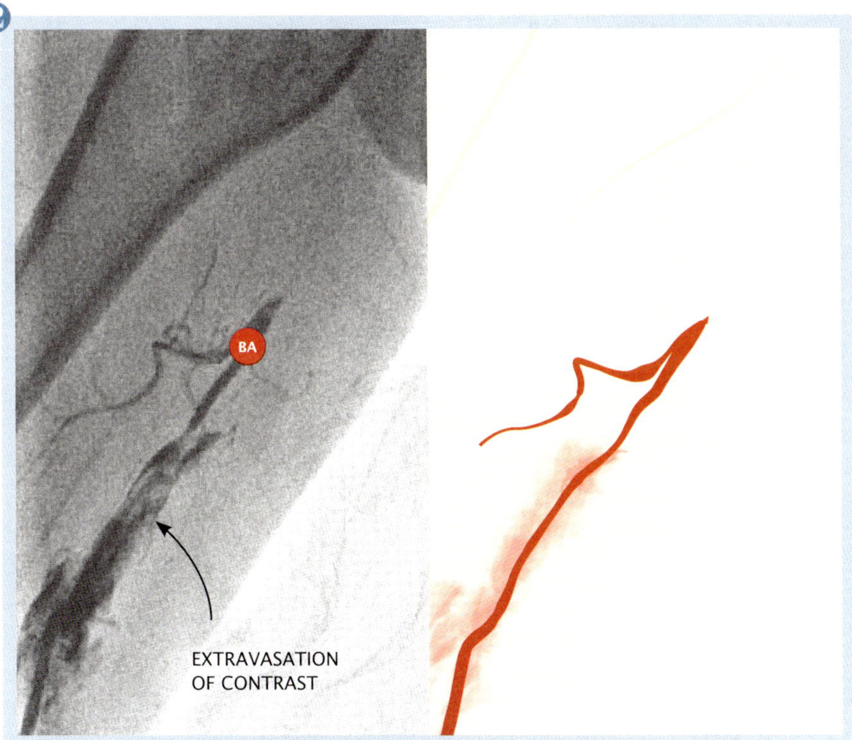

- Arteriovenous fistula
- Radial artery eversion during sheath removal
- Hand ischemia

Forearm Hematoma

Small hematoma involving the hand and forearm was present in only 2.5% of over 32,000 procedures. Note that the mechanism of J-tipped guidewires may induce small side-branch perforation. It may be a good idea to exercise a high index of suspicion regarding forearm pain and firmness, and immediate compression at the site. Ignoring the risk of compartment syndrome may have serious consequences. Forearm hematomas can be categorized using the easy hematoma classification system described by Bertrand et al.

EASY forearm hematoma classification system

- Grade I: local hematoma < 5 cm, no muscular infiltration
- Grade II: Hematoma 5–10 cm, with muscular hematoma
- Grade III: Hematoma >10 cm but not extending proximal to the elbow joint
- Grade IV: Hematoma extending above the elbow joint
- Grade V: Hematoma with ischemic threat (compartment syndrome)

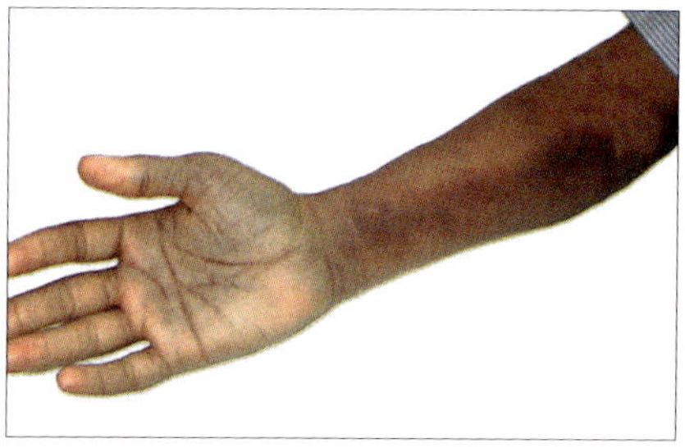

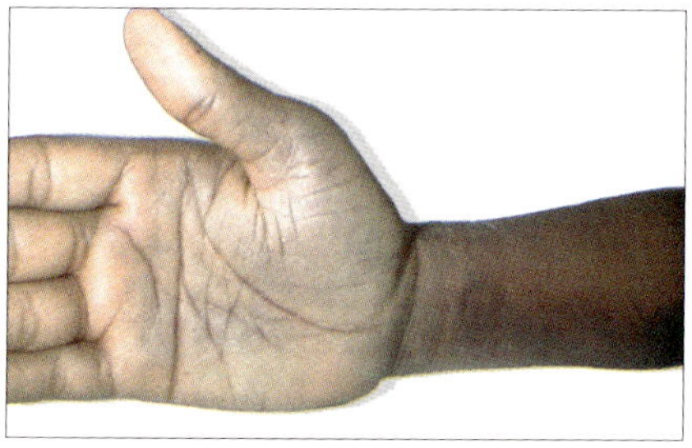

Remember

- Identify and evaluate a hematoma as soon as possible to prevent potential compartment-compression syndrome.
- A depigmented scar occurs due to very tight application of a radial artery closure device for a long time.
- Perforations of the radial artery or the brachial artery are rare. Try to maintain control of the arterial lumen as described in Chapter 5.
- Techniques to reduce the incidence of radial artery occlusion and methods to deal with this issue are detailed in Chapter 5.

Recommended Reading

1. Agostoni P, Biondi-Zoccai G, de Benedictis M, et al. Radial versus femoral approach for percutaneous coronary diagnostic and interventional procedures; Systematic overview and meta-analysis of randomized trials. J Am Coll Cardiol. 2004; 44 (2): 349-56.
2. Bazemore E, Mann T. Problems and complications of the transradial approach for coronary interventions: a review. J Invasive Cardiol. 2005; 17 (3): 156-59.
3. Behan M, Haworth P, Colley P, et al. Decreasing operators' radiation exposure during coronary procedures: the transradial radiation protection board. Catheter Cardiovasc Interv. 2010; 76 (1): 79-84.
4. Bertrand OF. Acute forearm muscle swelling post transradial catheterization and compartment syndrome: prevention is better than treatment! Catheter Cardiovasc Interv. 2010; 75 (3): 366-68.
5. Chase A, Fretz E, Warburton W, et al. Association of the arterial access site at angioplasty with transfusion and mortality: the M.O.R.T.A.L study (Mortality benefit Of Reduced Transfusion after percutaneous coronary intervention via the Arm or Leg). Heart. 2008; 94 (8): 1019-25.
6. Fagih B, Beaudry Y, Campeau L. Pseudo aneurysm a late complication of the transradial approach after coronary angiography. J Invasive Cardiol. 2000; 12 (4): 216-17.
7. Fang H, Wu C. Haemomediastinum, haemopericardium and haemothorax caused by elective transradial coronary angiography in a rare Kommerell's diverticulum. Eur J Cardiothorac Surg. 2010; 37 (4): 957.
8. Gilchrist I. Laissez-faire hemostasis and transradial injuries. Catheter Cardiovasc Interv. 2009; 73 (4): 473-74.
9. Hall I, Lo T, Nolan J. Deep vein thrombosis in the arm following transradial cardiac catheterization: an unusual complication related to hemostatic technique. Catheter Cardiovasc Interv. 2004; 62 (3): 346-48.
10. Hamon M, Gomes S, Clergeau M, et al. Risk of acute brain injury related to cerebral

microembolism during cardiac catheterization performed by right upper limb arterial access. Stroke. 2007; 38 (7): 2176-79.

11. Kiemeneij F, Laarman G, Odekerken D, et al. A randomized comparison of percutaneous transluminal coronary angioplasty by the radial, brachial and femoral approaches: the access study. J Am Coll Cardiol. 1997; 29 (6): 1269-75.
12. Kim J, Yoon J, Yoo B, et al. The effect of a eutectic mixture of local anesthetic cream on wrist pain during transradial coronary procedures. J Invasive Cardiol. 2007; 19 (1): 6-9.
13. Kozak M, Adams D, Ioffreda M, et al. Sterile inflammation associated with transradial catheterization and hydrophilic sheaths. Catheter Cardiovasc Interv. 2003; 59 (2): 207-13.
14. Lim J, Suri A, Chua T. Steroid-responsive sterile inflammation after transradial cardiac catheterisation using a sheath with hydrophilic coating. Heart. 2009; 95 (14): 1202.
15. Liou M, Tung F, Kanei Y, et al. Treatment of radial artery pseudoaneurysm using a novel compression device. J Invasive Cardiol. 2010; 22 (6): 293-95.
16. Pancholy S, Coppola J, Patel T, et al. Prevention of radial artery occlusion-patent hemostasis evaluation trial (PROPHET study): a randomized comparison of traditional versus patency documented hemostasis after transradial catheterization. Catheter Cardiovasc Interv. 2008; 72 (3): 335-40.
17. Pancholy S. Impact of two different hemostatic devices on radial artery outcomes after transradial catheterization. J Invasive Cardiol. 2009; 21 (3): 101-104.
18. Park K, Chung J, Chang S, et al. Two cases of mediastinal hematoma after cardiac catheterization: A rare but real complication of the transradial approach. Int J Cardiol. 2008; 130 (3): e89-92.
19. Patel T, Shah S, Sanghavi K, Pancholy S. Management of radial and brachial artery perforations during transradial procedures—a practical approach. J Invasive Cardiol. 2009; 21 (10): 544-47.
20. Politi L, Aprile A, Paganelli C, et al. Randomized clinical trial on short-time compression with kaolin-filled pad: a new strategy to avoid early bleeding and subacute radial artery occlusion after percutaneous coronary intervention. J Interv Cardiol. 2011; 24 (1): 65-72.
21. Rathore S, Stables R, Pauriah M, et al. A randomized comparison of TR band and radistop hemostatic compression devices after transradial coronary intervention. Catheter Cardiovasc Interv. 2010; 76 (5): 660-67.
22. Rhyne D, Mann T. Hand ischemia resulting from a transradial intervention: successful management with radial artery angioplasty. Catheter Cardiovasc Interv. 2010; 76 (3): 383-86.
23. Romagnoli E, Nasso G, Angeloni G, et al. Cardiovocal syndrome after transradial cardiac catheterization: An unusual complication. Int J Cardiol. 2008; 124 (3): e39-41.
24. Sasano N, Tsuda T, Sasano H, et al. A case of complex regional pain syndrome type II after transradial coronary intervention. J Anesth. 2004; 18 (4): 310-112.
25. Spence M, Byrne J, Haegeli L,et al. Rare access site complications following transradial coronary intervention. Can J Cardiol. 2009; 25 (6): e206.
26. Swaminathan R, Wong S. Radial access site inflammatory reaction to a recently available hydrophilic coated sheath. Catheter Cardiovasc Interv. 2011 (In Press).
27. Tharmaratnam D, Webber S, Owens P. Adverse local reactions to the use of hydrophilic sheaths for radial artery canulation. Int J Cardiol. 2010; 142 (3): 296-98.
28. Tizón-Marcos H, Barbeau G. Incidence of compartment syndrome of the arm in a large series of transradial approach for coronary procedures. J Interv Cardiol. 2008; 21 (5): 380-84.
29. Zellner C, Ports T, Yeghiazarians Y, et al. Sterile radial artery granuloma after transradial procedures: a unique and avoidable complication. Catheter Cardiovasc Interv. 2010: 76 (5): 673-76.

Radial and Brachial Regions: Understanding and Addressing the Issues

5

Tejas Patel, Sanjay Shah, Samir Pancholy, Rajnikant Radadiya and Alok Ranjan

In this chapter, the normal and relevant abnormal anatomy of the radial and brachial arteries will be discussed.

Classic examples of spasm, atherosclerosis, calcification, tortuosity, abnormal origin of the radial artery (from high brachial and axillary artery), radial artery (RA) perforation, RA occlusion, and types of loops and curvatures are shown.

Techniques to address these issues successfully are shown.

Normal Anatomy of Brachial and Radial Artery

The RA commences at the bifurcation of the brachial artery near the elbow, and passes along the radial side of the forearm to the wrist. The RA extends from the neck of the radius to the front of the styloid process. The upper part lies on the medial side of radius and the lower part lies on the bone. The upper part is deep and lies below the muscle (brachioradialis) in most cases. The lower part is superficial, covered by skin, and superficial and deep fascia. The RA is slightly smaller in caliber than the ulnar artery (UA).

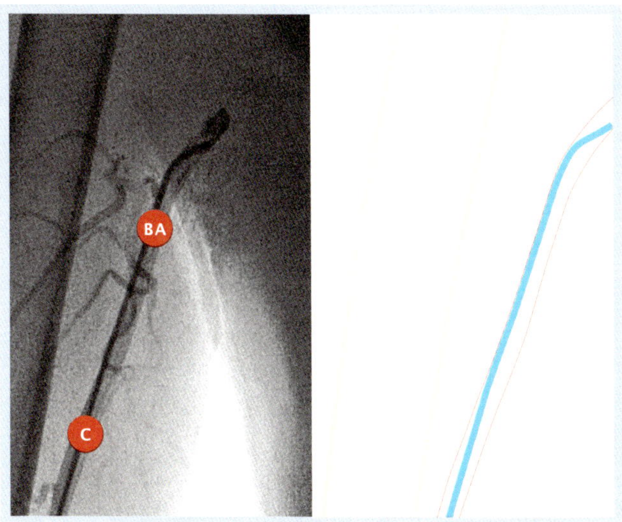

Normal brachial artery anatomy.

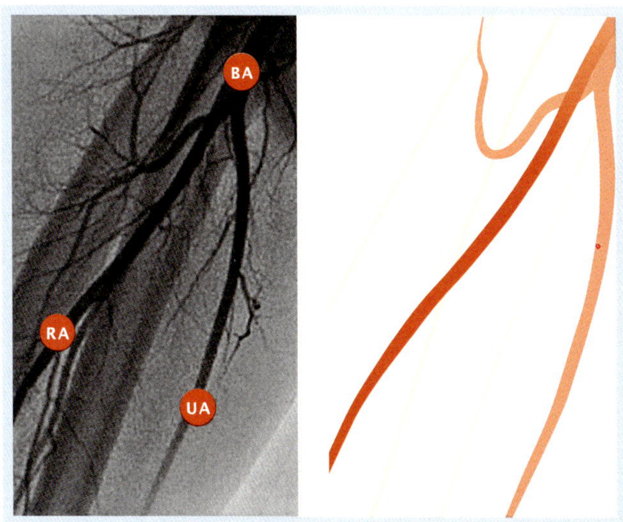

Normal anatomy of the radial artery and ulnar artery.

(A) RA Spasm

Beginning radialists have apprehension to deal with RA spasm. True RA spasm is not as common as most interventionalists think. The overall incidence in experienced hands is about 5.6%, 0.5% of whom have severe spasm. RA spasm can be broadly classified into focal and diffuse.

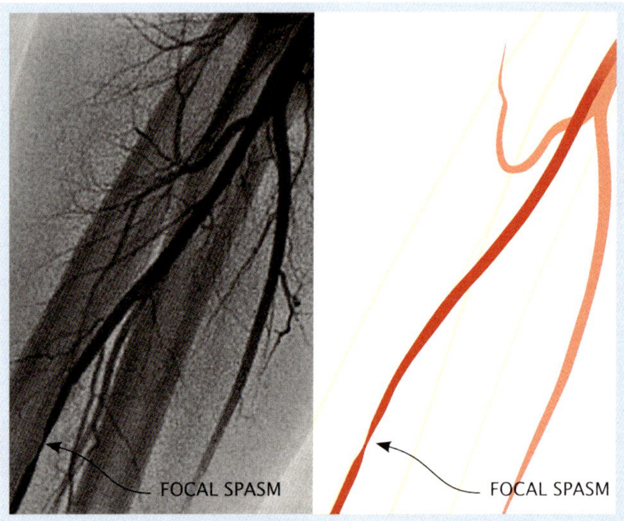

Focal spasm of the radial artery.

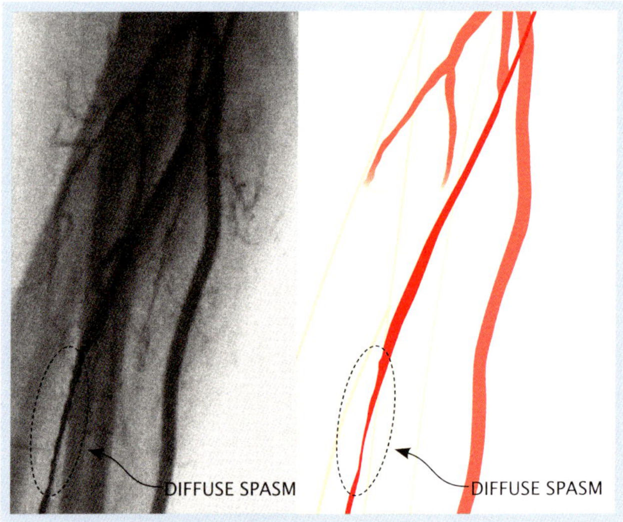

Diffuse spasm involving a segment length of 20 mm or more.

Identification

- If a patient complains of significant local pain in the region of RA during the passage of a guidewire and/or a catheter, RA spasm should be suspected.
- Perform a radial angiogram through the side port of the introducer sheath or through catheter itself, to define the anatomy and detect spasm.
- If RA spasm is confirmed, an additional dose of spasmolytic cocktail should be given and another radial angiogram should be performed after a short period (30 seconds to 1 minute) to confirm that spasm is relieved.

- If RA spasm contributes at this stage, the affected segment should be crossed carefully using a 0.025-inch J-shaped hydrophilic guidewire or a soft-tip 0.014-inch PTCA guidewire. Once it is done successfully, a diagnostic or a guide catheter should be negotiated over it. Instead of the usual pushing movement, use a slow, corkscrew movement to break the spasm. Once the tip of a catheter crosses the affected segment, the rest of the procedure can be completed in regular fashion.

- If spasm develops in RA with the initial catheter, downsizing the catheter (to a 4 Fr instead of a 5 Fr diagnostic catheter, or a 5 Fr instead of a 6 Fr guide catheter) helps to work past the spasm successfully.

- Beginners have relatively higher incidence of RA spasm. Multiple attempts for RA puncture is the most common cause. Sometimes the RA pulse becomes feeble or disappears because of severe spasm. Subcutaneous injection of nitroglycerin should be given; it helps return the RA pulse in most instances.

- Significant tortuosity, calcification or atherosclerosis of RA segment may create difficulty in passing a guidewire and/or catheter. Repeated push of the assembly against this resistance is usually counterproductive and can lead to reactive focal or diffuse RA spasm. Repeat cocktail and use of aforementioned steps to negotiate the assembly usually brings success.

- Anatomical variations of the RA, particularly anomalous origin of the RA from high brachial or axillary artery and radio-brachial loops, are most commonly misinterpreted as RA spasm. Whenever the RA has high brachial or axillary artery origin, its caliber is almost invariably small. This leads to significant resistance to passage of assembly through this segment. Downsizing the catheter resolves the problem to a great extent. The method of working through loops is discussed later in this chapter.

- Very rarely after completion of a diagnostic procedure or an intervention, the catheter is severely gripped in RA spasm segment. Even a gentle attempt to pull the catheter gives agonizing pain to the patient. In this rare situation, a short course of general anesthesia is helpful. Once the patient is anesthetized, the catheter can usually be easily removed without pain.

(B) RA Atherosclerosis

RA atherosclerosis is usually a part of a generalized atherosclerotic process. It is possible to perform an angiogram or an intervention successfully in this situation.

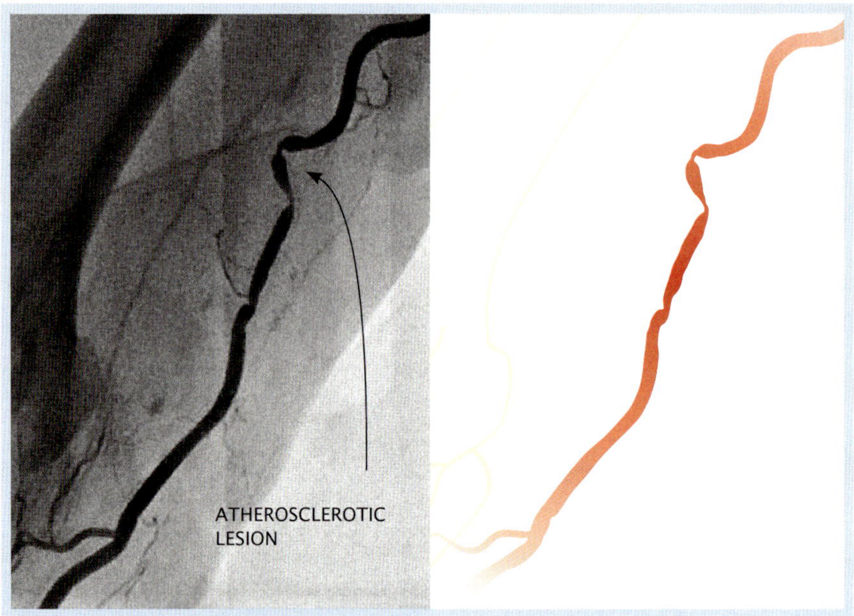

There was no change in the caliber of the radial artery after an additional dose of spasmolytic cocktail, proving that this was true atherosclerosis and not spasm.

Tips

- Atherosclerotic lesions in RA give resistance to the movement of a guidewire and/or a catheter.
- Once resistance is encountered, it is important to perform an RA angiogram.
- If an RA angiogram reveals an atherosclerotic lesion, it is important to define its severity (mild to moderate, or severe).
- If the obstruction is mild, careful passage of the assembly through the affected segment under fluoroscopic guidance should help the operator perform and complete the procedure successfully.
- If it is a severe stenotic lesion, it is advisable to dilate the lesion with a PTCA catheter, then work through the affected segment.
- In both situations, a repeat dose of spasmolytic cocktail facilitates the passage of the assembly.

(C) RA Calcification

Although uncommonly seen, it is important to identify this issue. RA calcification can be patchy or diffuse.

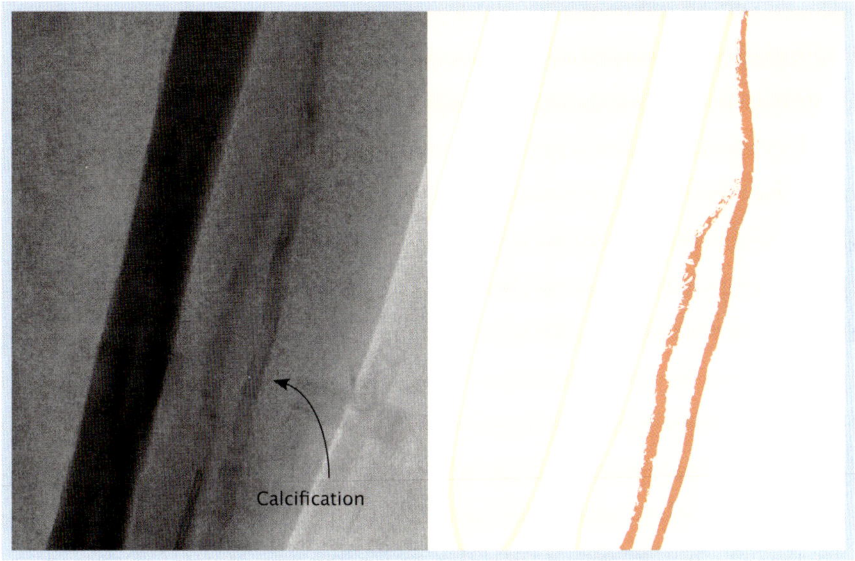

Radial and ulnar artery calcification seen on fluoroscopy.

Tips

- Patchy calcification offers mild resistance to the passage of a guidewire and/or a catheter. However, it is easy to work through it using the standard technique.
- Diffuse calcification creates significant resistance to the passage of a guidewire and/or a catheter. Instead of using the standard push of the catheter over the wire, a slow corkscrew movement is recommended. This technique decreases the friction in the affected segment. Once the segment is crossed by the initial part of the catheter, the resistance disappears or decreases markedly, and the rest of the diagnostic or interventional procedure can be completed in the regular fashion.

(D) Tortuosity

It is an important issue to understand. Tortuosity is more common in patients above 70 years, long-standing diabetics and females.

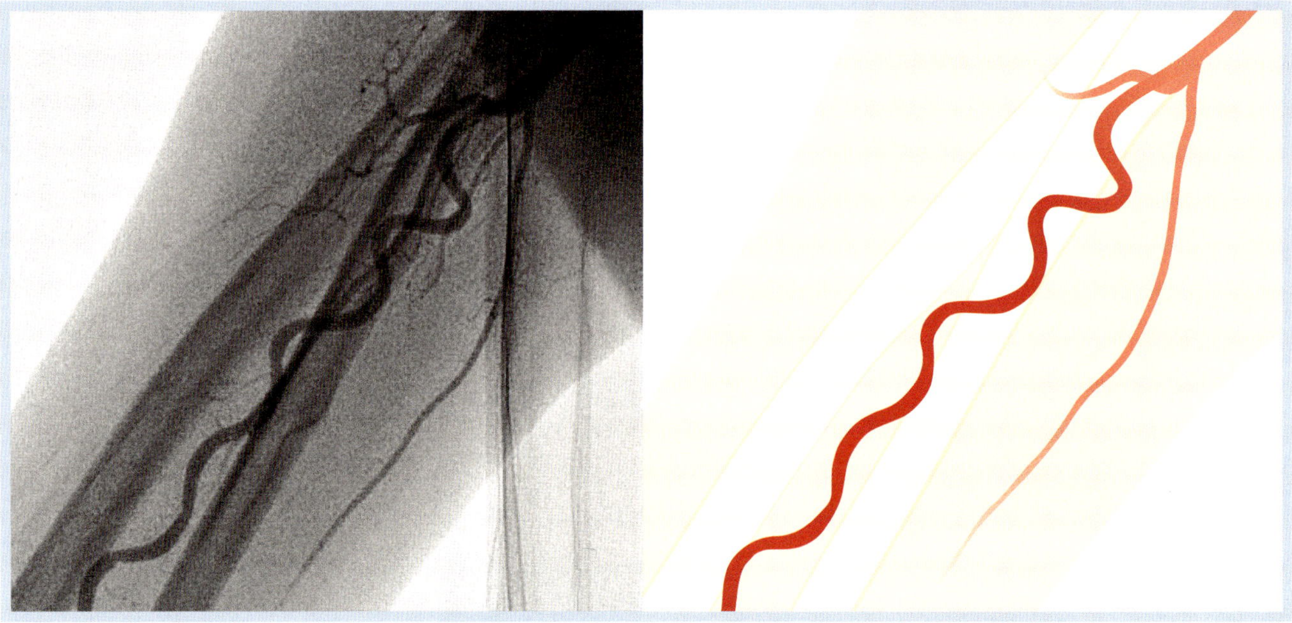

Tortuosity of the radial artery.

Tips

- Tortuosity is an major cause of resistance to the movement of a guidewire and/or a catheter.
- RA angiogram reveals the severity and extent of tortuosity.
- If the RA diameter is big, negotiate the assembly through it.
- If the RA diameter is small and the tortuous segment long, it should be crossed using a 0.025-inch or 0.032-inch J-shaped hydrophilic guidewire or a 0.014-inch soft-tip PTCA guidewire. Carefully negotiate a catheter over the wire using a slow corkscrew movement under fluoroscopic guidance. Once the segment is crossed with the assembly, the rest of the procedure can be finished in the usual fashion.
- Direct push of the catheter is not recommended in this situation as it can induce reactive spasm. Spasm in a tortuous RA segment is painful both for patient and operator.
- Repeat dose of cocktail may help working through a small caliber of RA and tortuous segment with or without spasm.

(E) High Origin of RA From a High Brachial or Axillary Artery

These common anatomical variants are important to recognize. The caliber of RA in this situation is almost invariably small.

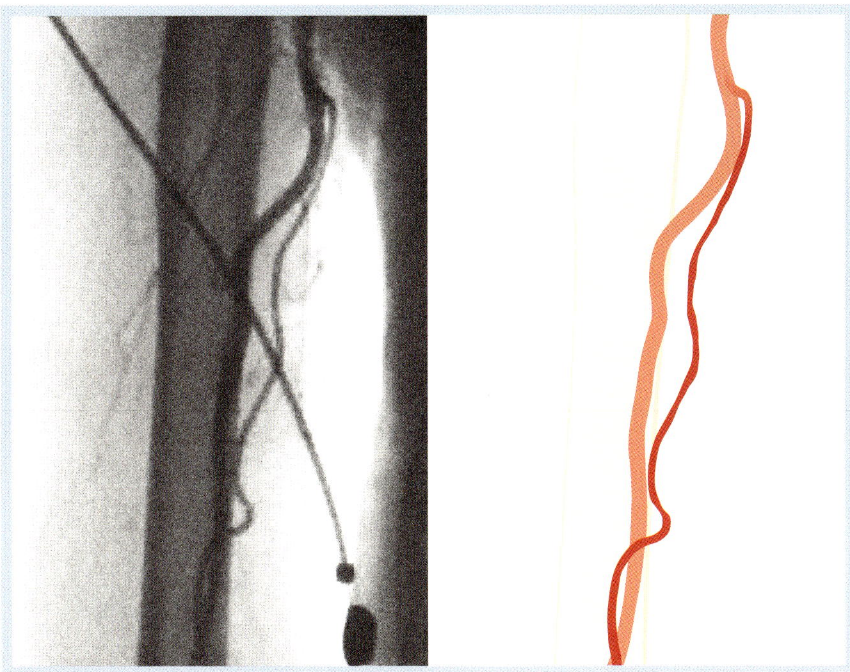

High origin of the radial artery from the brachial artery.

Tips

- High origins of the RA are a major cause of resistance to the movement of a catheter.
- It is commonly misinterpreted as RA spasm.
- RA angiogram reveals the diagnosis.
- Downsizing the catheter and administering a repeat dose of the cocktail helps reduce the resistance in the passage of a catheter.

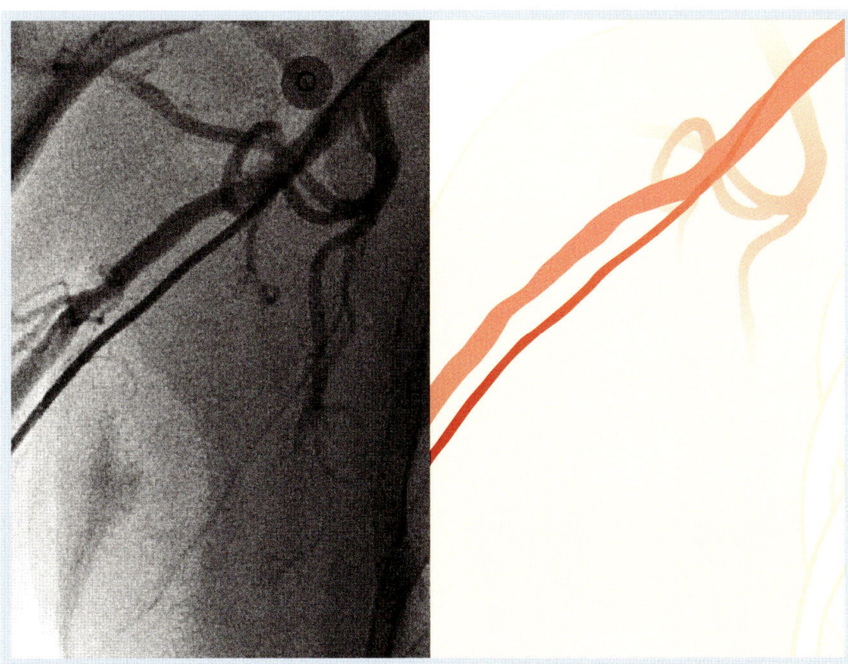

High origin of the radial artery from the axillary artery.

(F) Radial-Brachial Artery Perforation

This complication needs to be identified and managed immediately. It is the most common cause of forearm hematoma. The incidence is about 0.1% in large series.

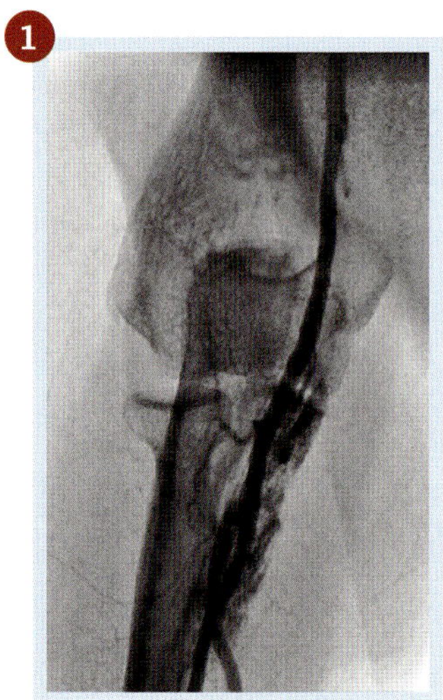

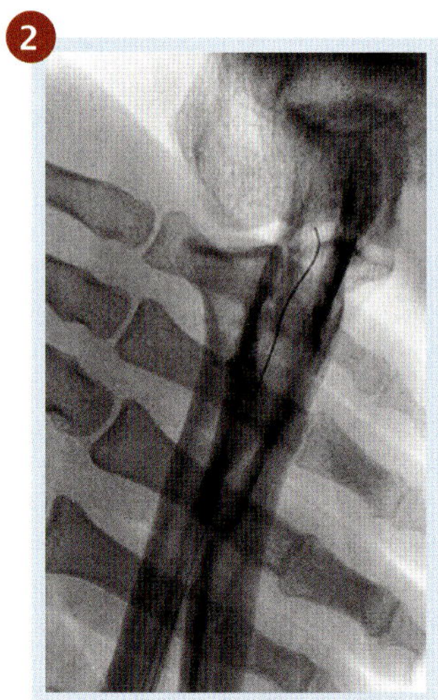

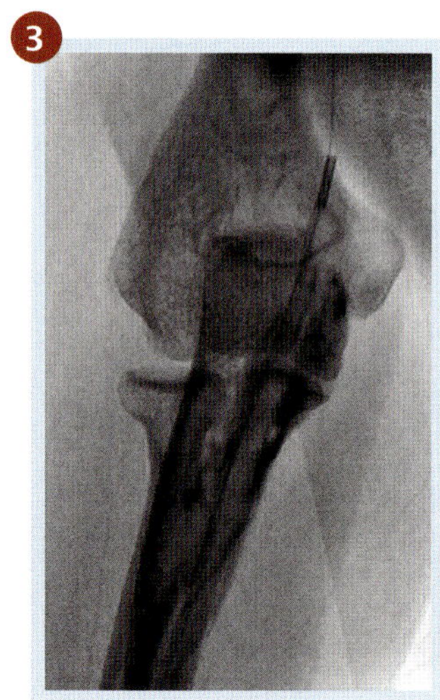

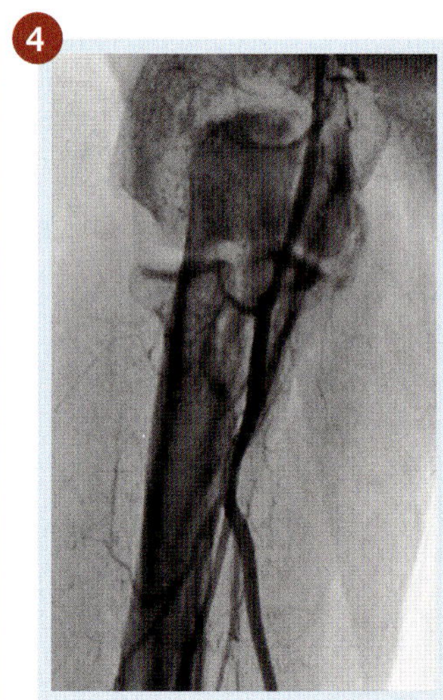

1. An example of a guidewire induced perforation at radio-brachial junction. Significant extravasation of contrast is seen.
2. A soft tip 0.014-inch PTCA guidewire was used to cross the perforated segment successfully.
3. A soft tip 0.014-inch PTCA guidewire was used to cross the perforated segment successfully.
4. After successful completion of coronary angiogram, contrast injection through the catheter revealed sealed perforation and no extravasation of contrast.

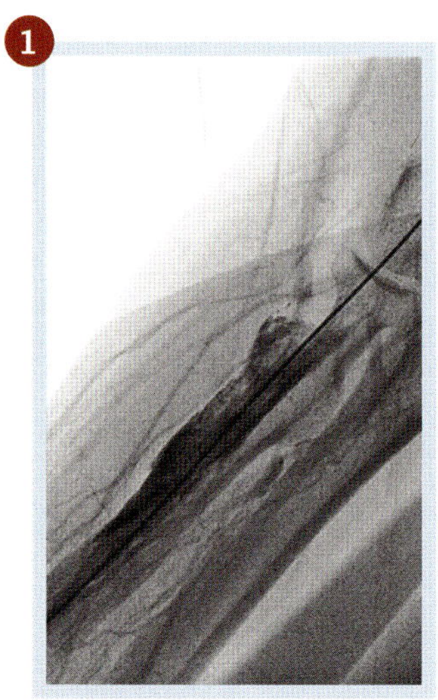

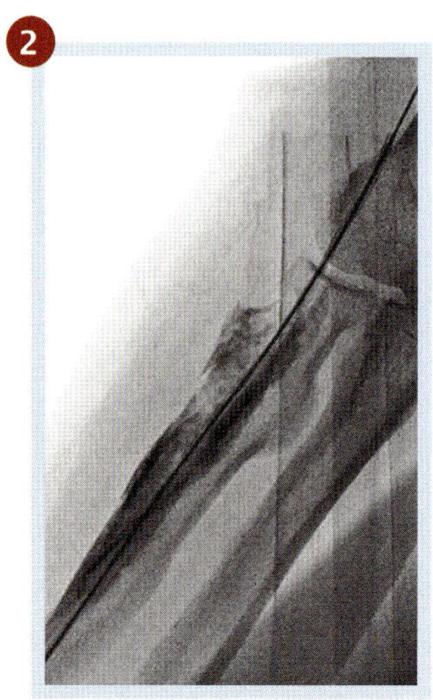

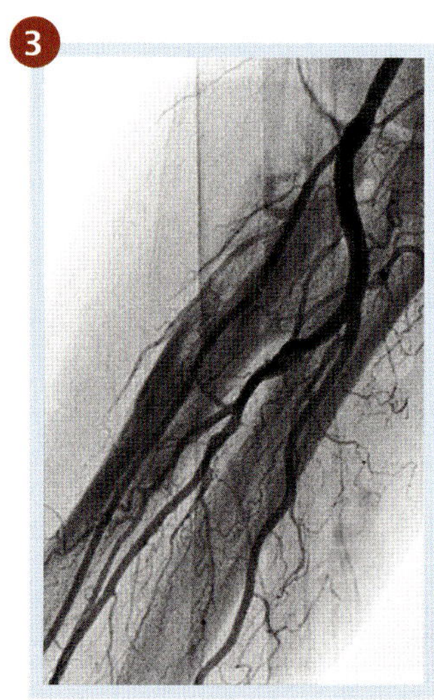

1. Another example of radial artery perforation. Extravasation of contrast is seen and a 0.025" hydrophilic guidewire has been negotiated across the affected segment.
2. The catheter has been negotiated over the wire across the affected segment.
3. Post-procedure injection at the local site revealed proper sealing of perforation and no extravasation.

Tips

- Excessive resistance in the passage of a guidewire and/or a catheter felt by the operator, associated with complaint of significant local pain in the radial and/or brachial region from the patient, with or without development of an expanding hematoma makes the diagnosis.
- Immediately removing the assembly and injection of the diluted contrast through the side port of an introducer sheath confirms the site and size of perforation.
- A beginning radialist may be apprehensive about working through perforation. One may be inclined to abandon the procedure, reverse the effect of heparin and give manual compression at the local site for a sufficiently long time to prevent a hematoma. The procedure may be completed after several hours or the next day, using a contralateral radial or a femoral route.
- Experience has shown that control of the artery and continuation of the procedure after crossing the perforation is the preferred technique rather than abandoning the artery and prolonging the procedure.

These are the steps:

1. Identify the site and size of perforation by injecting diluted contrast through the side port of introducer sheath.
2. Use a floppy-tip 0.014-inch PTCA wire and carefully cross the affected area. Park the wire higher in the brachial or axillary region.
3. Negotiate a diagnostic or a guide catheter over the wire and stop when the tip of the catheter reaches the perforated segment.
4. Gently negotiate the catheter using a slow corkscrew movement (instead of the usual push) to reduce friction in the perforated segment. Once the tip crosses the affected segment, the movement of the catheter becomes smooth, and the procedure can be completed in usual fashion.
5. If there is resistance to the movement of the catheter tip at the perforation site, remove the catheter immediately and downsize it (i.e., to a 4 Fr diagnostic catheter instead of 5 Fr, or a 5 Fr guide catheter instead of 6 Fr). This strategy facilitates the successful crossing of affected segment with less friction.
6. Once the diagnostic or interventional procedure is over, the catheter is pulled back over the wire and diluted contrast is injected through the side port of the introducer sheath to confirm appropriate sealing of the perforated segment. It is important to understand that the catheter functions as an internal hemostatic device to help seal the perforated segment.

(G) Loops and Curvatures

These are other important anatomical variations to understand. There is typically no resistance when advancing guidewires and catheters up to the ascending aorta. Resistance to movement of a wire and/or a catheter is most commonly interpreted as RA spasm. Most often, what initially appears to be RA spasm is actually an anatomical variation in the form of tortuosity, loop or curvature. Once again, a low threshold for performing an RA angiogram is critical, as it defines the anatomy and helps define a working solution through the vast majority of these challenges.

Loops and curvatures are to be expected, and a radialist needs to have a plan to work through these challenges. A consistent plan will reduce the apprehension of a beginning radialist and give additional confidence to an experienced operator. A successful approach is outlined on the following pages.

Important steps to remember

❶ Define the task

When resistance is encountered in the movement of a wire and/or a catheter, inject diluted contrast to define the anatomy. If a simple loop is identified, it can be worked through under fluoroscopic guidance. If the loop is complex, take multiple views (i.e., RAO and LAO, cranial or caudal angulations). Identify the view that best defines the loop. The chosen view can then be used as a map for working through the loop.

❷ Downsize the guidewire

If resistance is encountered in the passage of a standard 0.032-inch or 0.035-inch guidewire while working through the loop, remove the wire; repeated attempts to negotiate against the resistance can lead to perforation, spasm and severe local pain. A flexible guidewire (e.g., a 0.014-inch soft-tip PTCA guidewire or 0.025-inch hydrophilic guidewire) should be used in place of a standard guidewire to cross the loop. The tip of a guidewire (especially of a 0.014-inch PTCA wire) can be shaped to the angle of the loop to facilitate crossing. When the guidewire crosses the loop, its tip is parked as high as possible (e.g., high brachial, axillary or subclavian region). Then the catheter can be advanced over it. Sometimes, when these guidewires do not adequately support the advancement of the catheters, the strategy should be changed (discussed in the next part).

❸ Use of buddy wire(s)

When a single 0.014-inch PTCA guidewire provides inadequate support for a catheter to cross the loop, using an additional one or two such guidewires should facilitate the advancement of the catheter by adding support.

❹ Straightening of the loop

Usually the catheter can easily be negotiated over the wire across a loop without disturbing the shape of the loop. When there is resistance in passage of the catheter while working through the loop, the following technique is useful.

Push the catheter as far as possible into the loop, keeping the wire tip as high as possible (e.g., in the high brachial, axillary or subclavian region). Then pull the entire assembly (the catheter along with the guidewire) slightly back. This maneuver opens and straightens the loop. At this stage, advancement of the catheter across the loop becomes easy.

❺ Exchanging the guidewire

This technique is helpful in addressing the most difficult loops. It is used if the catheter is partly inside the loop, but has not crossed the entire loop and is difficult to advance any farther.

Advance the catheter into the loop as far as possible. Exchange the thin guidewire with another guidewire to provide extra support. A 0.014-inch PTCA guidewire can be exchanged with a 0.025-inch hydrophilic guidewire, and a 0.025-inch hydrophilic guidewire can be exchanged with a standard 0.035-inch guidewire, if necessary. Then advance the catheter on the new wire. Avoid using a super-stiff guidewire unless the loop has been crossed and the catheter tip is well-advanced into the higher segment (e.g., high brachial, axillary or subclavian region). This technique is useful in working through a difficult radio-cubital trunk and a 360° loop with very small diameter.

Here are few examples of the types of loops.

- Simple loop

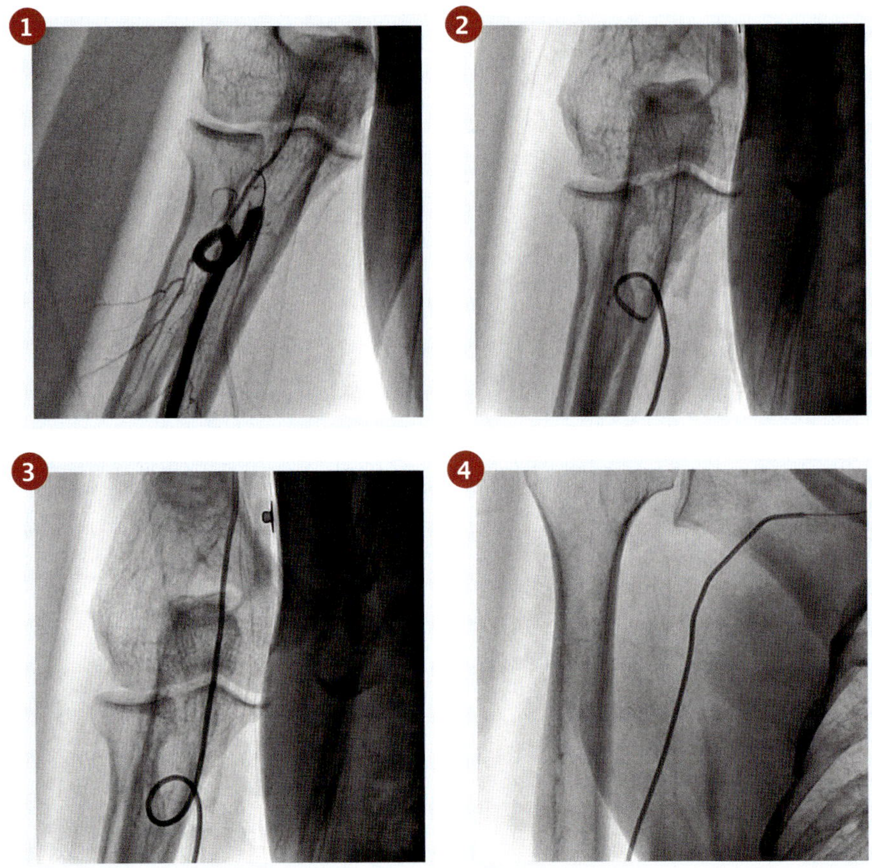

1. This is an example of a simple loop.
2. A 0.014-inch PTCA guidewire was used to negotiate the loop, and the catheter was advanced halfway into the loop.
3. The catheter was advanced beyond the loop, farther in the brachial artery, and the PTCA guidewire was removed.
4. The 0.014-inch PTCA guidewire was exchanged with a hydrophilic 0.025-inch guidewire, and the procedure was completed without unfolding the loop.

More challenging loop

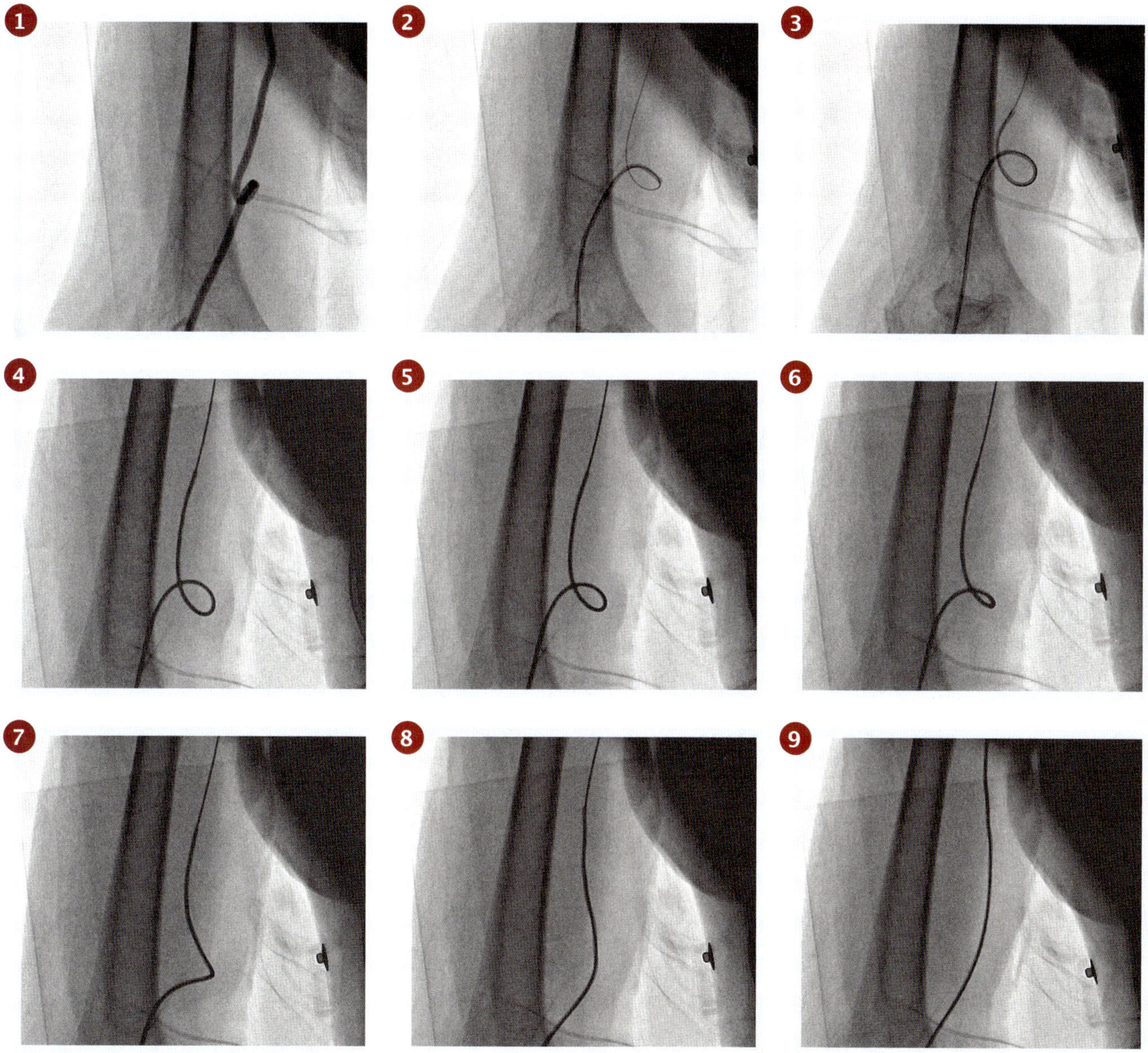

1. This is an example of a more challenging loop of the radial artery (high origin).
2. A 0.014-inch PTCA guidewire was negotiated through the loop, and a 4 Fr diagnostic catheter was advanced over the guidewire.
3. The catheter was advanced farther into the loop.
4. The catheter tip crossed the loop and entered the brachial artery but refused to advance further.
5. To straighten the loop, the entire assembly was pulled back.
6. The loop started straightening.
7. The loop further straightened.
8. The loop was successfully straightened.
9. The catheter could be easily advanced over the guidewire.

Examples of the most challenging loops

Double-hairpin loop

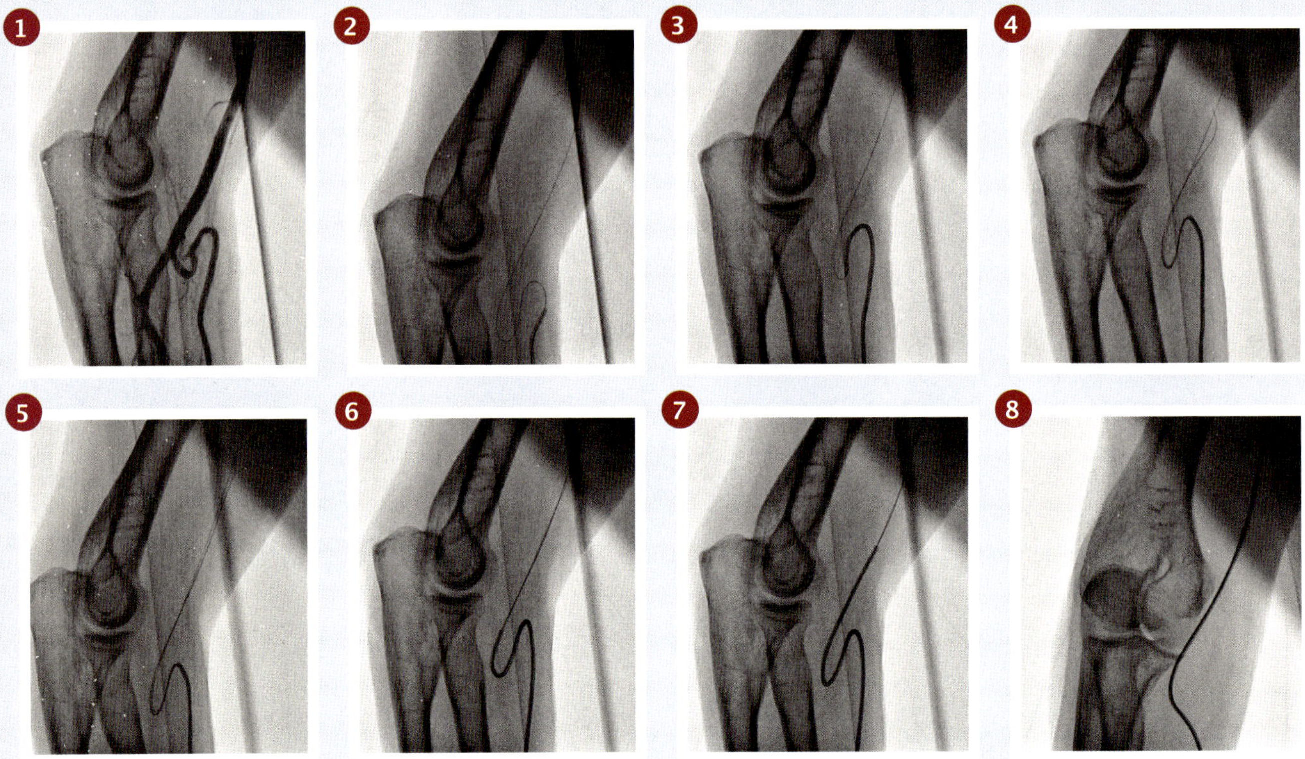

1. This is an example of a double-hairpin loop.
2. A 0.014-inch PTCA guidewire was used to negotiate the loop.
3. A 5 Fr diagnostic catheter negotiated the first hairpin turn of the loop, but refused to budge any farther.
4. Another 0.014-inch PTCA guidewire (buddy wire) was used.
5. The buddy wire was advanced farther.
6. This allowed the catheter to cross the second hairpin turn.
7. The catheter was advanced into the brachial artery.
8. A gentle pullback of the entire assembly straightened the loop and made further advancement of the catheter easier.

Radio-cubital trunk

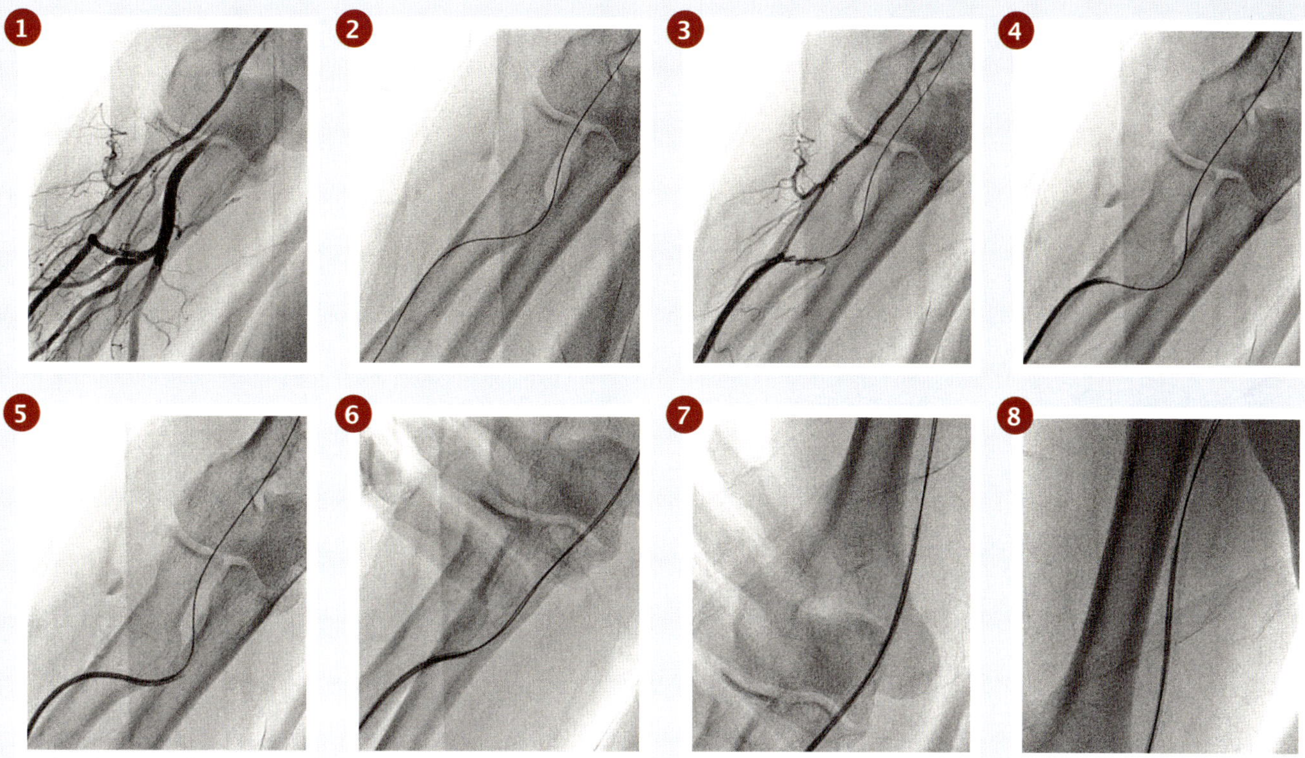

1. This is an example of a complex radiocubital trunk.
2. A 0.014-inch PTCA guidewire was used to negotiate the loop.
3. An angiogram confirmed the position of the 0.014-inch PTCA guidewire in the distal part of the brachial artery across the loop.
4. An attempt was made to advance a 5 Fr diagnostic catheter over the 0.014-inch PTCA guidewire.
5. The catheter would not budge beyond mid-loop.
6. At this point, a second 0.014-inch PTCA guidewire (buddy wire) was used to provide adequate support, and the catheter was advanced over the two 0.014-inch PTCA guidewires.
7. The catheter crossed the loop successfully.
8. The catheter was advanced easily in the brachial artery.

A complex 360⁰ loop

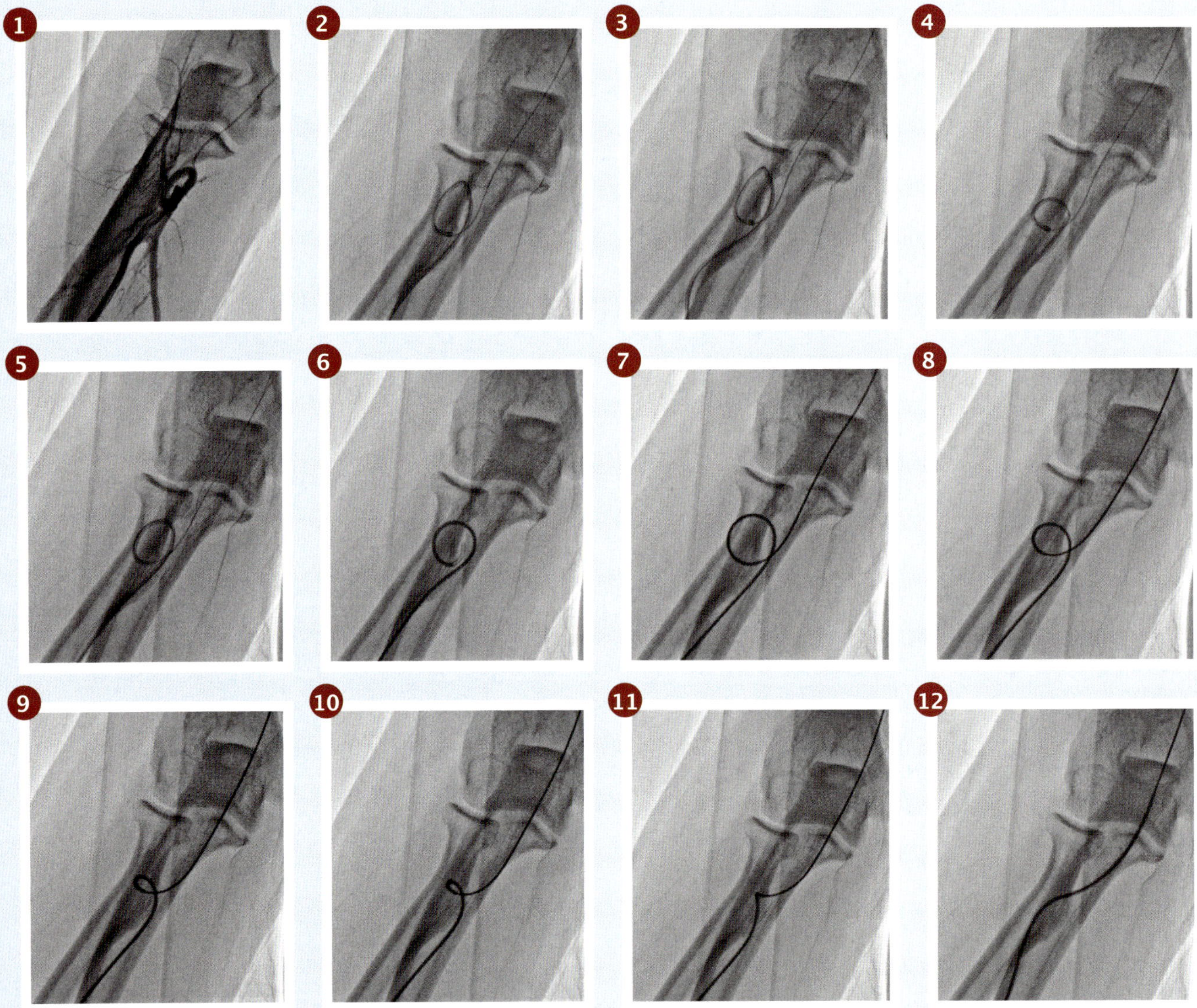

1. This is an example of a very small diameter 360° loop.
2. Two 0.014-inch PTCA guidewires were negotiated through the loop into the brachial artery; a 5 Fr Opti-torque TIG catheter was advanced into the loop.
3. It refused to budge beyond halfway.
4. The catheter was removed and exchanged for a 5 Fr pigtail catheter.
5. The pigtail catheter also refused to budge beyond halfway.
6. Both the PTCA guidewires were removed.
7. A 0.035-inch standard guidewire was negotiated through the loop into the brachial artery.
8. We started to pull back the whole assembly.
9. The loop started straightening.
10. The loop straightened further.
11. The loop straightened almost completely.
12. The catheter could be negotiated easily into the brachial artery.

Loop with perforation

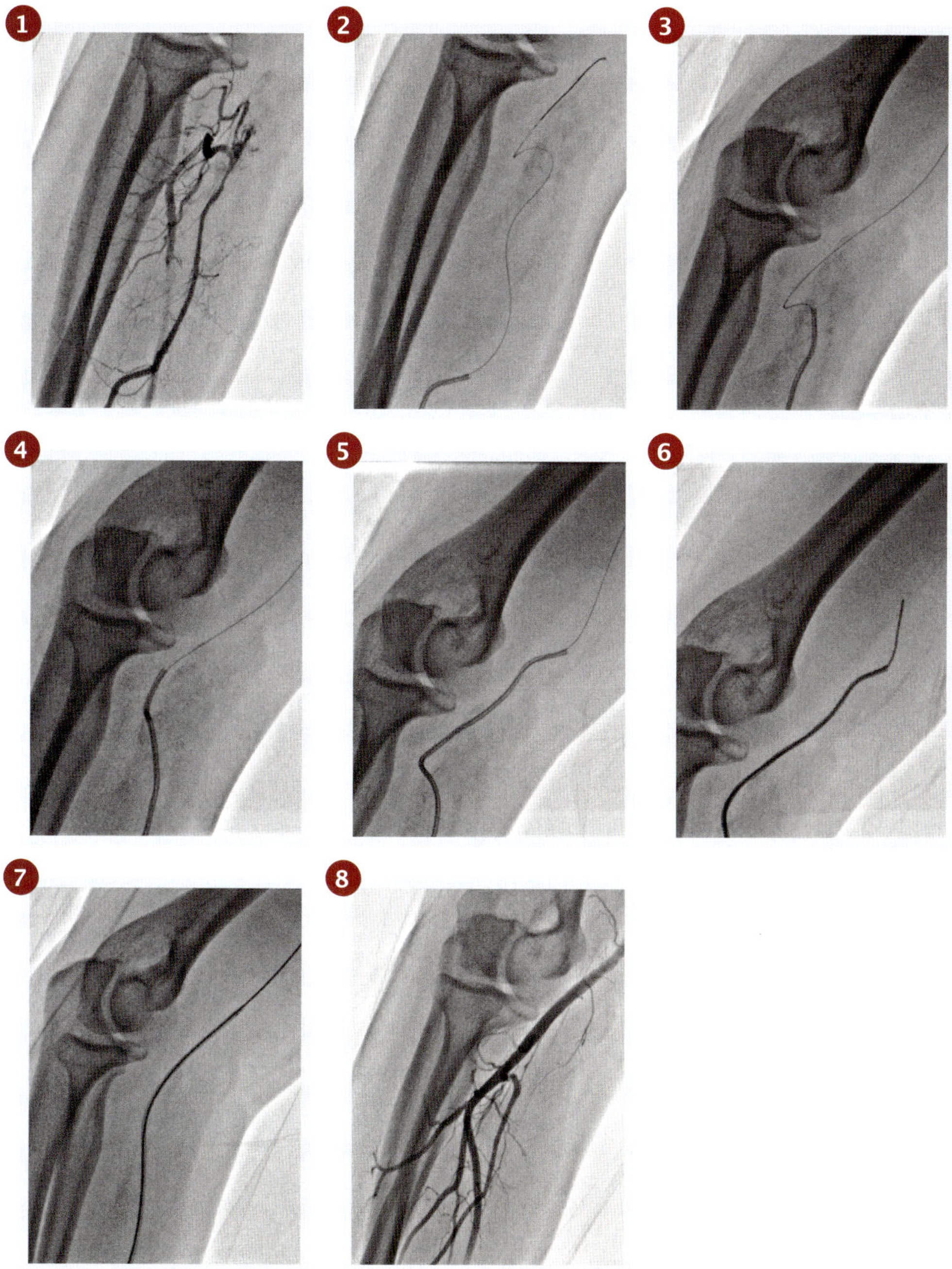

1. This is an example of a loop complicated by perforation.
2. A 0.014-inch PTCA guidewire was carefully negotiated through the perforated segment.
3. A 5 Fr diagnostic catheter was advanced carefully over the wire.
4. The perforated segment was crossed by gentle corkscrew maneuvering of the catheter over the PTCA guidewire.
5. The perforated segment was crossed by the catheter.
6. The PTCA guidewire was replaced by a 0.035-inch standard guidewire.
7. The catheter was negotiated further over a standard 0.035-inch guidewire.
8. Radial angiogram at the end of the procedure revealed a sealed perforation.

Hidden loop (mimicking spasm)

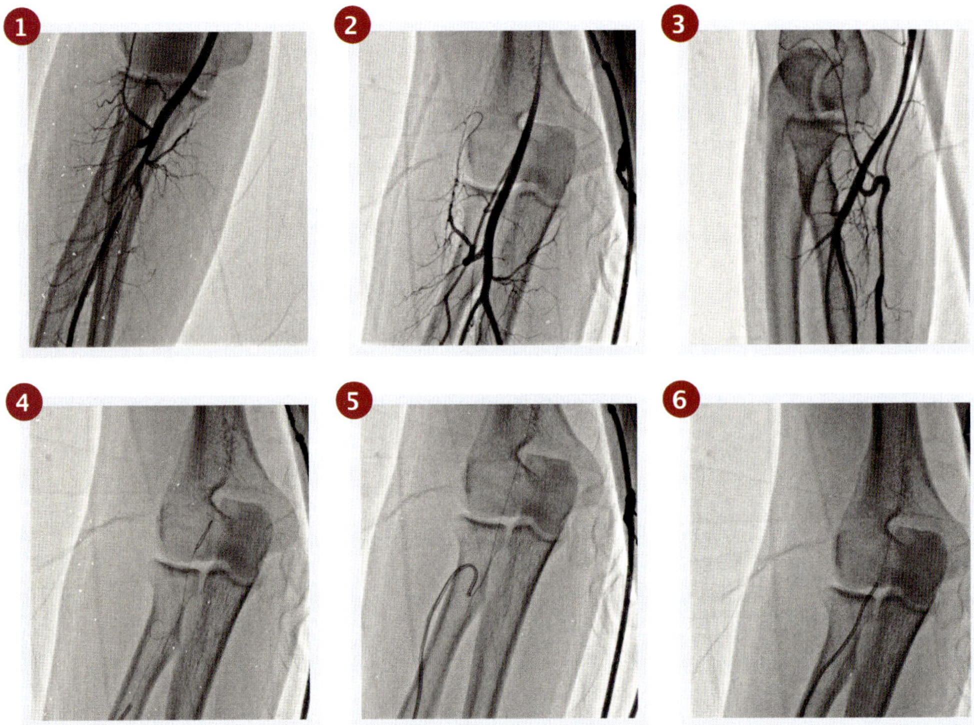

1. An example of a "hidden loop" and associated segmental spasm of radial artery.
2. An RA angiogram was done by injecting contrast through the side port of the introducer sheath; RAO view revealed a loop.
3. The loop is shown in an LAO view.
4. The 0.014-inch PTCA guidewire was carefully negotiated through the loop.
5. The catheter was negotiated over the 0.014-inch PTCA guidewire.
6. The catheter crossed the loop and entered the brachial artery.

Very low radial loop

Example 1

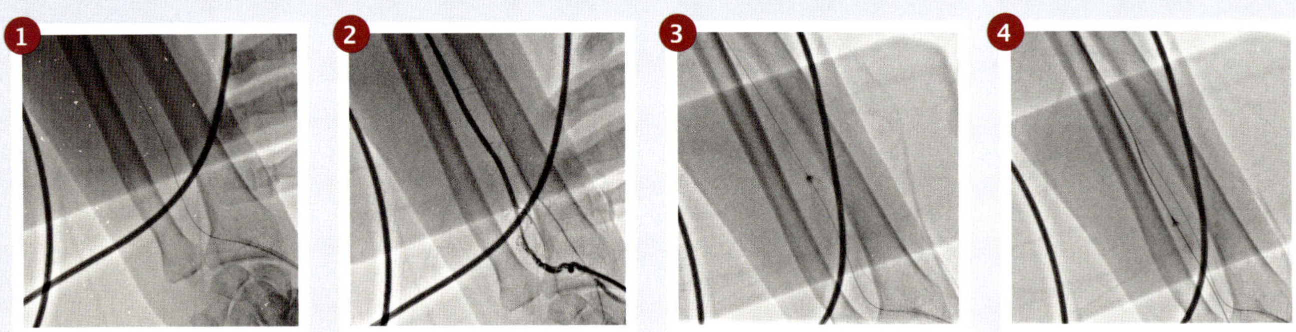

1. This is an example of a very low radial loop. A 0.014-inch PTCA guidewire could be negotiated in the RA, but the introducer sheath refused to budge beyond a particular point. The patient started complaining of severe local pain.
2. Contrast injected through the side port revealed a 360° loop in a very low segment of the RA. The higher segment of the RA had a straight course and a good diameter.
3. The RA was punctured in the higher segment, keeping the PTCA guidewire as a roadmap.
4. The guidewire could easily be negotiated, and the sheath was introduced to complete the procedure.

Example 2

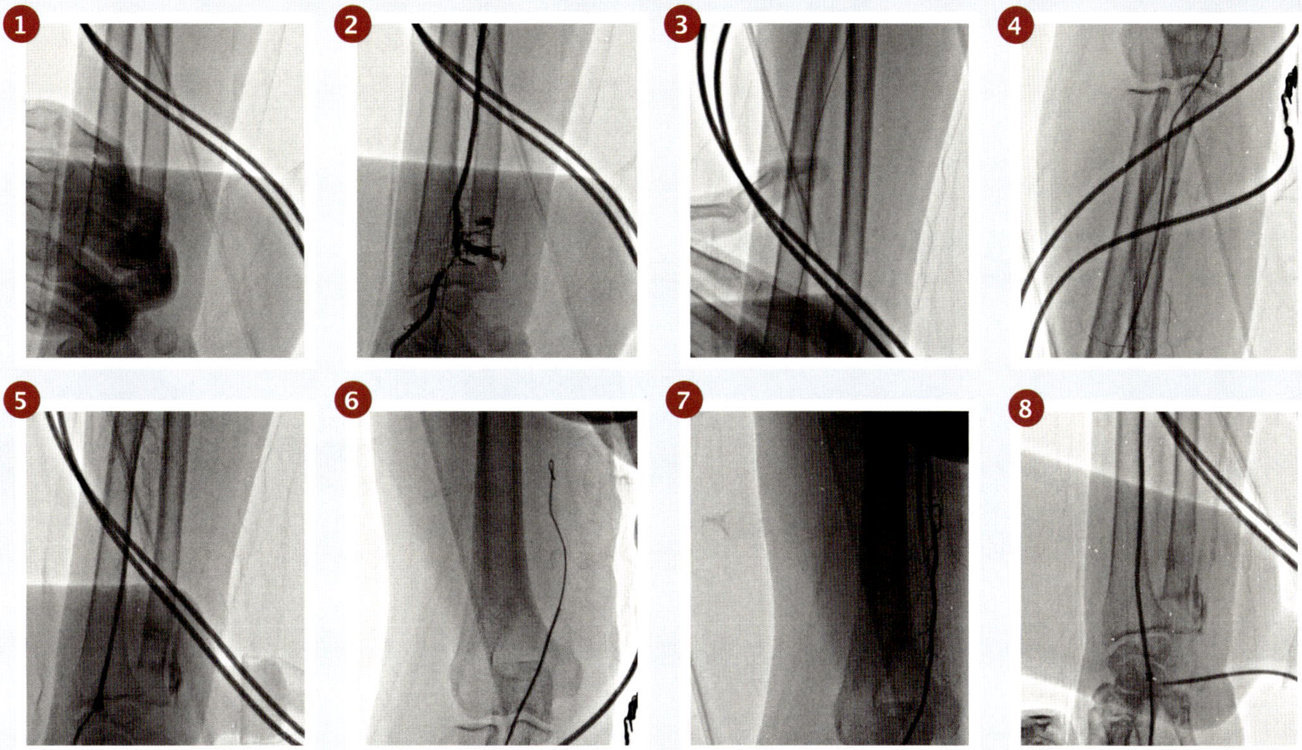

1. This is an example of a very low radial loop complicated by perforation. There was a good backflow of blood from the cannula of the puncture needle, but a hydrophilic 0.025-inch guidewire and 0.014-inch PTCA guidewire each failed to progress farther.
2. An injection of contrast through the cannula revealed a complex radial loop in the lower segment that was complicated by perforation. However, the higher RA segment was straight with a good diameter.
3. After removal of the cannula and compression of the local part, the RA was punctured in the higher segment and a 5 Fr introducer sheath was deployed. A 0.014-inch PTCA guidewire was negotiated through it.
4. Injection of contrast through the cannula revealed an RA of a very small caliber arising from the axillary artery directly.
5. A 5 Fr introducer sheath is pictured in situ.
6. The procedure was completed in the usual fashion.
7. A post-procedure angiogram of the RA revealed its small caliber and high origin from the axillary artery.
8. The procedure was completed successfully, and the perforation was sealed.

Algorithm

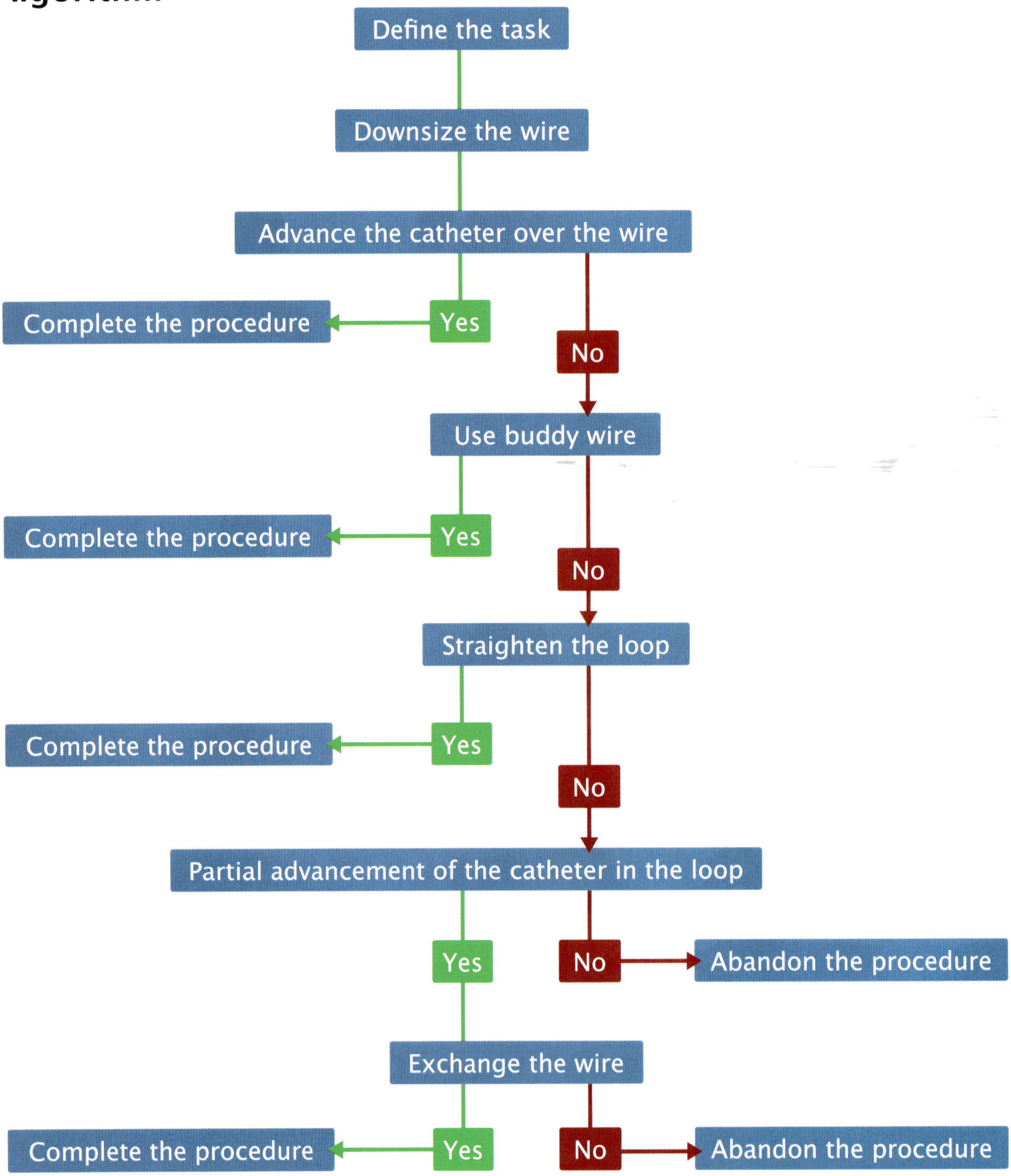
Define the task
Downsize the wire
Advance the catheter over the wire
Complete the procedure
Yes
No
Use buddy wire
Complete the procedure
Yes
No
Straighten the loop
Complete the procedure
Yes
No
Partial advancement of the catheter in the loop
Yes
No
Abandon the procedure
Exchange the wire
Complete the procedure
Yes
No
Abandon the procedure

Balloon-assisted Tracking of a Catheter:
A must-learn technique

Sometimes, the operator encounters a radial artery with a smaller caliber, extreme tortuosity or atherosclerotic lesions — each of which can lead to difficult tracking of a diagnostic or a guide catheter. Repeated attempts to negotiate a catheter increase the chances of spasm, pain, discomfort and perforation, potentially leading to hematoma. An effective technique to work through this complexity is called "balloon-assisted tracking of a catheter."

For balloon-assisted tracking, define anatomy by contrast injection through the side port of the introducer sheath. Cross the segment with a 0.014-inch floppy-tip PTCA guidewire. A PTCA catheter of 1.5 mm, 2.0 mm or 2.5 mm diameter should be selected, depending on the inner lumen of the diagnostic or guide catheter (5 Fr, 6 Fr or 7 Fr). The distal 4-5 mm segment of balloon should protrude outside the mouth of the catheter. The catheter is kept in the proximal segment. The balloon is inflated to 4-5 atmospheres of pressure, and the assembly is tracked through the segment. Once the segment is crossed, the procedure is finished in usual fashion. This technique has the subtle advantage of avoiding friction and the razor effect while working through small and tortuous radial segments.

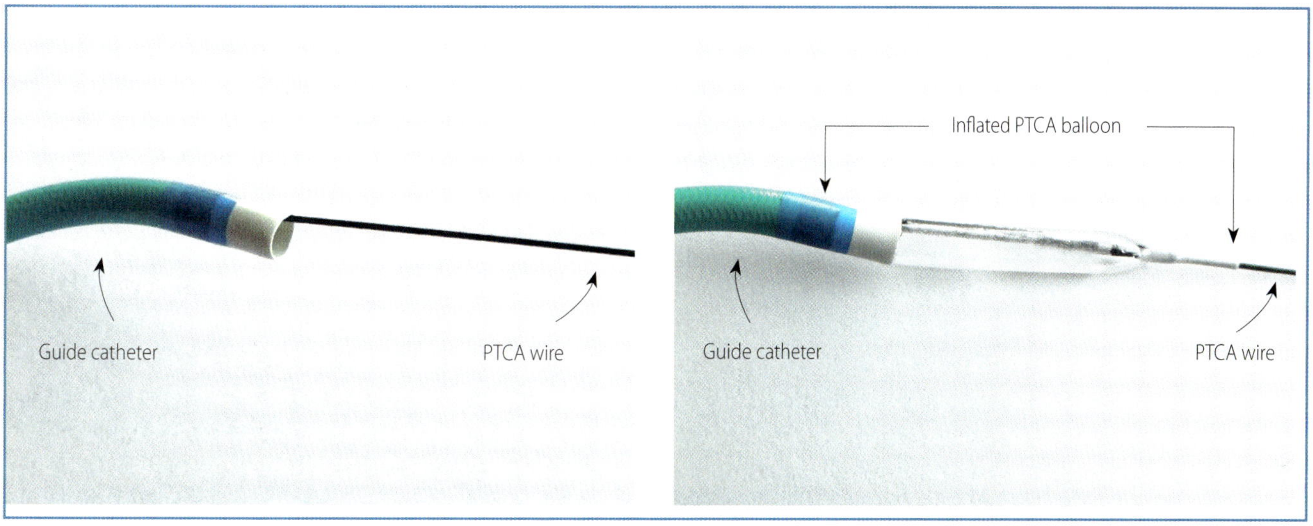

In vitro demonstration of the technique

Example of balloon-assisted tracking of a catheter

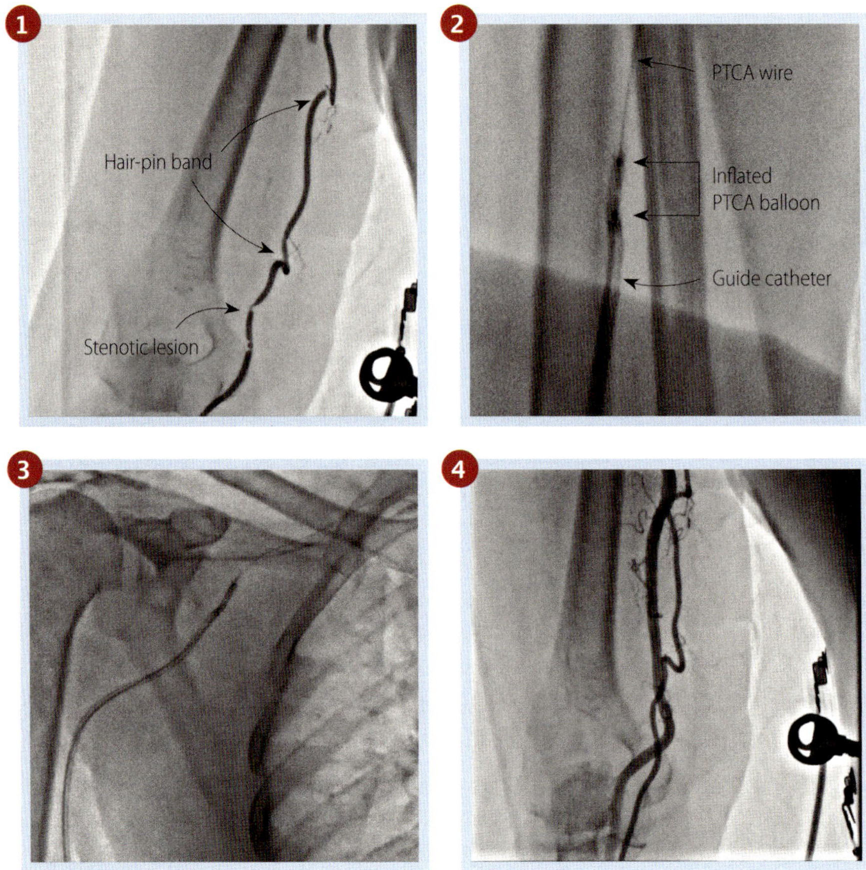

1. Contrast injection revealed an anomalous RA arising from the axillary artery and having atherosclerotic lesions and two sharp, hair-pin bands.
2. Balloon-assisted tracking is shown in progress.
3. The segment is crossed successfully.
4. Post-procedure injection revealed no damage to the RA.

Recommended Reading

1. Barbeau G. Radial loop and extreme vessel tortuosity in the transradial approach: advantage of hydrophilic-coated guidewires and catheters. Catheter Cardiovasc Interv. 2003; 59 (4): 442-50.
2. Behan M, Haworth P, Colley P, et al. Radial artery occlusion- a limitation of transradial catheterization. Catheter Cardiovasc Interv. 2010; 76 (5): 659.
3. Calviño-Santos R, Vázquez-Rodríguez J, Salgado-Fernández J, et al. Management of iatrogenic radial artery perforation. Catheter Cardiovasc Interv. 2004; 61 (1): 74-78.
4. Coppola J, Patel T, Kwan T, et al. Nitroglycerin, nitroprusside, or both, in preventing radial artery spasm during transradial artery catheterization. J Invasive Cardiol. 2006; 18 (4): 155-58.
5. Dawson E, Rathore S, Cable N, et al. Impact of introducer sheath coating on endothelial function in humans after transradial coronary procedures. Circ Cardiovasc Interv. 2010; 3 (2): 148-56.
6. Dehghani P, Mohammad A, Bajaj R, et al. Mechanism and predictors of failed transradial approach for percutaneous coronary interventions. JACC Cardiovasc Interv. 2009; 2 (11): 1057-64.
7. Fujii T, Masuda N, Toda E, et al. Analysis of right radial artery for transradial catheterization by quantitative angiography - anatomical consideration of optimal radial puncture point. J Invasive Cardiol. 2010; 22 (8): 372-76.
8. Gilchrist I. Transradial technical tips. Catheter Cardiovasc Interv. 2000; 49 (3): 353-54.
9. Kiemeneij F. Prevention and management of radial artery spasm. J Invasive Cardiol. 2006; 18 (4): 159-60.
10. Lo T, Nolan J, Fountzopoulos E, et al. Radial artery anomaly and its influence on transradial coronary procedural outcome. Heart. 2009; 95 (5): 410-15.
11. Louvard Y, Lefèvre T. Loops and transradial approach in coronary diagnosis and intervention. Catheter Cardiovasc Interv. 2000; 51 (2): 250-52.
12. Patel T, Shah S, Sanghavi K, et al. Management of radial and brachial artery perforations during transradial procedures--a practical approach. J Invasive Cardiol. 2009; 21 (10): 544-47.
13. Ruiz-Salmerón R, Mora R, Masotti M, et al. Assessment of the efficacy of phentolamine to prevent radial artery spasm during cardiac catheterization procedures: a randomized study comparing phentolamine vs. verapamil. Catheter Cardiovasc Interv. 2005; 66 (2): 192-98.
14. Saito S, Ikei H, Hosokawa G, et al. Influence of the ratio between radial artery inner diameter and sheath outer diameter on radial artery flow after transradial coronary intervention. Catheter Cardiovasc Interv. 1999; 46 (2): 173-78.
15. Sakai H, Ikeda S, Harada T, et al. Limitations of successive transradial approach in the same arm: the Japanese experience. Catheter Cardiovasc Interv. 2001; 54 (2): 204-208.
16. Staniloae C, Mody K, Sanghvi K, et al. Histopathologic changes of the radial artery wall secondary to transradial catheterization. Vasc Health Risk Manag. 2009; 5 (3): 527-32.
17. Valsecchi O, Vassileva A, Musumeci G, et al. Failure of transradial approach during coronary interventions: anatomic considerations. Catheter Cardiovasc Interv. 2006; 67 (6): 870-78.

18. Varenne O, Jégou A, Cohen R, et al. Prevention of arterial spasm during percutaneous coronary interventions through radial artery: the SPASM study. Catheter Cardiovasc Interv. 2006; 68 (2): 231–35.

19. Wu S, Galani R, Bahro A, et al. 8 french transradial coronary interventions: clinical outcome and late effects on the radial artery and hand function. J Invasive Cardiol. 2000; 12 (12): 605–09.

20. Yokoyama N, Takeshita S, Ochiai M, et al. Anatomic variations of the radial artery in patients undergoing transradial coronary intervention. Catheter Cardiovasc Interv. 2000; 49 (4): 357–62.

Subclavian, Innominate and Aortic Arch Regions: Understanding and Addressing the Issues

6

Tejas Patel, Sanjay Shah and Rajnikant Radadiya

Normal Anatomy of Subclavian and Axillary Arteries

The anatomy differs on the right and left sides as far as the subclavian artery is concerned. On the right side, the subclavian artery arises from the innominate artery. On the left side, it arises from the arch of the aorta. While the subclavian arteries differ in length, direction, and their relationship to neighboring structures in their proximal locations, both share common pathways distally (described in Chapter 5) as they extend down the forearm.

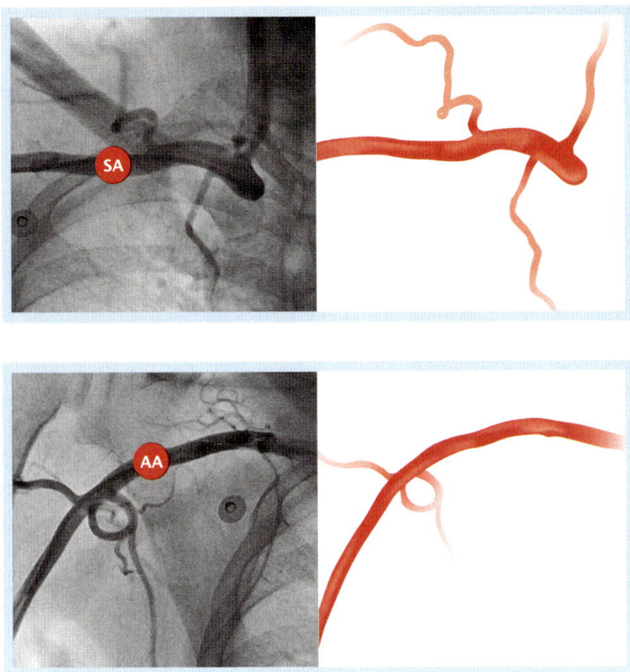

Normal right subclavian and axillary arteries

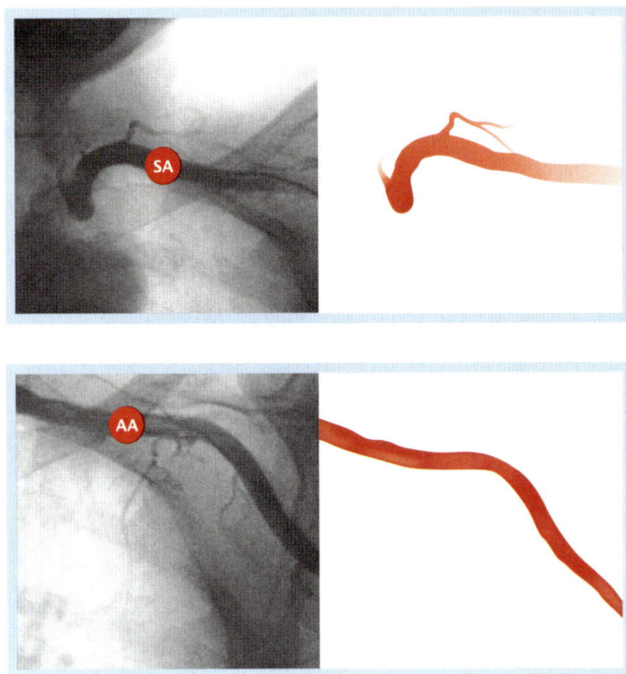

Normal left subclavian and axillary arteries

Normal Innominate-Aortic Arch Junction Anatomy

The innominate aortic arch junction is unique to transradial procedures. Here the catheters and guidewires must take an obtuse angle turn to enter the ascending aorta.

In cases of normal anatomy, the turn is smooth and does not pose obstacles to performing diagnostic or interventional procedures. In cases of abnormal anatomy due to dilation and/ or distortion of the aorta, the procedure requires judicious use of guidewires (0.025-inch or 0.032-inch hydrophilic guidewires, standard 0.035-inch guidewires, and super-stiff guidewires) and catheters (unusual curves, if necessary) to complete the procedure.

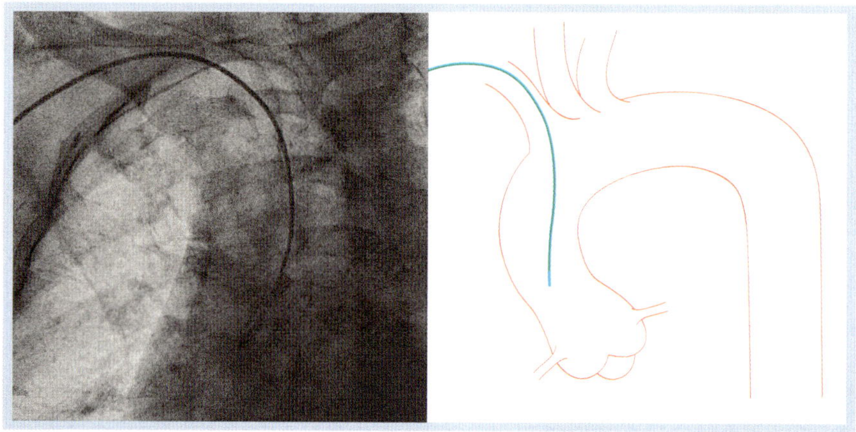

Normal anatomy of the innominate-arch junction (Note the smooth curve at the junction.)

(A) Subclavian Artery Stenosis

(1) Total occlusion of subclavian artery

It is a rare issue. Usually it occurs as a result of atherosclerotic process or aortoarteritis.

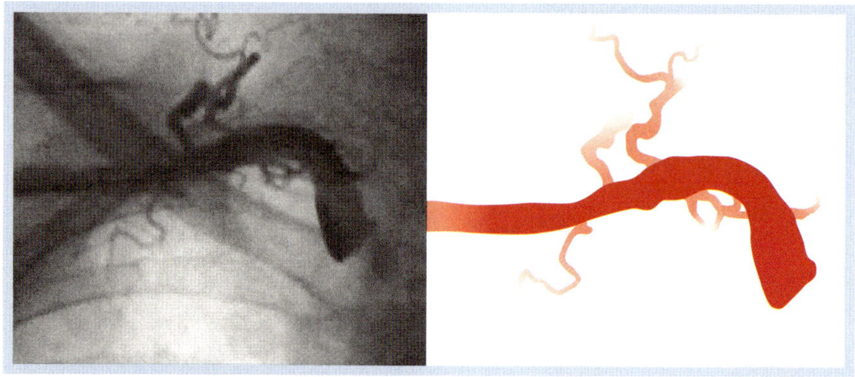

Total occlusion of right subclavian artery. (This patient had a normal Modified Allen's Test.)

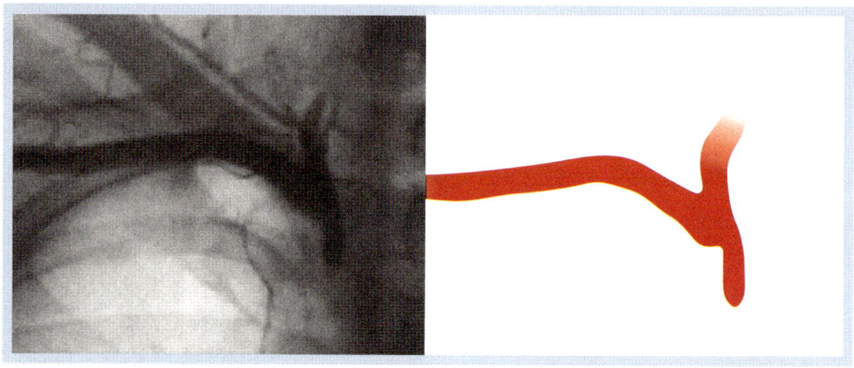

Total occlusion of the distal part of the right innominate artery

Identification

- Whenever there is resistance in the passage of a standard 0.032-inch guidewire, a 0.025-inch hydrophilic guidewire or a 0.014-inch soft-tip PTCA guidewire, this problem should be suspected.
- Hand injection of contrast in this region reveals the diagnosis.
- A feeble or absent radial pulse gives a clue for this diagnosis. However, in most instances, the radial pulse is normal with an Allen's Test because of development of extensive collaterals.

Tips

- Once the diagnosis is established, crossover to the contralateral radial or femoral approach is safest.
- Working through a subclavian occlusion may lead to dissection and/or damage to important structures in the vicinity (e.g., carotid, vertebral or internal mammary artery ostia).

(2) **Subtotal or partial stenosis of subclavian artery**
This is also an uncommon issue. Normally it is of atherosclerotic origin.

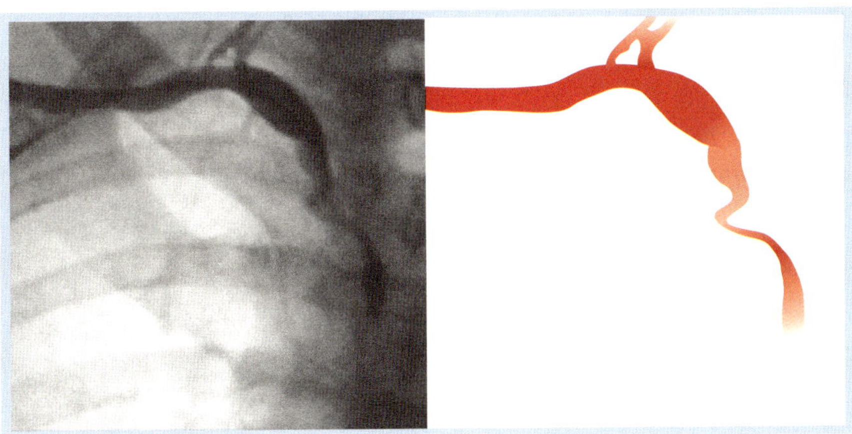

Long-segment stenosis in the proximal part of the right subclavian artery

Identification and Management

- Whenever resistance is encountered with the movement of a standard 0.032-inch or 0.035-inch guidewire and/or a catheter, this problem should be suspected.
- Hand injection with contrast in this region establishes the diagnosis.

- At times, more than one view in different angulations may be needed to define the diagnosis.
- Once the diagnosis is complete, use a 0.025-inch or 0.032-inch hydrophilic guidewire to cross the stenosis and enter the ascending or descending aorta.
- At times, using a soft-tip 0.014-inch PTCA guidewire may also bring success.
- Once the stenosis is crossed with the guidewire, use a diagnostic or guide catheter to enter the ascending or descending aorta to complete a coronary or a peripheral procedure.
- Always use fluoroscopic guidance while working through this region to prevent damage to carotid, vertebral or internal mammary artery ostia.
- Most subclavian stenosis can be treated with PTA and stenting (discussed in Chapter 15).

(B) Mild Tortuosity in the Subclavian Region

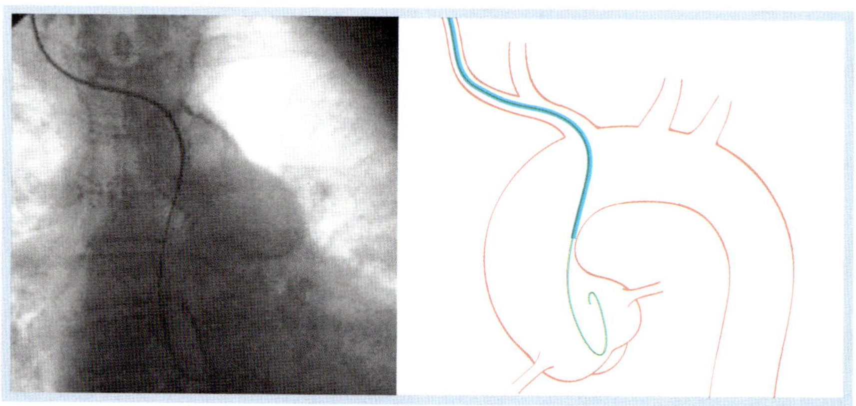

An example of simple tortuosity of the right subclavian artery

Identification and Management

- Resistance to the movement of a guidewire and/or a catheter in this region should prompt consideration of this problem.

- Gentle movement of the assembly should bring successful entry into the ascending aorta.

- Normally mild tortuosity does not create any challenges for a diagnostic or an interventional procedure.

- Avoid using a super-stiff wire, unless the ascending or descending aorta has been entered, as it can create injury and dissection in this region.

- At times, deep inspiration facilitates the entry of guidewire and catheter in the ascending aorta.

(C) Severe Tortuosity in Subclavian Region

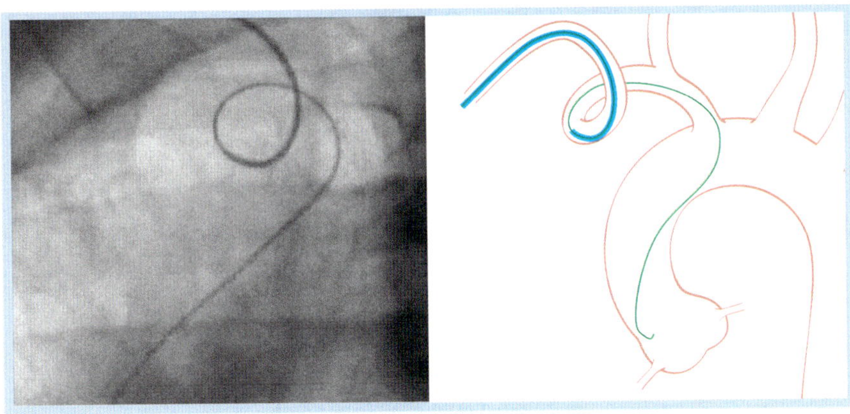

An example of severe tortuosity of the subclavian artery

Identification and Management

- Basic protocol is the same as that of mild tortuosity.

- However, at times, despite a having guidewire optimally positioned in the ascending aorta, the catheter movement encounters severe resistance in subclavian-innominate artery junction.

- At this stage, instead of pushing the catheter further over the wire, pulling it slightly back along with the guidewire straightens the tortuosity, allowing for smooth entry of a catheter in the ascending aorta.

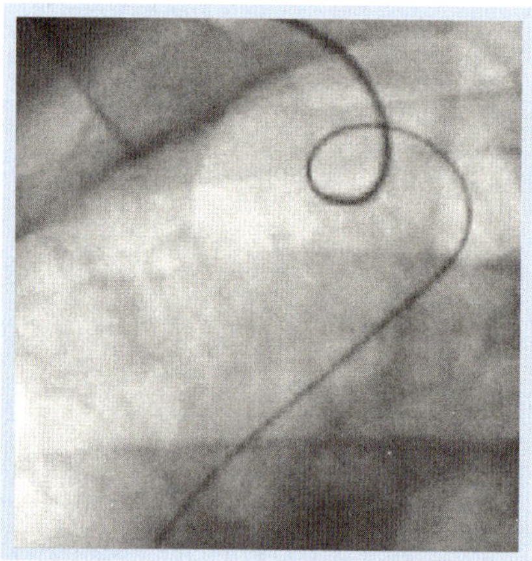

An attempt was made to advance the catheter over the guidewire, but it refused to budge.

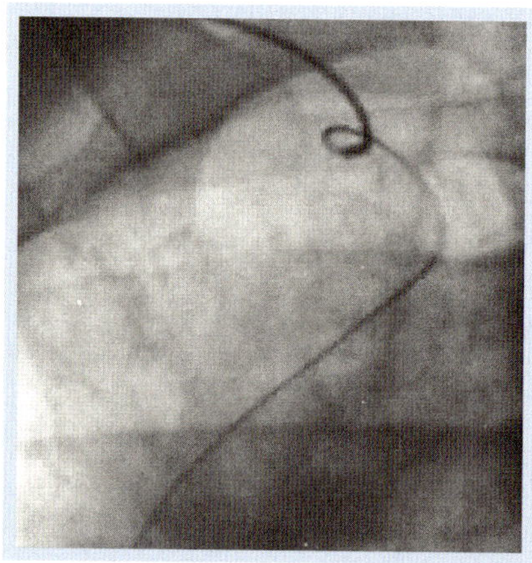

We pulled back the entire assembly to straighten the guidewire.

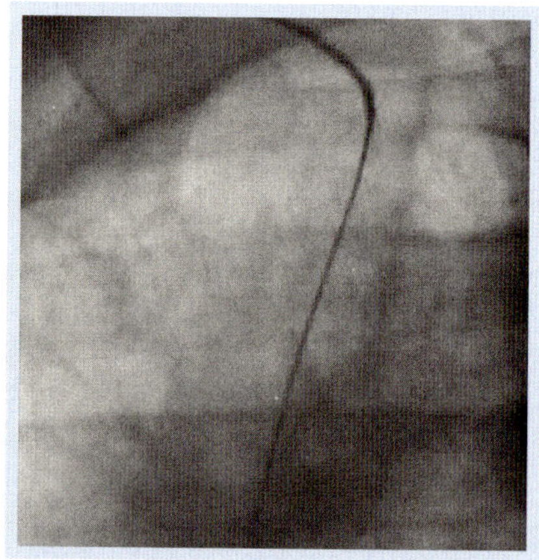

The catheter was easily advanced over the guidewire and the procedure was completed in the usual fashion.

- At times, deep inspiration facilitates the entry of the guidewire and catheter in the ascending aorta.

Before discussing the issues related to a severely dilated and distorted aortic route and arteria lusoria, it is important to understand the catheter's entry into ascending aorta while working through the right and left radial approaches.

Entering the Ascending Aorta Through Right Radial Approach

In the majority of cases, the diagnostic catheter and the guidewire enter the ascending aorta effortlessly. However, they sometimes selectively enter the descending aorta. The angiograms and schematic drawings demonstrate how to enter the ascending aorta in such cases.

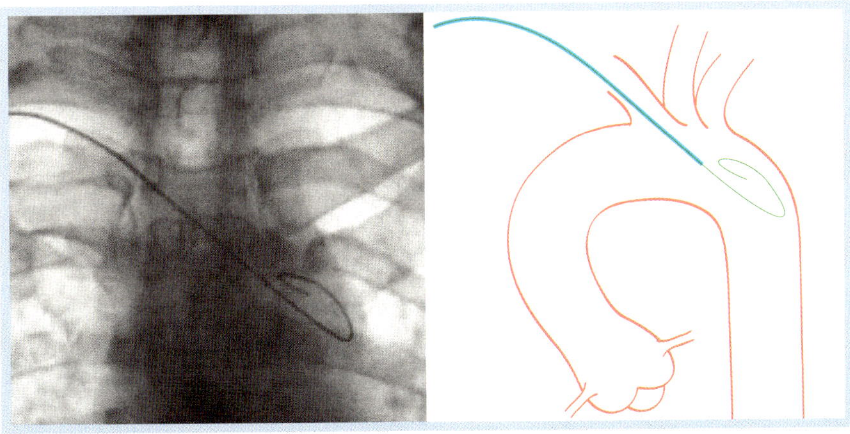

A diagnostic catheter and a standard 0.035-inch guidewire inside the descending aorta.

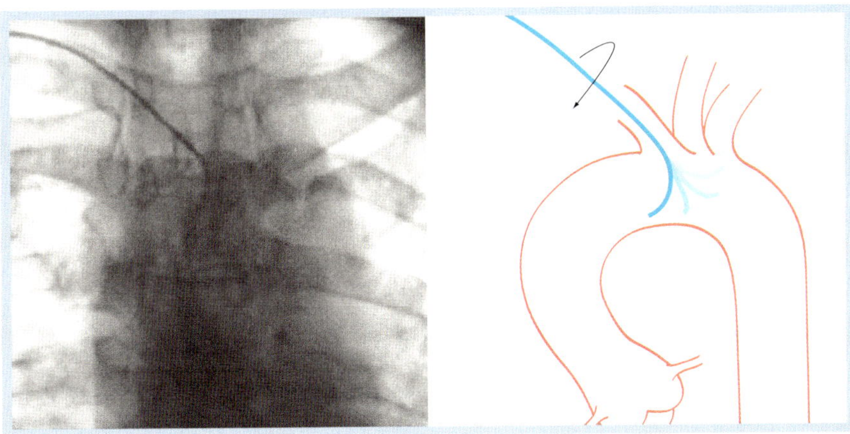

We pulled the guidewire inside the catheter, then pulled the entire assembly into the aortic arch. We asked the patient to take a deep breath. We rotated the tip of the catheter toward the ascending aorta.

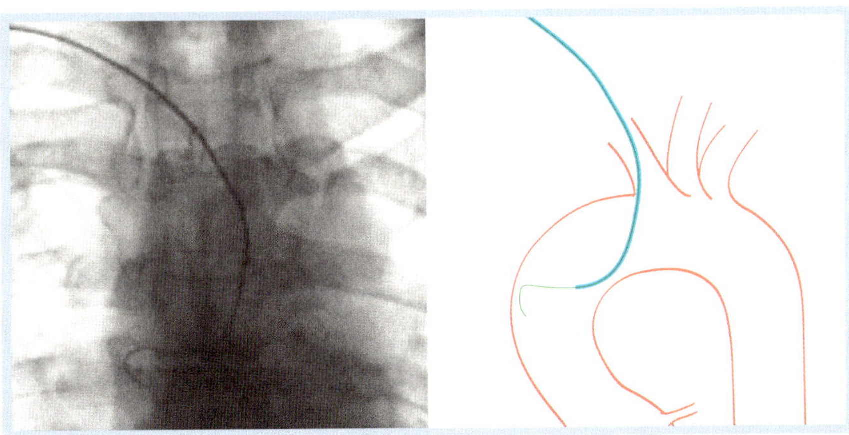

We gently pushed the guidewire into the ascending aorta and advanced the catheter over the guidewire. (In case of difficulty, an LAO 40-degree view helps to enter the ascending aorta.)

Entering the Ascending Aorta Through the Left Radial Approach

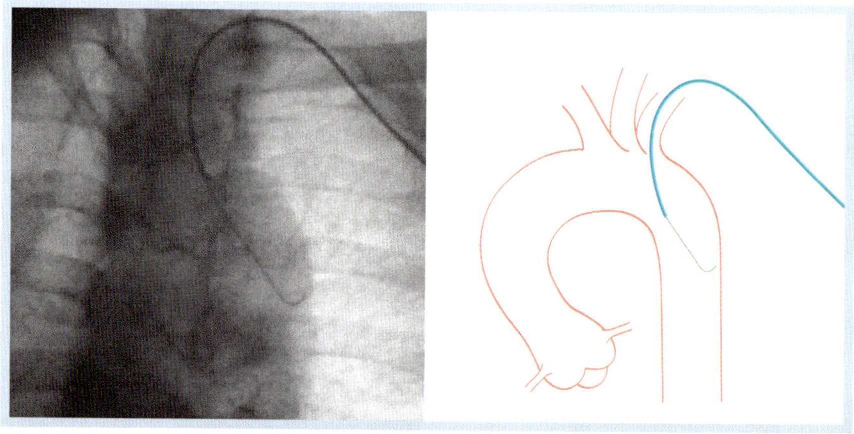

In this case, the procedure was performed from the left radial route. The catheter and the guidewire entered the descending aorta.

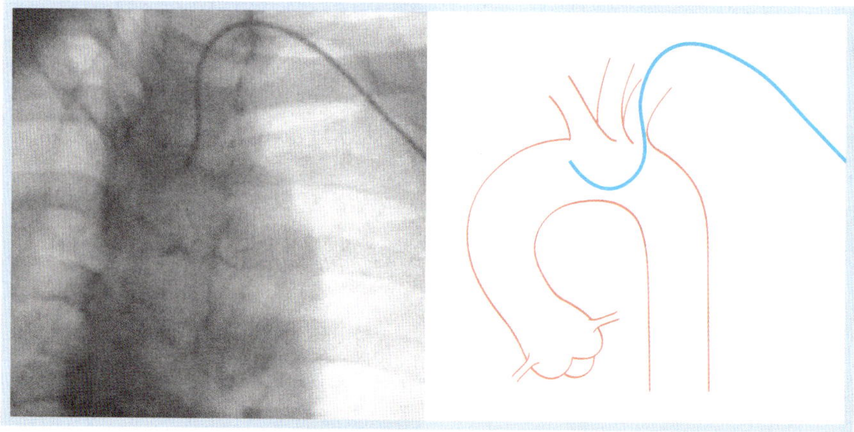

We pulled the guidewire inside the catheter, then pulled the entire assembly into the aortic arch. We asked the patient to take a deep breath. We rotated the tip of the catheter toward the ascending aorta.

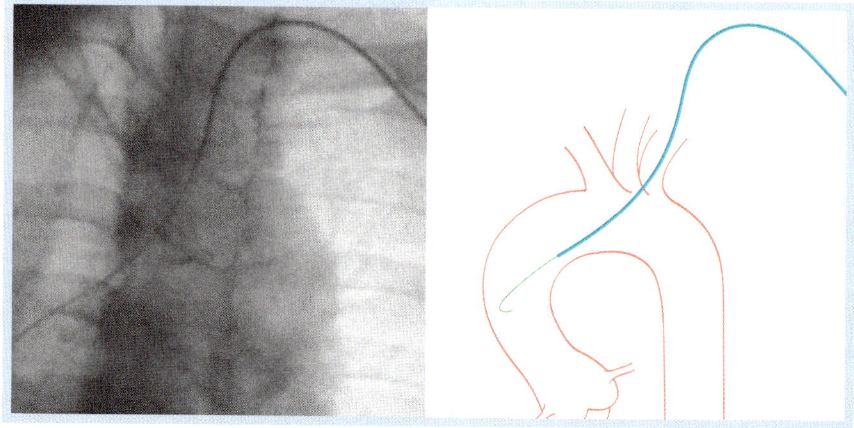

We gently pushed the guidewire into the ascending aorta and advanced the catheter over the guidewire. (In case of difficulty, an LAO 40 degree view helps to enter the ascending aorta).

(D) Severely Dilated And Distorted Aortic Route
(PSEUDO-ARTERIA LUSORIA)

Identification and Management

- Severe dilatation and distortion of the aortic route occurs due to long-standing hypertension, severe aortic stenosis or chronic severe aortic regurgitation.
- It leads to change in the anatomy, particularly distances of the origin of aortic-arch branches.
- The catheter traverses through a wider angle, leading to certain acquired loops (e.g., a small Z-loop or a small roller-coaster loop).
- Entering the ascending aorta is not difficult; however, wider catheter curves may be needed for coronary cannulation.
- If the catheter has tendency to slip toward the descending aorta, deep inspiration helps to enter the ascending aorta.

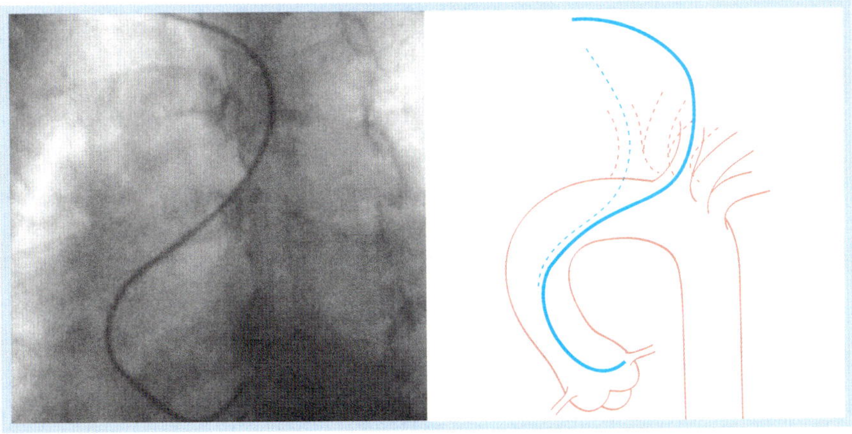

A Z-Loop of the catheter due to dilation and distortion at the innominate-arch junction; dotted lines show the normal anatomy.

(E) Dilated and Distorted Aortic Route Working Through Left Radial Approach

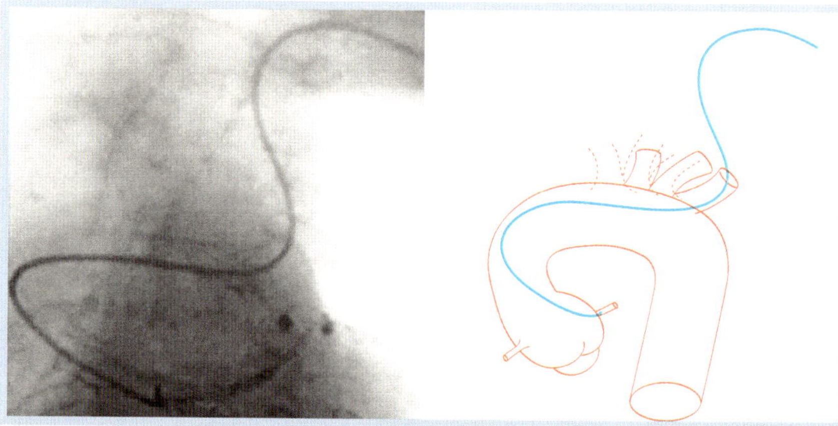

A sigma loop on the left-radial artery approach due to abnormal anatomy

Identification and Management

- Catheter traverses through a wider angle, leading to a sigma loop.
- Entry in the ascending aorta is easy. However, wider catheter curves may be needed for coronary cannulation.
- If the catheter tends to slip into the descending aorta, deep inspiration helps to enter ascending aorta.

(F) Working Through Arteria Lusoria: The Right Transradial Approach

Arteria lusoria is a congenital anomaly of the right subclavian artery characterized topographically as follows: The artery originates below the left subclavian artery as the fourth main branch of the aortic arch and turns to the right behind the esophagus, in front of the vertebral column. In over 32,000 transradial procedures done by us, only 45 (0.14%) arteria lusoria have been objectively documented, as it is a rare anomaly.

Arteria Lusoria

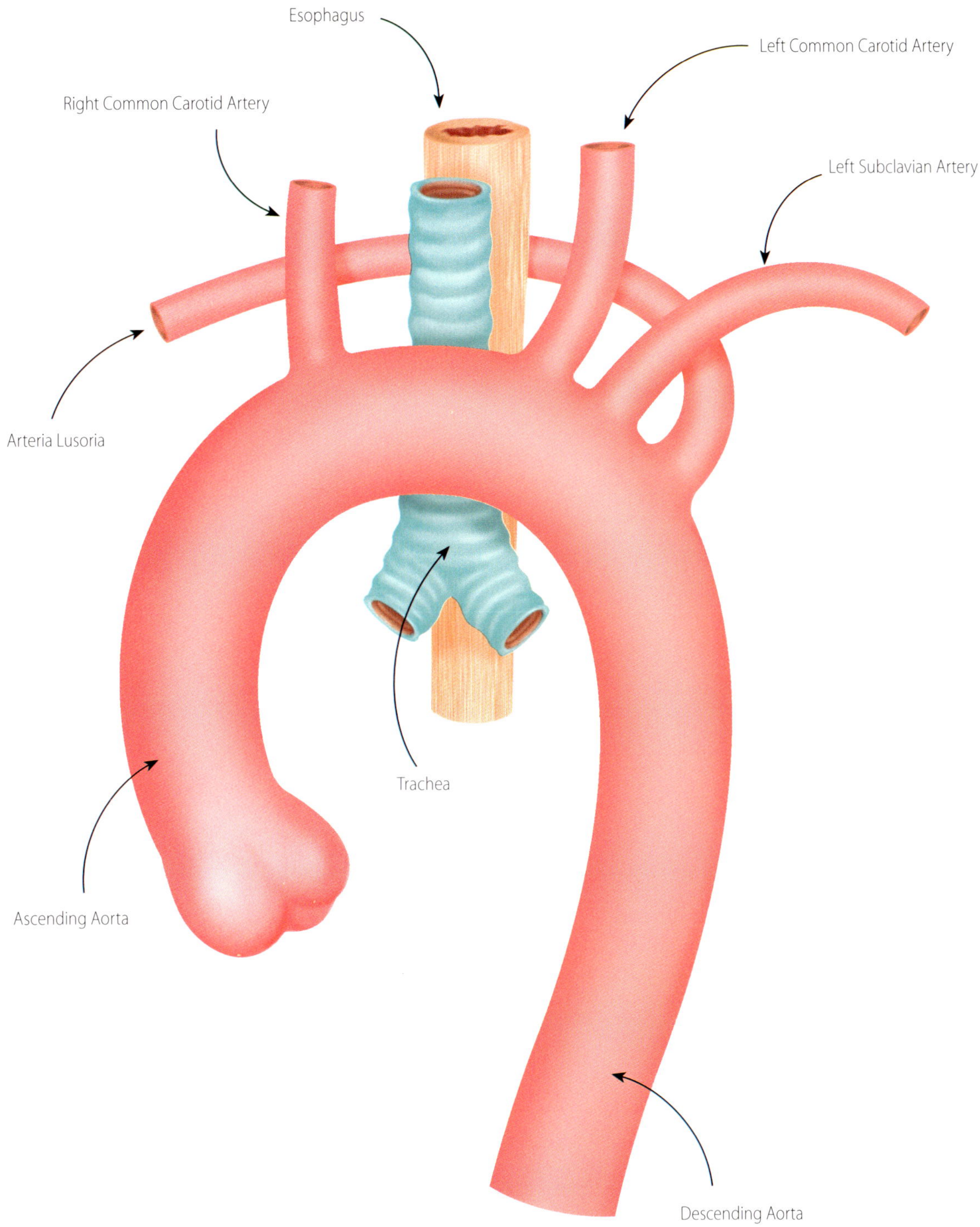

While crossover to an alternative arterial site is reasonable, the following protocol has worked to pass through this anomaly. It is divided into two parts: (1) entering the ascending aorta through arteria lusoria and (2) the cannulation of the coronary arteries.

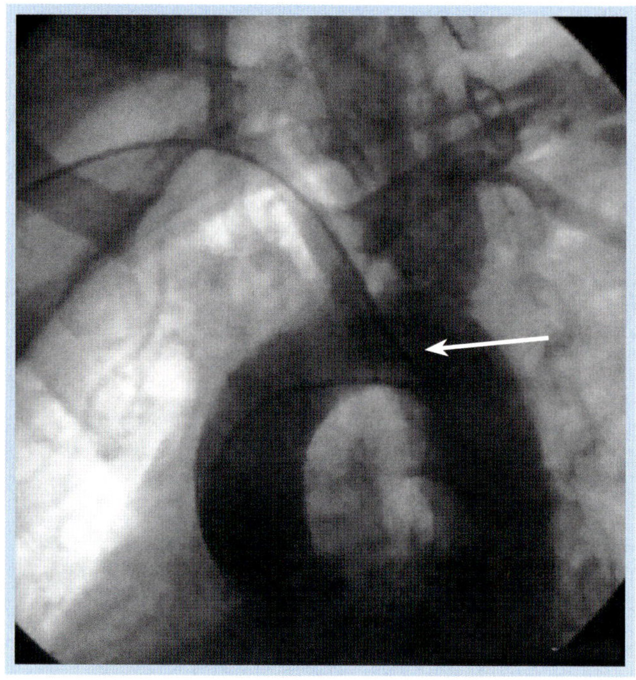

1. Entering the ascending aorta

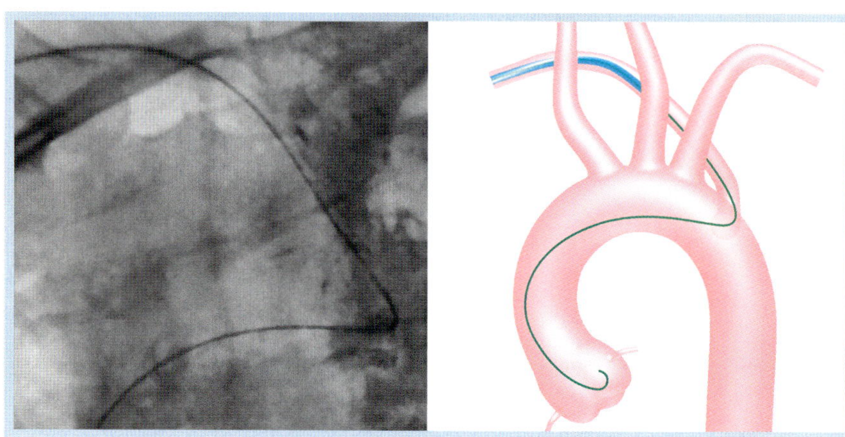

A 0.035-inch standard guidewire is positioned in the ascending aorta.

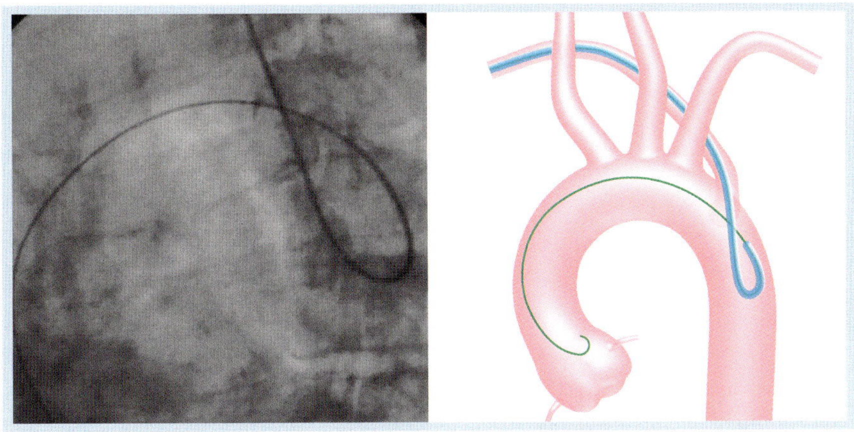

The catheter is negotiated over the wire to enter the ascending aorta.

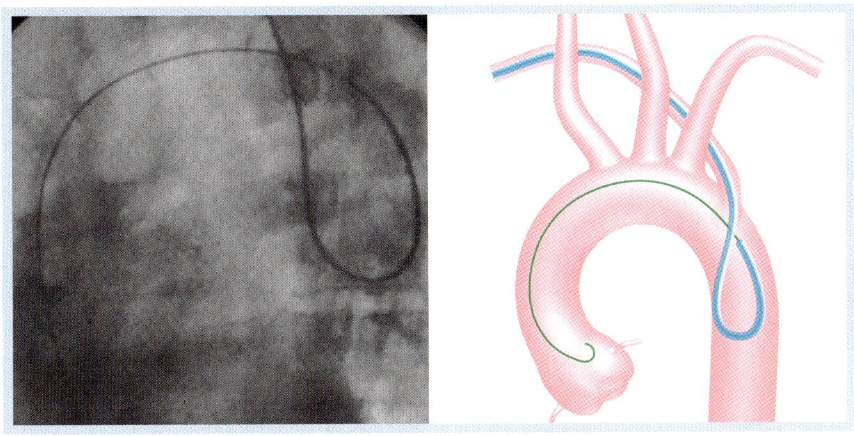

While pushing the catheter over the wire, it has a tendency to enter the descending aorta, along with the guidewire loop.

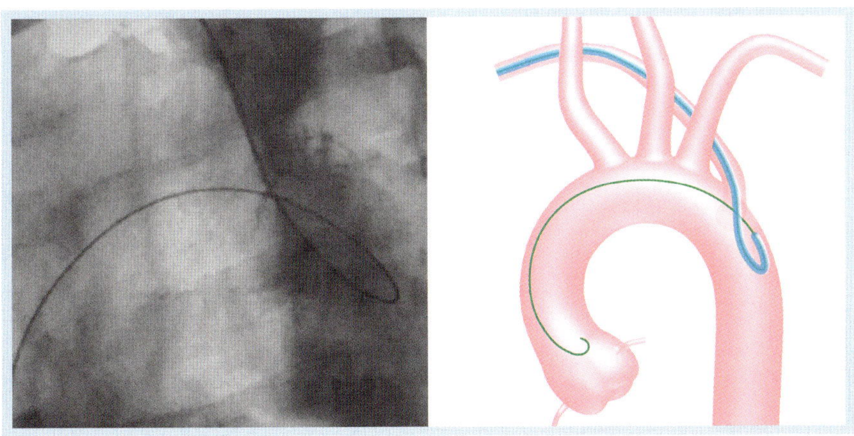

The whole assembly is gently pulled back.

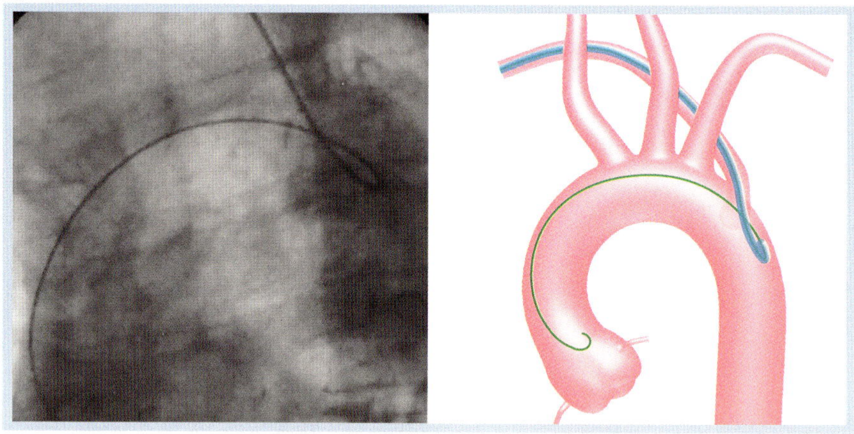

The process continues.

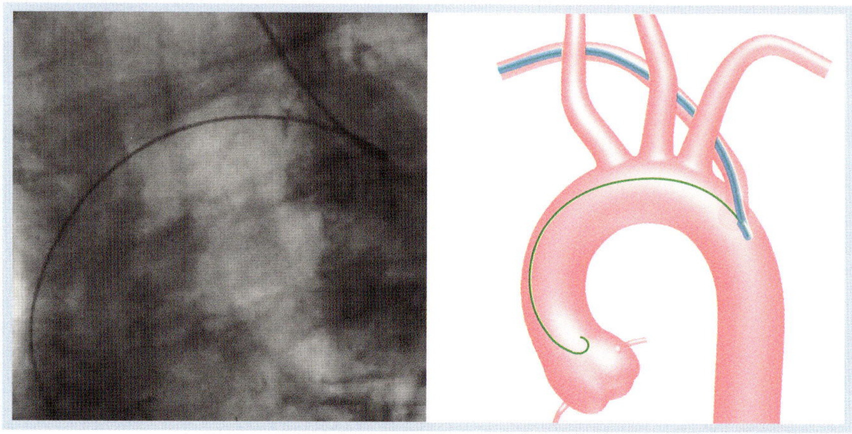

The process continues.

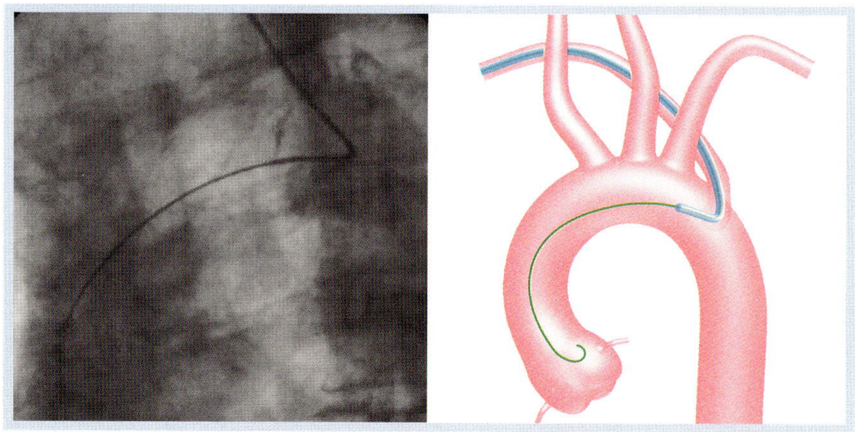

The catheter is slowly pushed over the wire to enter the ascending aorta.

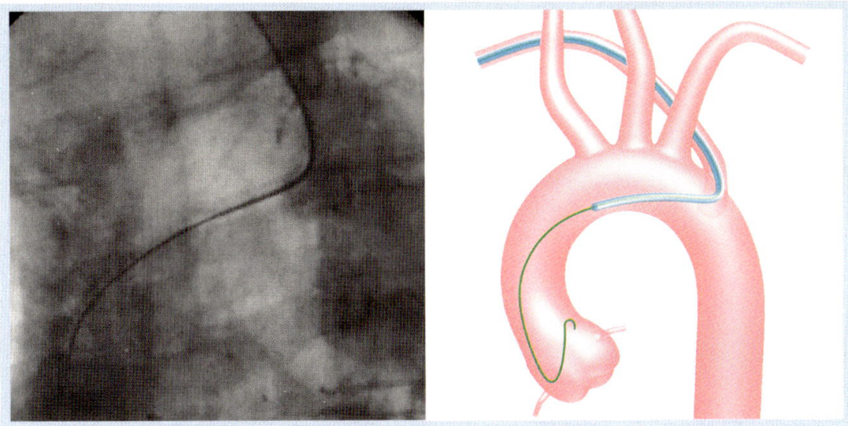

The catheter enters the ascending aorta.

Tips

Step 1

The catheter and guidewire have a tendency to enter the descending aorta. If this happens, withdraw the catheter and the guidewire together, as an assembly.

After asking the patient to take deep breath, gently push the 0.035-inch standard guidewire. If the guidewire enters the ascending aorta effortlessly, slide the catheter over the guidewire up into the ascending aorta.

Step 2

If Step 1 is not successful, keep the guidewire in the descending aorta. Remove the Judkins right or left catheter, or the first catheter tried. Take a 5 Fr IMA diagnostic catheter, put it into the descending aorta and over the guidewire, and try the Step 1 maneuver. In many cases, this approach will be successful for entry into the ascending aorta.

Step 3

If the IMA catheter fails, then a 5 Fr Simmon catheter can be used to enter the ascending aorta.

Step 4

If the 0.035-inch standard guidewire has a tendency to slip into the descending aorta, the second choices are a 0.032-inch or a 0.025-inch hydrophilic guidewire. The slippery character of a hydrophilic guidewire facilitates entry into the ascending aorta in challenging situations.

Note:

- Working in the 40-degree LAO view is preferable.
- Do not use super-stiff guidewires unless the ascending aorta has been entered.

2. Cannulation of the Coronary Arteries

Once the guidewire and the catheter are in the ascending aorta, cannulate the left or right coronaries in the usual fashion.

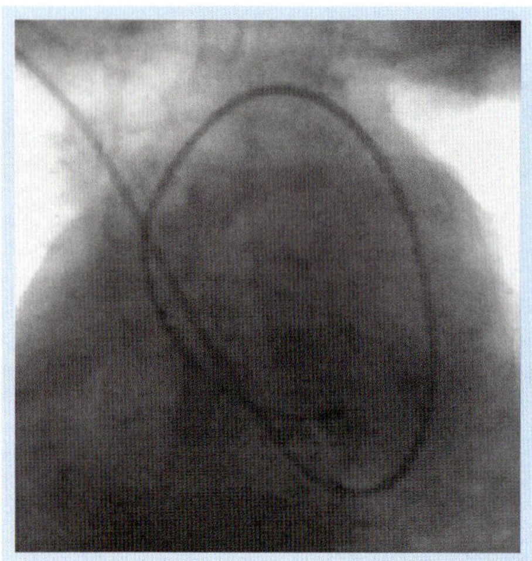

Cannulation of LCA

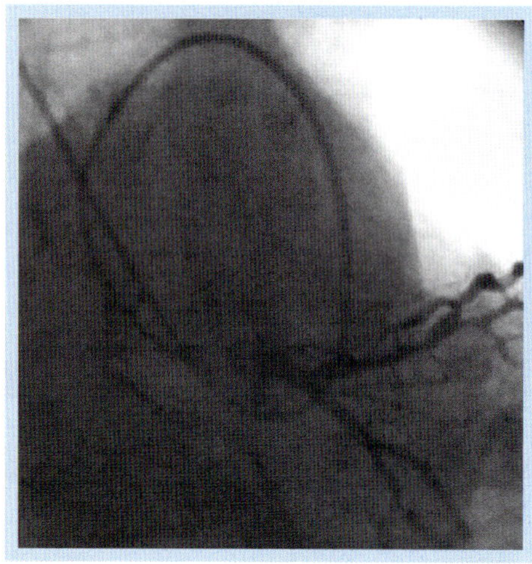

Left coronary angiogram working through arteria lusoria

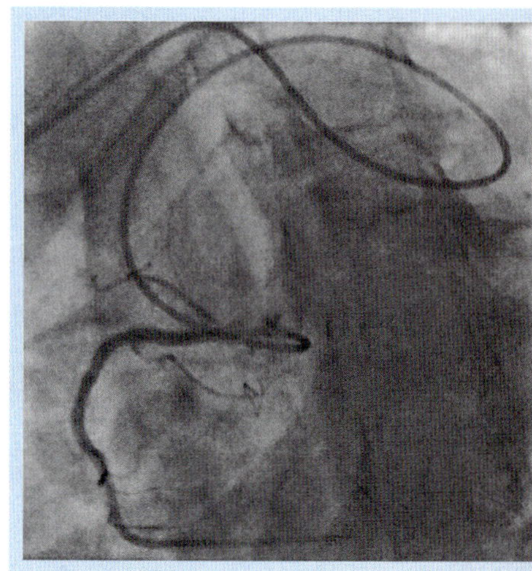

Cannulation of the RCA, and right coronary angiogram working through arteria lusoria

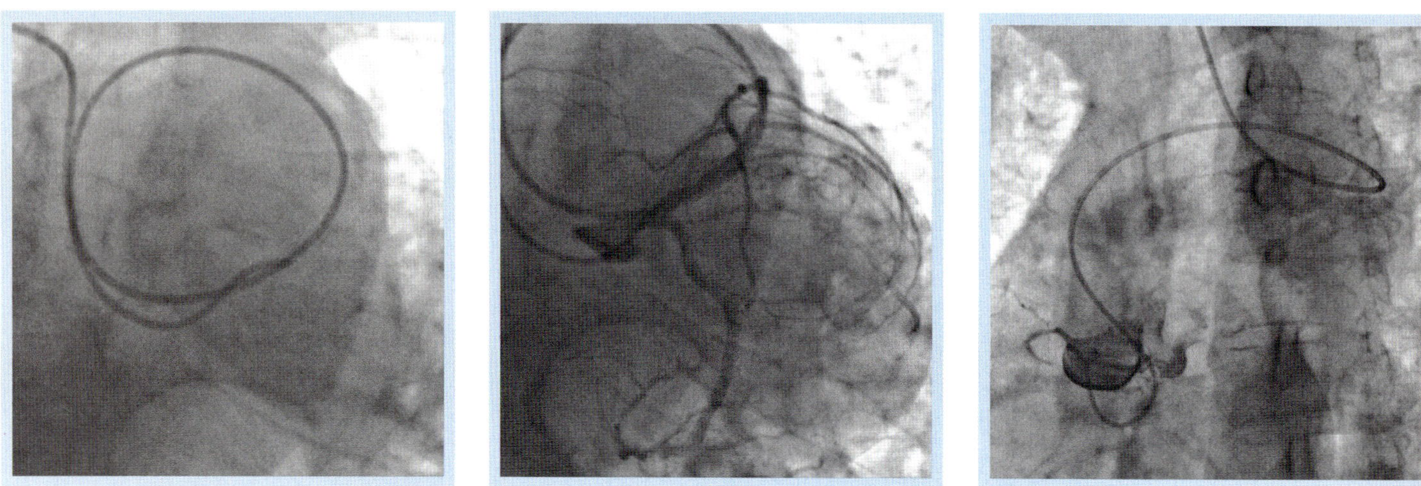

LCA & RCA cannulation using a 5 Fr AL-1 diagnostic catheter in a complex arteria lusoria situation

It is relatively easy to cannulate the coronaries. If there is a challenge, follow these steps:

Tips

Step 1

Remove the standard 0.035-inch guidewire or the hydrophilic guidewire, keeping the catheter in the ascending aorta.

Step 2

Using a 0.035-inch super-stiff guidewire, make a loop of wire in the ascending aorta. Slowly slide the catheter over it so that the assembly (catheter and guidewire) can traverse the aortic loop.

Step 3

Slowly pull the guidewire slightly inside the mouth of the catheter and pull the assembly back. This usually cannulates the left coronary artery.

For cannulation of the right coronary artery, slowly and gently rotate the assembly clockwise.

For diagnostic procedures, use a Judkins left, Optitorque TIG or an Amplatz left catheter to cannulate the left coronary ostium. Sometimes, a 5 Fr extra back-up (EBU) guide catheter is useful for cannulating the left coronary ostium. Use a Judkins right, Amplatz right or Amplatz left catheter to cannulate the right coronary ostium.

For intervention in the left coronary arteries, choose any EBU guide catheter as a first choice. If this is not successful, use a Judkins left or an Amplatz left guide catheter.

For intervention in the right coronary arteries, an Amplatz right catheter is a good first choice. If this does not succeed, a Judkins right or an Amplatz left catheter is used.

Note

- At any stage during cannulation of the coronary ostium, do not push too much or the assembly may flip into the descending aorta.

3. Intervention Through Arteria Lusoria

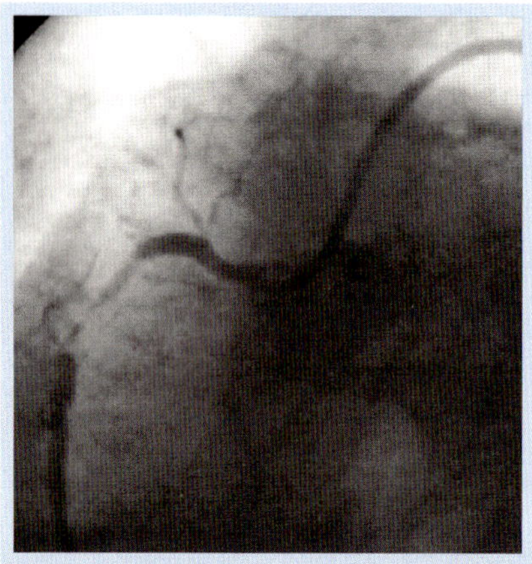

A right coronary intervention works through arteria lusoria. The RCA is cannulated using a 6 Fr AR1 guide catheter, and injection reveals critical RCA stenosis.

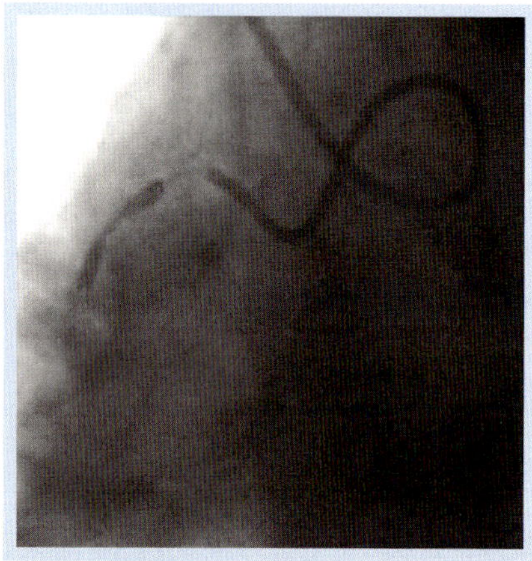

Stent implantation is in progress. Note a classical cobra loop.

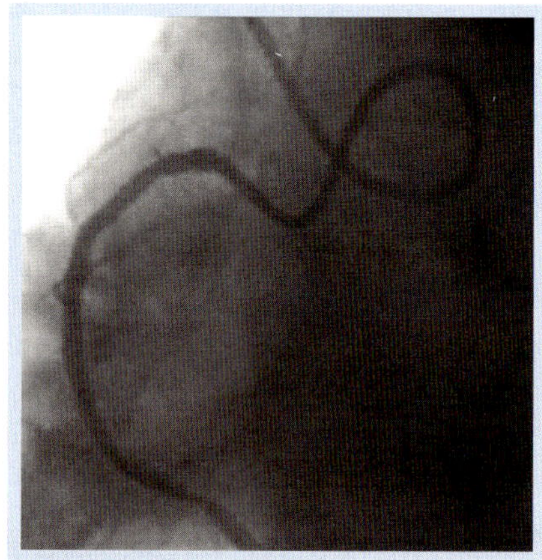

Final result

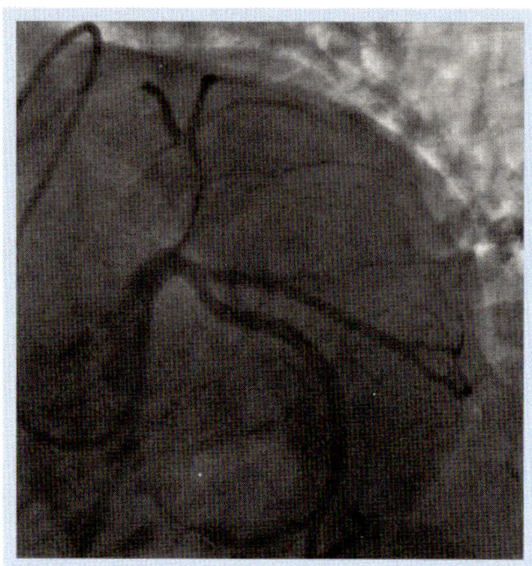

A left coronary intervention works through arteria lusoria. The LCA is cannulated using a 5 Fr EBU 3.5 guide catheter, and injection reveals a critical LAD stenosis.

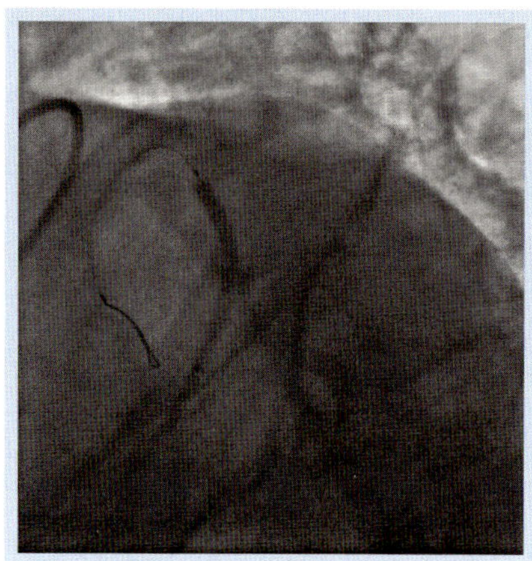

Stenting is shown in progress.

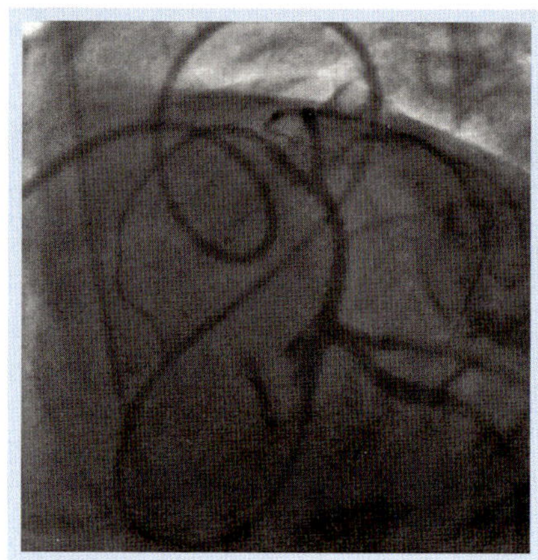

Final result

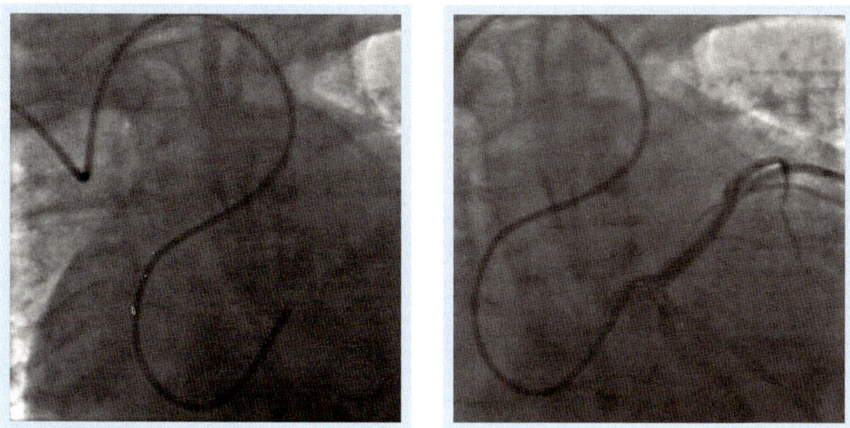

Note the very severe subclavian tortuosity and arteria lusoria.

SUMMARY

These steps may seem complicated, but arteria lusoria is very rare, and patience and perseverance can help complete the procedure in the usual fashion. If the first few attempts to enter the ascending aorta are unsuccessful, gracefully switch to the left radial or to the femoral route. Do not get discouraged. One day the learning curve will be overcome, and successfully completing the procedure via this approcah will be feasible.

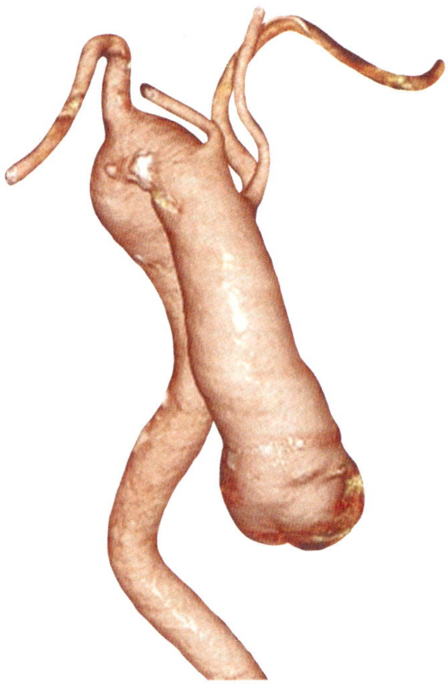

Right Aortic Arch

Working Through Right Aortic Arch: The Right TRA

Right aortic arch (RAA) is a developmental anomaly of arch of aorta. The common variant is mirror-image RAA. In the general adult population, the incidence is 0.1% and in cynotic congenital heart disease — particularly in the Tetralogy of Fallot population — the incidence is up to 25%.

In this patient, the catheter has a tendency to dive into the descending aorta, maintaining a right paraspinal position. It can easily be misinterpreted as entry to the right atrium through the superior vena cava. An angiogram with pigtail catheter confirms the right paraspinal position of the descending thoracic aorta. Another angiogram in arch position confirms the innominate artery origin at an acute angle from the right aortic arch. Keeping curvilinear calcification as a roadmap, the ascending aorta was entered. An aortic route angiogram was done. Selective LCA injection was also performed.

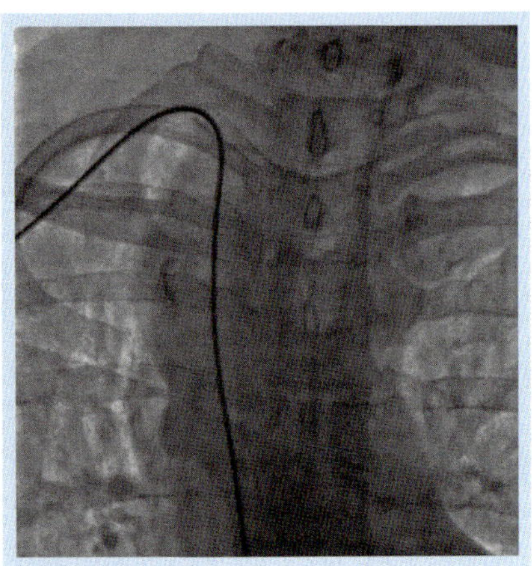

A 0.035-inch standard guidewire had a tendency to enter the descending thoracic aorta.

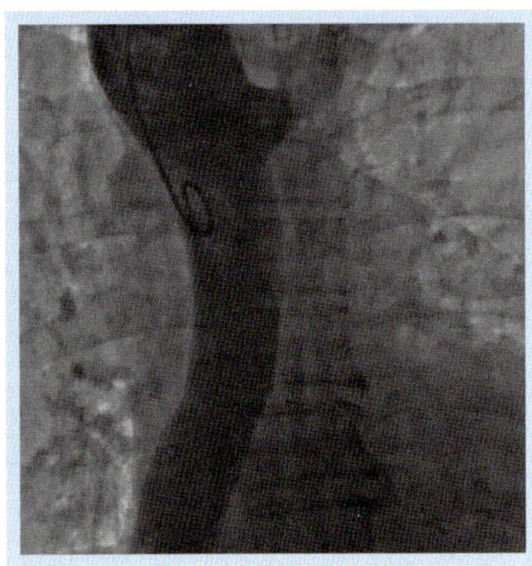

An angiogram revealed the right paraspinal position of the descending thoracic aorta.

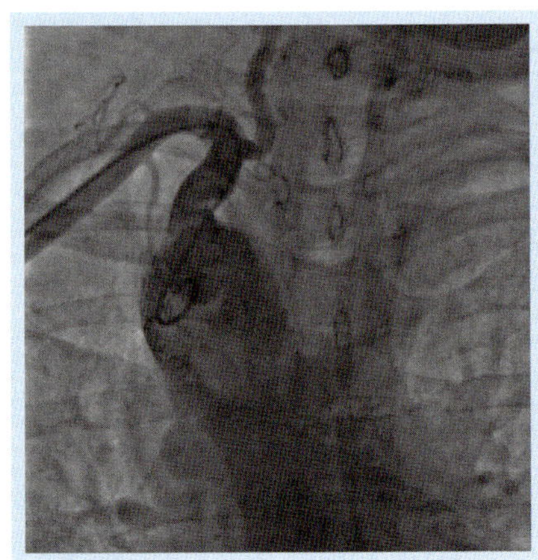

An aortic arch angiogram faintly opacified the ascending aorta.

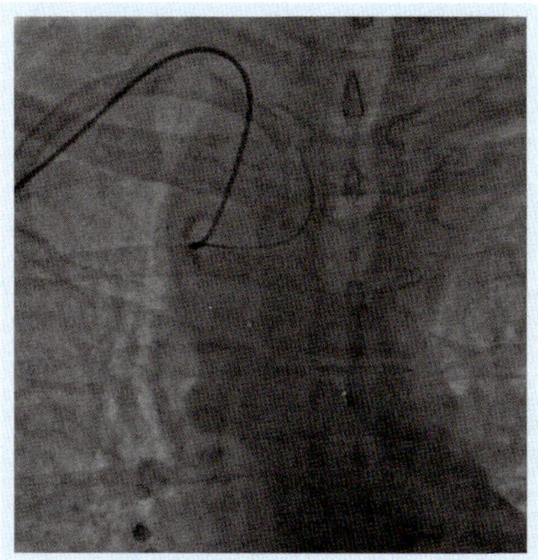

Keeping the curvilinear calcification of the arch of aorta as a roadmap, the guidewire was negotiated into the ascending aorta.

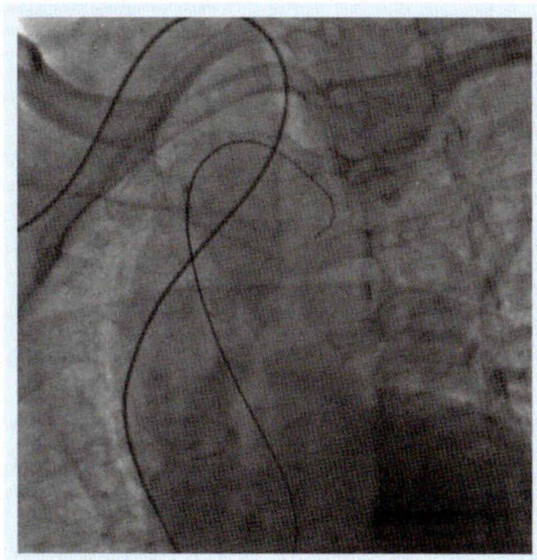

The guidewire was in the ascending aorta, and a catheter was negotiated over it.

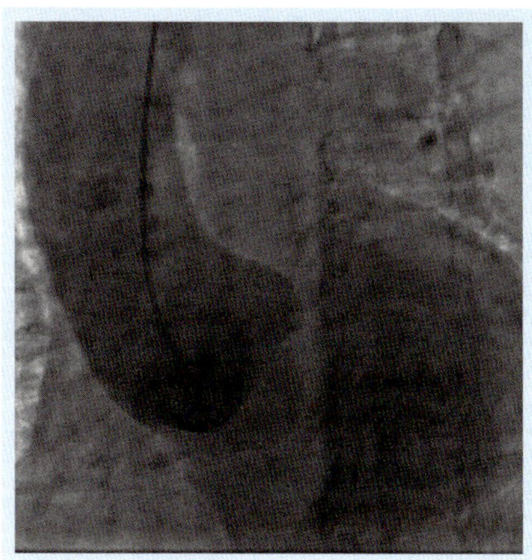

Aortic route angiogram faintly opacified the RCA.

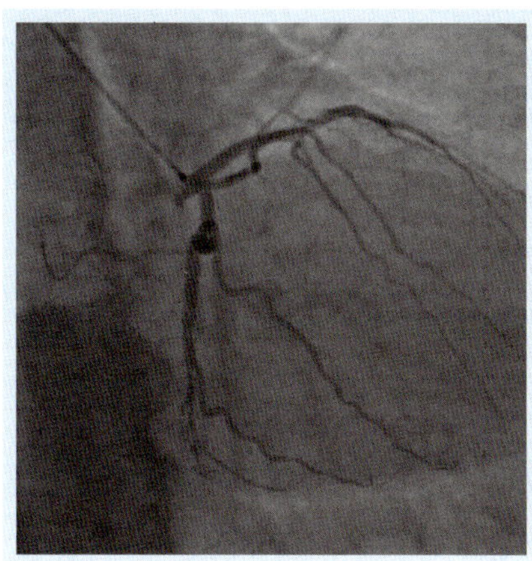

The left coronary angiogram is done.

Although uncommon, RAA is an important variant to understand for a radialist because, while working through TRA, entry to the ascending aorta is challenging because of the acute angle of the innominate artery with the RAA. This leads to selective diving of the catheter in the descending thoracic aorta. The problem is quite similar to that encountered while working through arteria lusoria during right TRA. However, anatomically with the left aortic arch, the descending thoracic aorta usually traverses in front of the spinal column, while in mirror-image RAA it traverses in continuity with the right paraspinal region. This is a subtle point to differentiate between RAA and arteria lusoria.

Tips

- The loops occurring in this region are usually acquired loops due to dilation and/or distortion of the aorta — except for arteria lusoria, which is a congenital condition.
- In most cases, loops are easy to tackle if the operator has patience and perseverance.
- Beginning radialists should avoid working through arteria lusoria.
- Repeated entry of a guidewire or a catheter in the descending aorta while working through right TRA should prompt an operator to rule out arteria lusoria or RAA.

Recommended Reading

1. Abhaichand R, Louvard Y, Gobeil J, et al. The problem of arteria lusoria in right transradial coronary angiography and angioplasty. Catheter Cardiovasc Interv. 2001; 54 (2): 196-201.
2. Caputo R, Simons A, Giambartolomei A, et al. Transradial cardiac catheterization in elderly patients. Catheter Cardiovasc Interv. 2000; 51 (3): 287-90.
3. Cha K, Kim M, Kim H. Prevalence and clinical predictors of severe tortuosity of right subclavian artery in patients undergoing transradial coronary angiography. Am J Cardiol. 2003; 92 (10): 1220-22.
4. Dehghani P, Mohammad A, Bajaj R, et al. Mechanism and predictors of failed transradial approach for percutaneous coronary interventions. JACC Cardiovasc Interv. 2009; 2 (11): 1057-64.
5. Gilchrist I. Transradial technical tips. Catheter Cardiovasc Interv. 2000; 49 (3): 353-54.
6. Grollman Jr. J. The many faces of the anomalous left aortic arch. Catheter Cardiovasc Interv. 2001; 54 (2): 202-03.
7. Hamon M, Gomes S, Clergeau M, et al. Risk of acute brain injury related to cerebral microembolism during cardiac catheterization performed by right upper limb arterial access. Stroke. 2007; 38 (7): 2176-79.
8. Klinke W, Hilton J, Warburton R, et al. Comparison of treatment outcomes in patients > or =80 years undergoing transradial versus transfemoral coronary intervention. Am J Cardiol. 2004; 93 (10): 1282-85.
9. Louvard Y, Benamer H, Garot P, et al. OCTOPLUS study group. Comparison of transradial and transfemoral approaches for coronary angiography and angioplasty in octogenarians (the OCTOPLUS study). Am J Cardiol. 2004; 94 (9): 1177-80.
10. Patel T. Right trans-radial approach-working through arteria lusoria. Indian Heart J. 2006; 58 (4): 301.
11. Patel T, Shah S, Pancholy S. Coronary cannulation through mirror-image right aortic arch during right transradial approach: A rare case report with review of literature. J Invasive Cardiol. 2012; (in press).
12. Valsecchi O, Vassileva A, Musumeci G, et al. Failure of transradial approach during coronary interventions: anatomic considerations. Catheter Cardiovasc Interv. 2006; 67 (6): 870-78.
13. Yiu K, Chan W, Jim M, et al. Arteria lusoria diagnosed by transradial coronary catheterization. JACC Cardiovasc Interv. 2010; 3 (8): 880-81.

Cannulation of the Coronary Ostia

7

Tejas Patel, Sanjay Shah, Charanjit Rihal and Rajiv Gulati

The device industry has designed the perfect hardware to cannulate the coronary ostia through the femoral route. Unfortunately, this is not yet true for the radial route, although several experienced radialists have designed diagnostic and guide catheters with differently shaped curves.

In this chapter, we show coronary cannulation using commonly used catheters including the Optitorque TIG (Terumo) catheter, Judkins catheters, and extra back-up (EBU) guide catheters.

Understanding the Catheter's Course: Radial Versus Femoral

With transfemoral intervention, it does not matter whether the right or the left femoral artery is used for coronary cannulation. But with transradial intervention, there are subtle differences between the right and the left approaches, shown in the following schematic drawings.

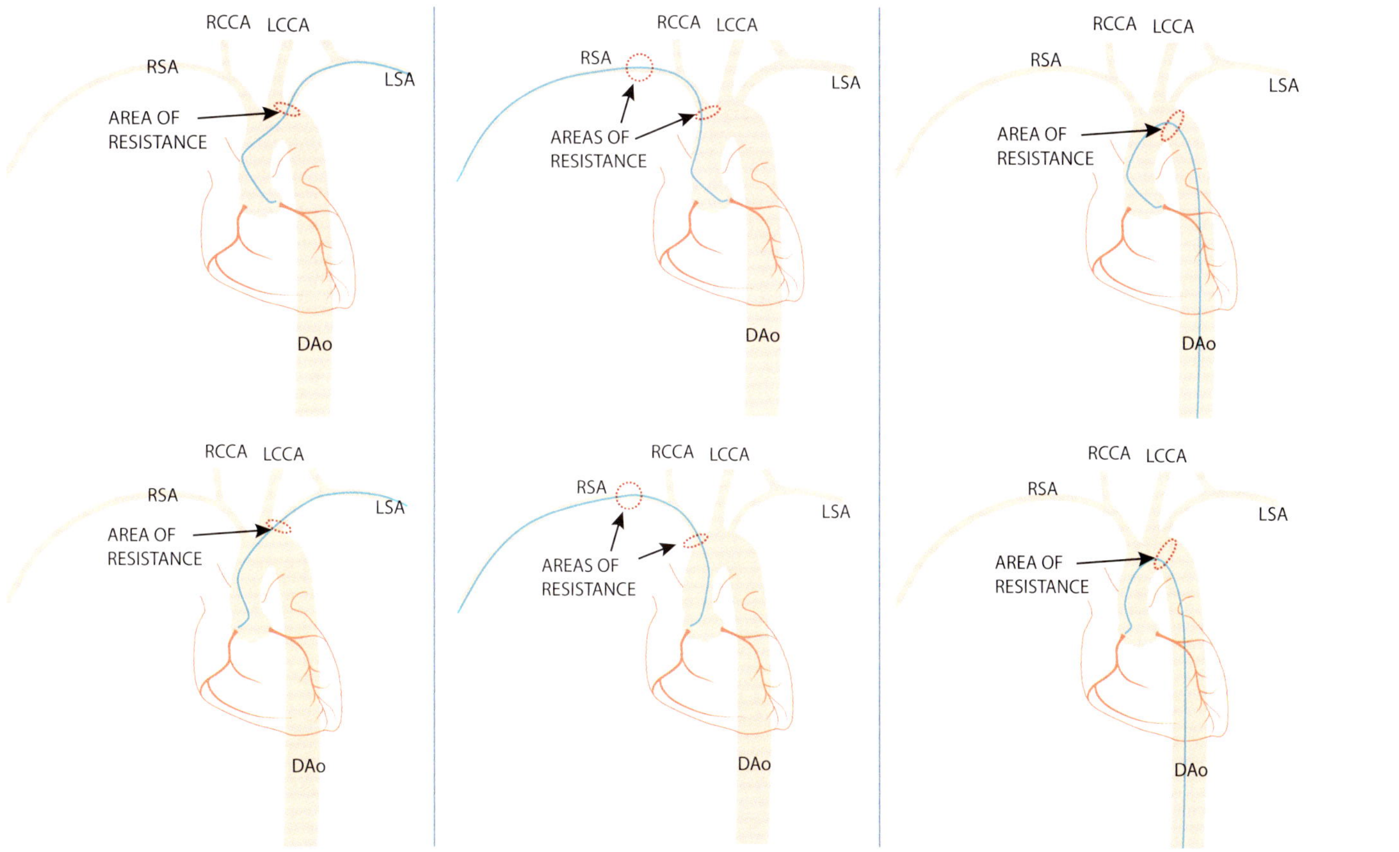

These six, self-explanatory drawings depict the course of the catheter via the transfemoral and the transradial (right and left) approaches. You can see the sites of resistance in the passage of catheters and guidewires through these approaches. These sites of resistance explain the different maneuvers needed to cannulate the coronary arteries. These maneuvers determine the torqueability and steerability of catheters and guidewires through the various angles of the arterial system.

Eye-Hand Coordination

For the femoral and the left-radial approach, there is only one level of resistance that affects the torque of the catheter. For the right radial approach, there are two levels of resistance. In routine cases with no significant tortuosities of the subclavian artery and no dilation and/or distortion of the arch, torque may not be a major issue, and the operator can cannulate the coronary ostia without much effort. However, eye-hand coordination is very useful if there is significant dilation, distortion and/or tortuosity at the subclavian level, which can lead to arteria lusoria or loops at the arch level.

This means that, rather than being fussy about whether to perform a clockwise or a counterclockwise rotation, the operator should simply look at the screen and direct the catheter's tip toward the coronary ostia.

We actually advise that new radial operators play video games regularly to improve eye-hand coordination.

Diagnostic Catheters

Various diagnostic catheters are used by operators to cannulate coronary arteries. The 5 Fr Optitorque TIG catheter is our first choice for coronary cannulation. This catheter cannulates both the left and right coronary arteries; a left ventriculogram is also possible with this catheter because it has an additional side hole.

The Judkins catheter is popular for diagnostic studies and it is successful in most cases. However, it requires two catheters —

left and right Judkins — to cannulate the left and right coronary arteries, respectively. Each catheter must be exchanged over a double-length, standard 0.035-inch guidewire. In rare cases, we use different catheters for abnormal anatomy (e.g., Amplatz, multi-purpose).

1. Optitorque TIG (Terumo)
2. Judkins left
3. Amplatz left
4. Judkins right
5. Amplatz right
6. Pa-Pa Curve (Medtronic)

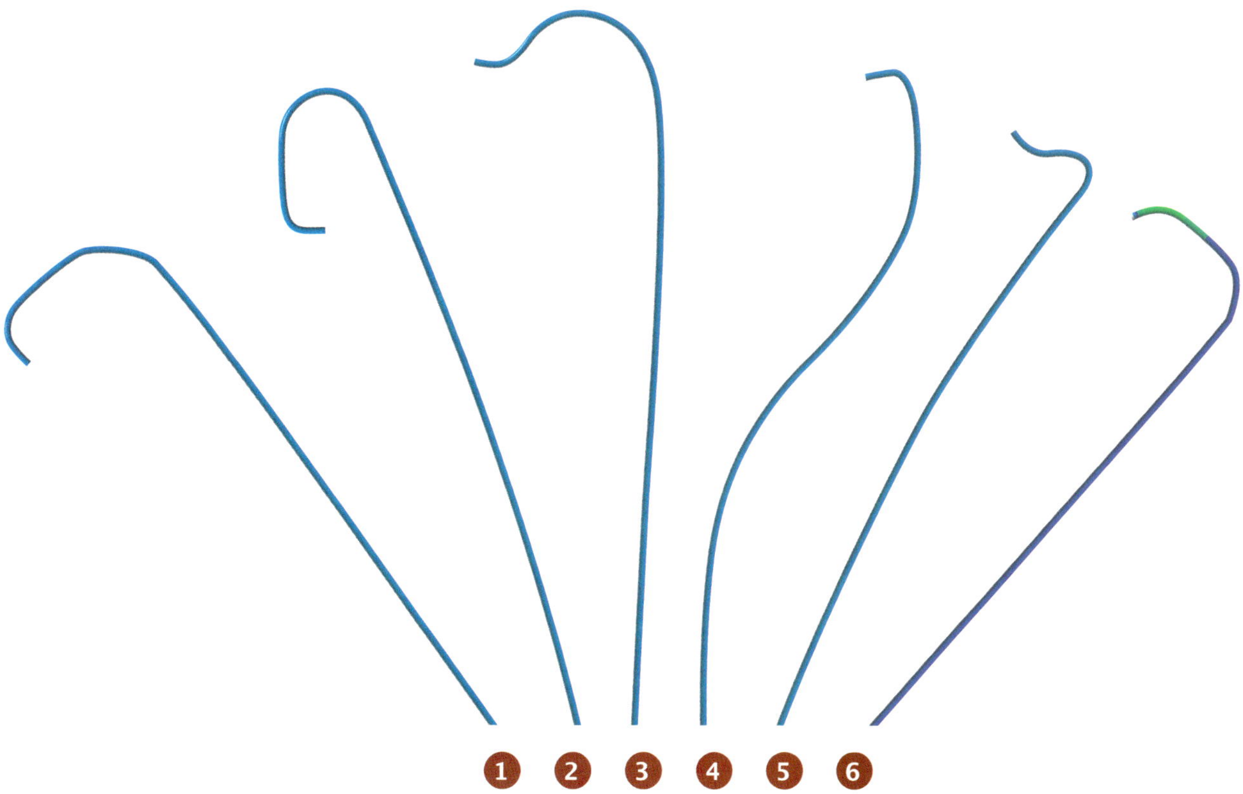

Cannulation With Diagnostic Catheters

Optitorque TIG (Terumo)

Left Coronary Cannulation

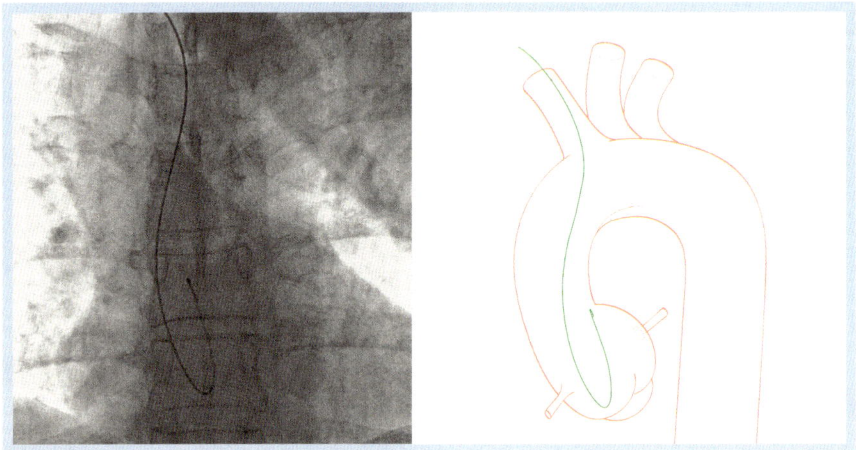

We made a loop of the standard 0.035-inch guidewire in the aortic root.

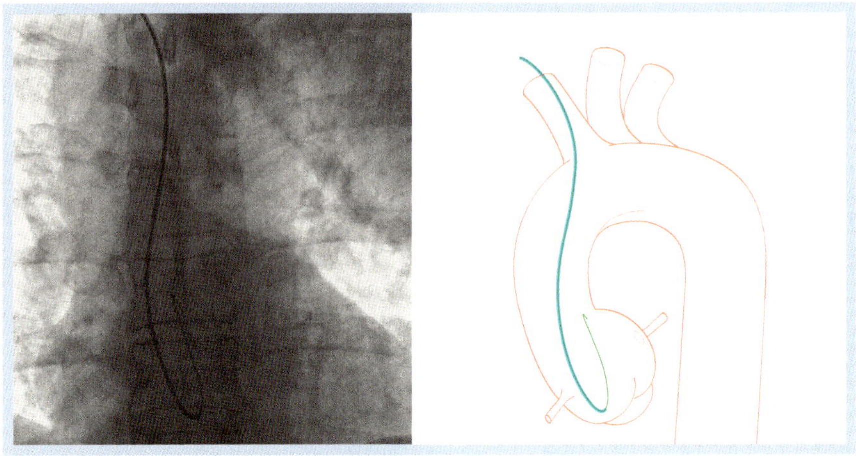

The catheter was advanced over the guidewire.

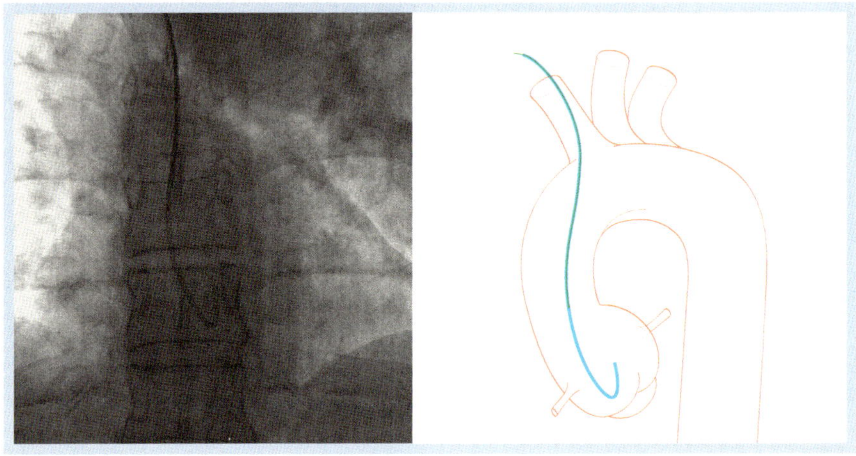

The guidewire was removed.

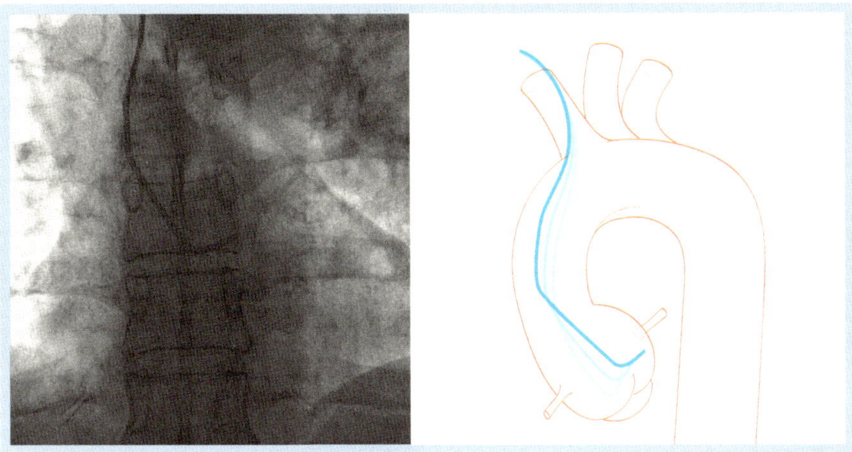

The catheter was pulled back and rotated gently clockwise and/or counterclockwise.

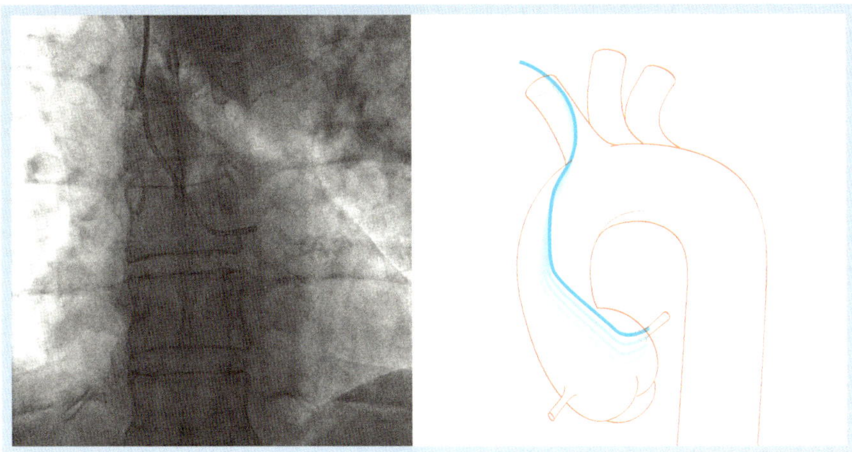

We continued the same movement.

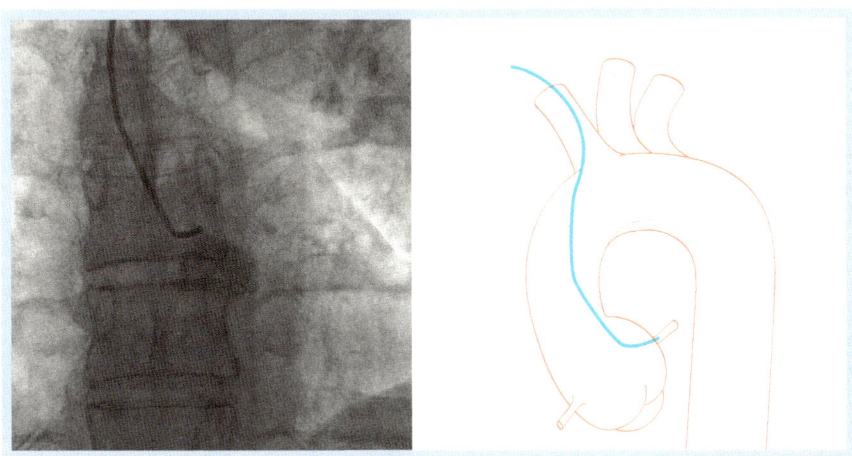

The catheter moved closer to the coronary ostia.

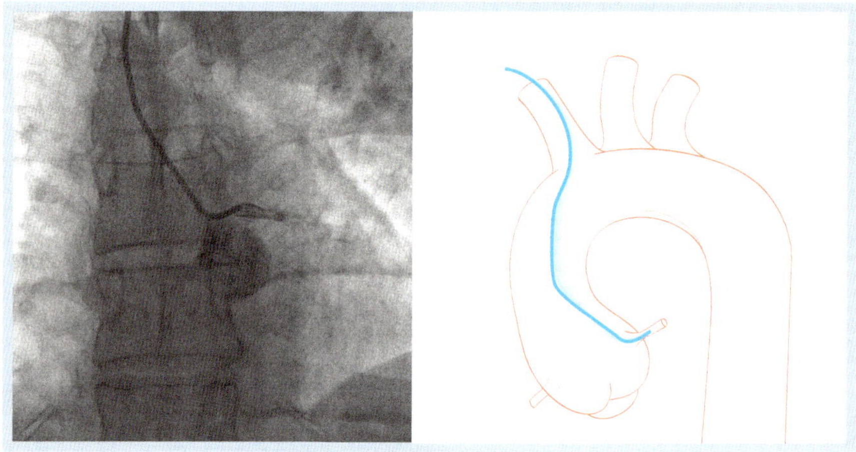

The catheter tip entered the LCA ostium.

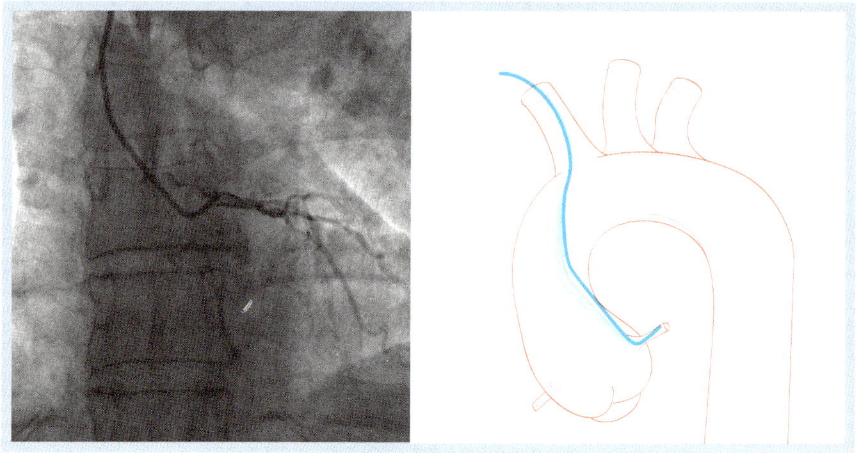

The left coronary artery was cannulated.

Optitorque TIG (Terumo) Right Coronary Cannulation

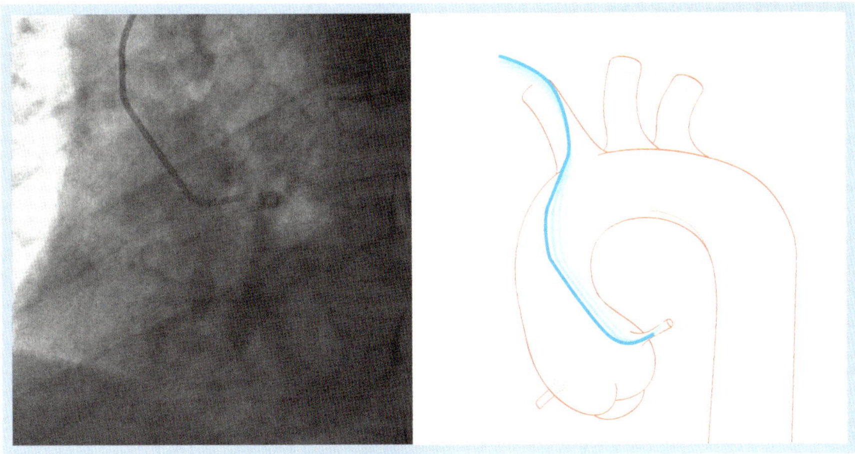

We started disengaging the catheter from the left coronary artery.

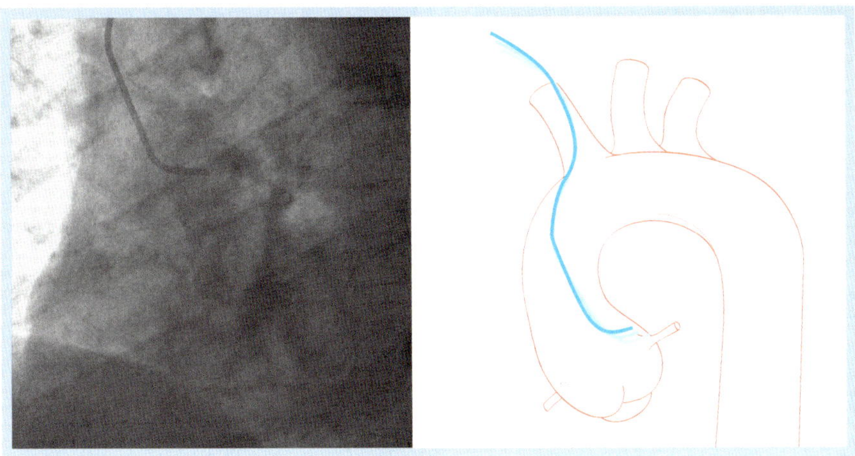

The catheter was disengaged from the left coronary artery.

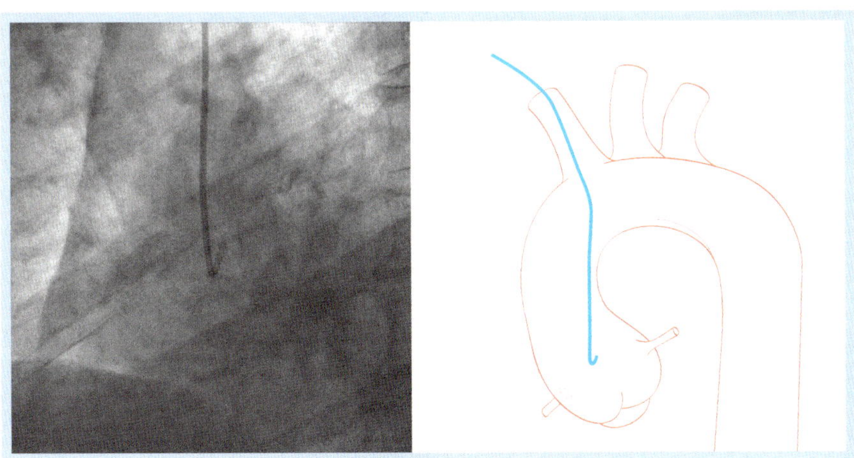

We rotated the catheter clockwise.

We gently pushed the catheter down toward the aortic valve.

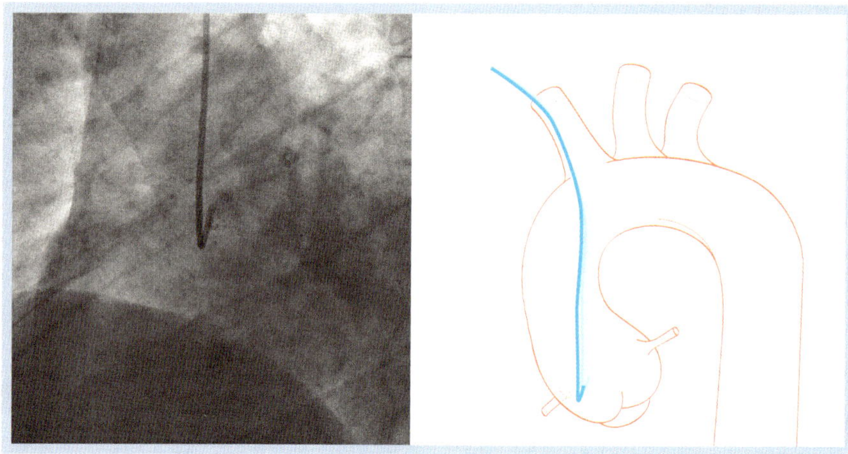

The catheter was pulled back gently and rotated clockwise to cannulate the right coronary artery ostium.

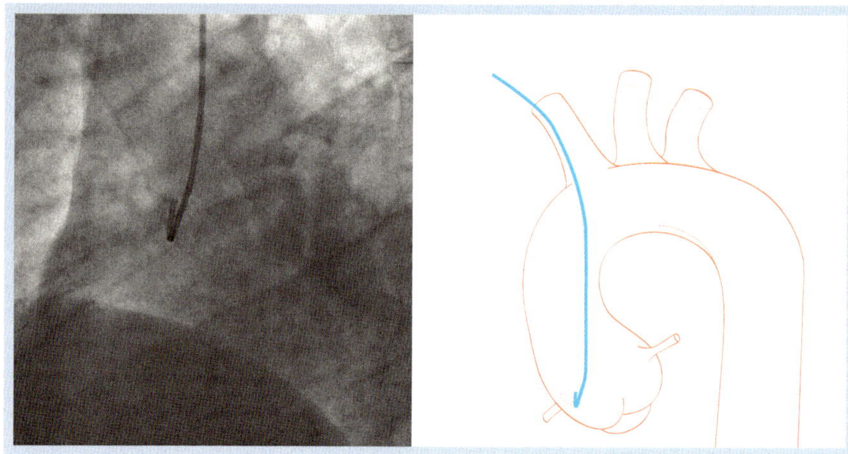

Simultaneous clockwise rotation and gentle pullback resulted in cannulation of the right coronary artery.

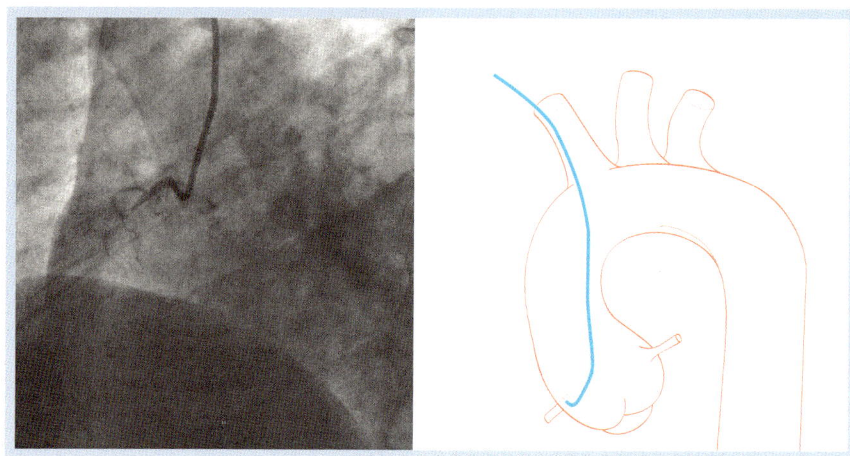

Judkins Left
Left Coronary Cannulation

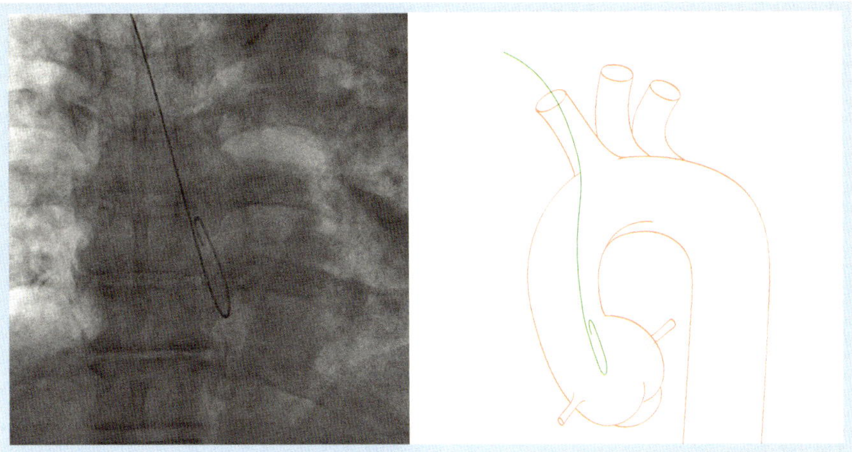

We made a loop of a standard 0.035-inch guidewire in the aortic root.

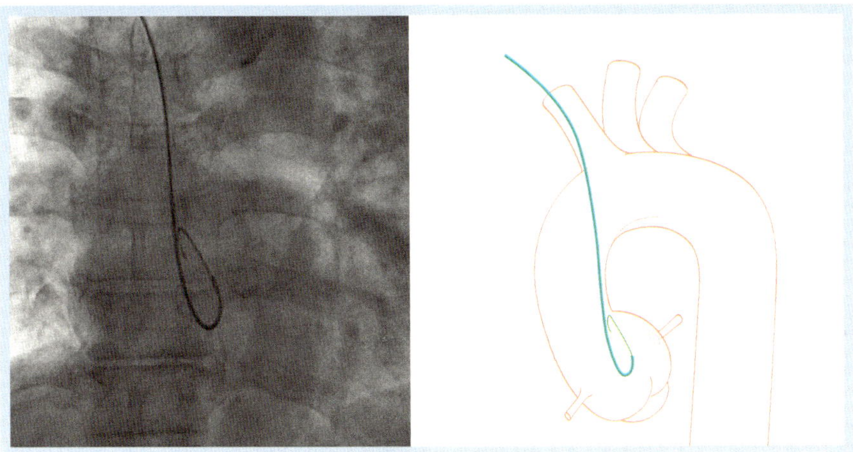

The catheter was advanced over the guidewire.

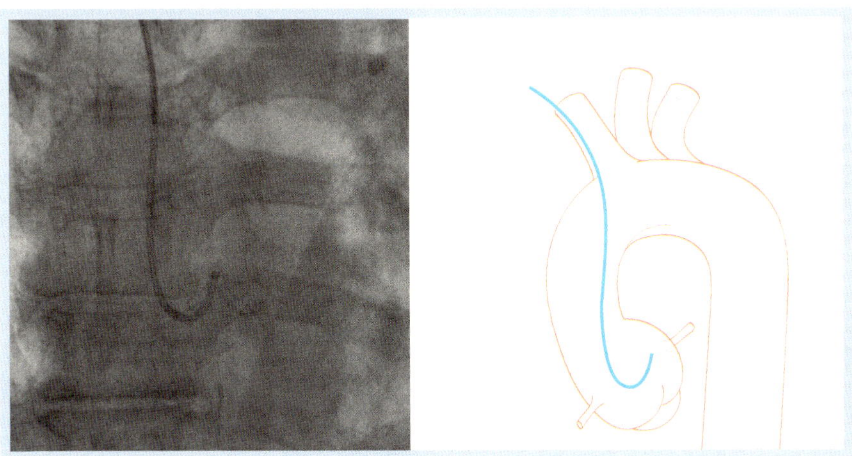

The guidewire was removed.

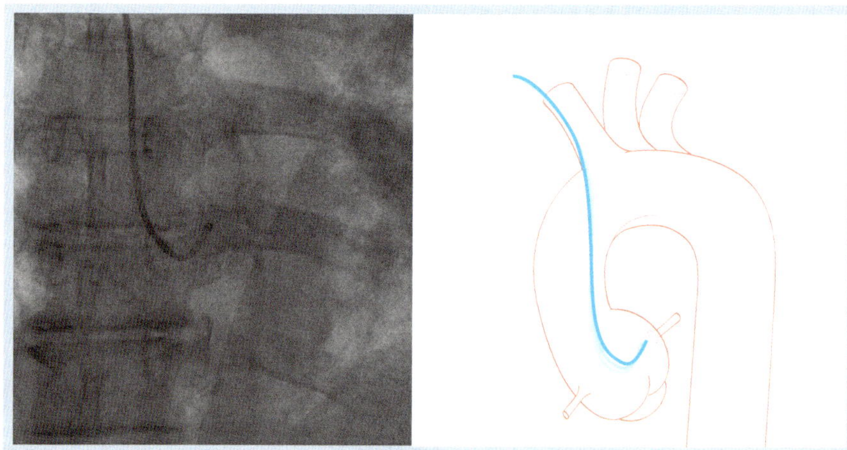

The catheter was pulled back gently and rotated clockwise.

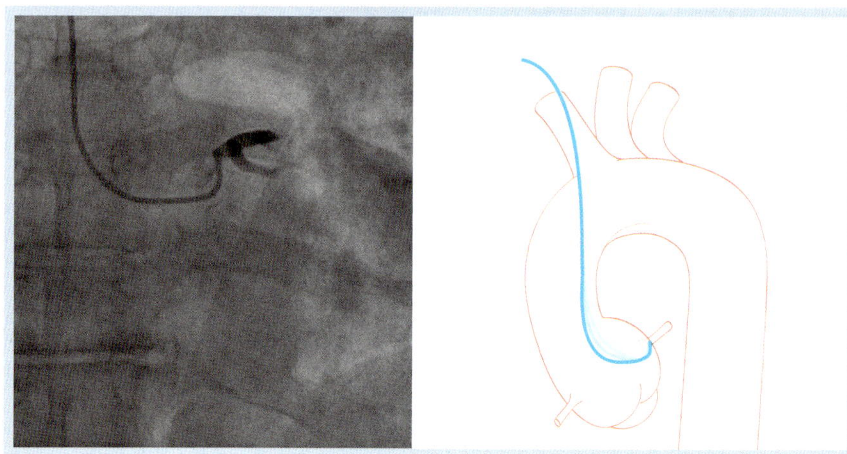

The left coronary artery was cannulated.

Judkins Right
Right Coronary Cannulation

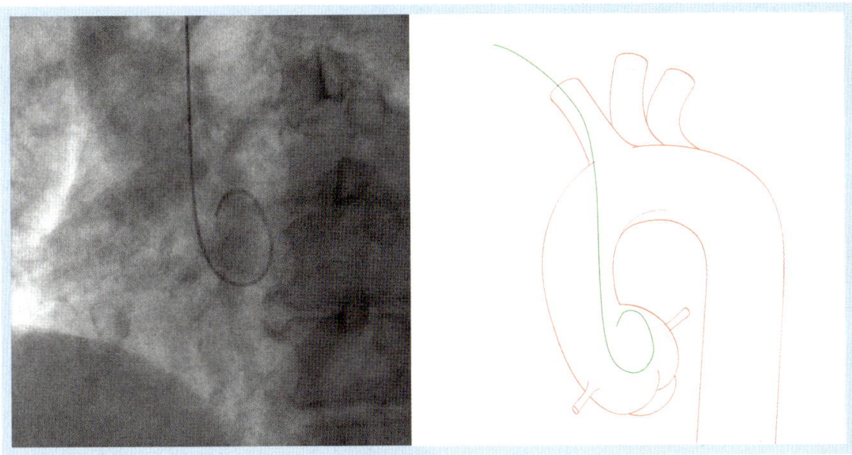

We made a loop of standard 0.035-inch guidewire in the aortic root.

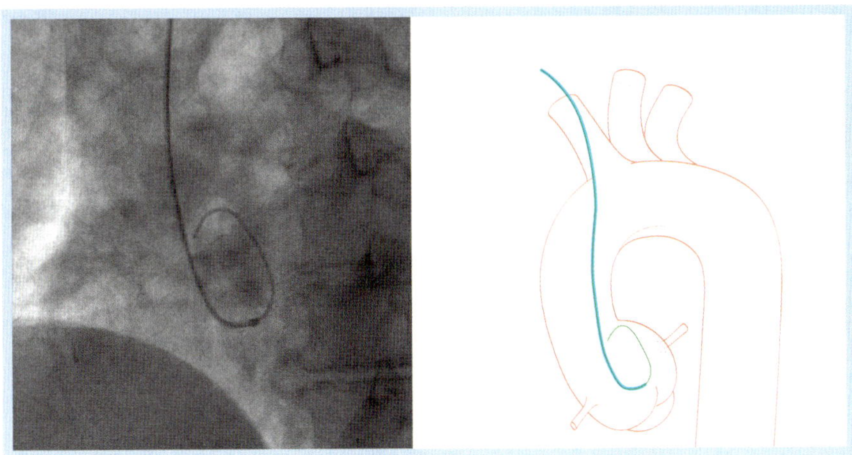

The catheter was advanced over the guidewire.

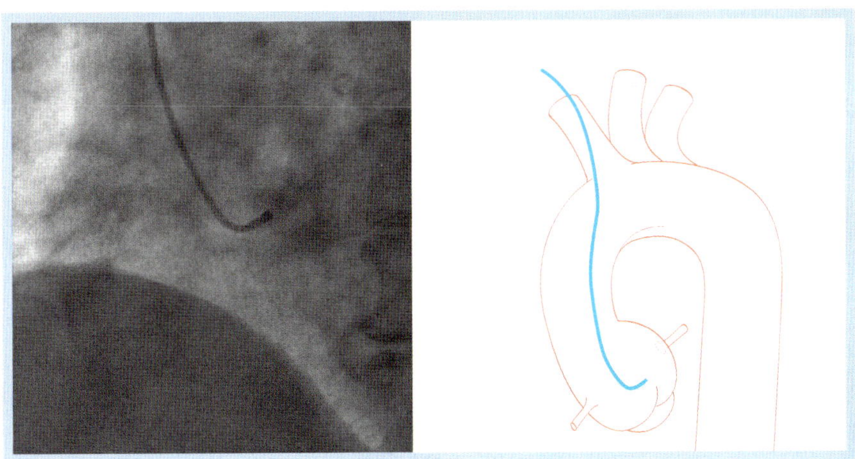

The guidewire was removed.

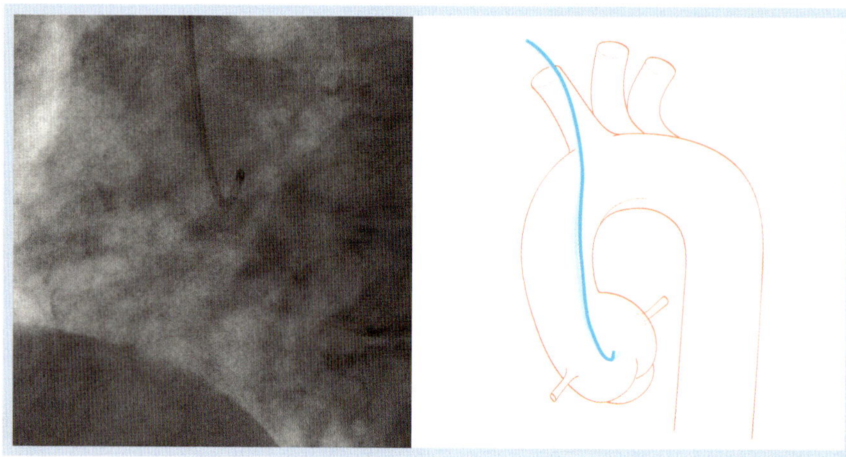

The catheter was pulled back gently and rotated clockwise.

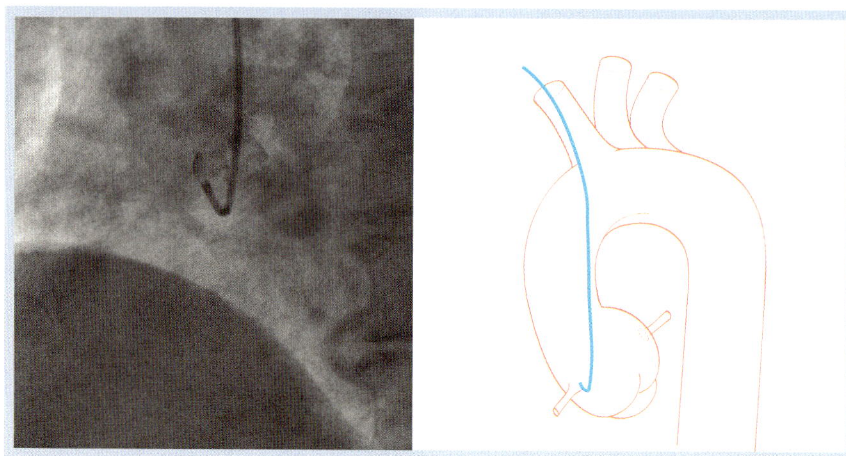

The catheter was facing toward the right coronary cusp.

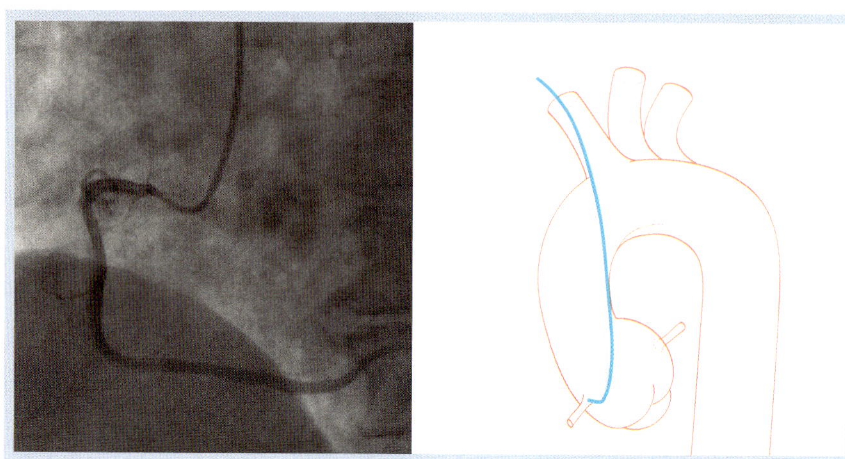

The right coronary artery was cannulated.

Guide Catheters

Various guide catheters are used by operators to cannulate coronary arteries. The EBU, XB, and Voda catheters are our first choices for left coronary cannulation.

A second choice for left coronary cannulation is a Judkins left guide catheter.

For right coronary artery cannulation, a Judkins right or Pa-Pa Curve catheter is the preferred curve. In selected situations, an Amplatz right, multipurpose, or Amplatz left catether can be used.
Examples of guide catheters are below.

1. EBU
2. XB
3. Voda
4. Judkins left
5. Amplatz left
6. Pa-Pa Curve (Medtronic)
7. Judkins right

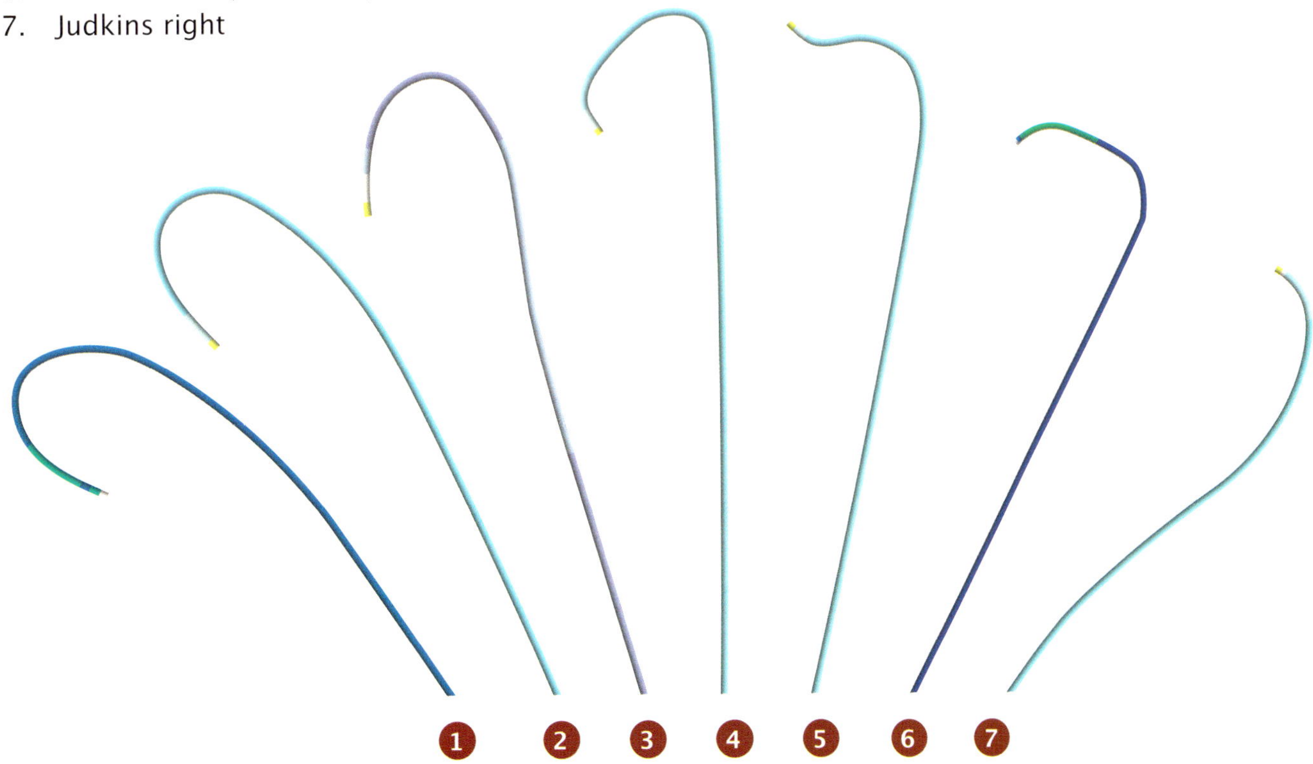

Cannulation With Guide Catheters

EBU Catheters

Left Coronary Cannulation

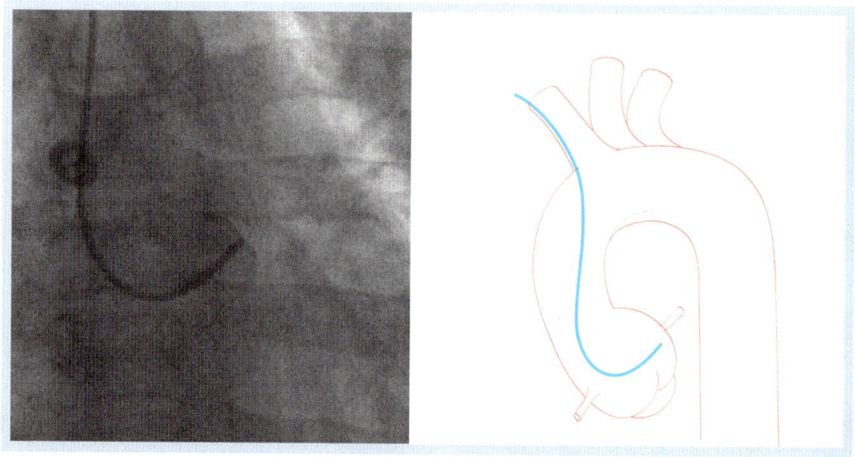

We advanced the guide catheter over a standard 0.035-inch guidewire to keep it in the left coronary cusp with the tip facing left.

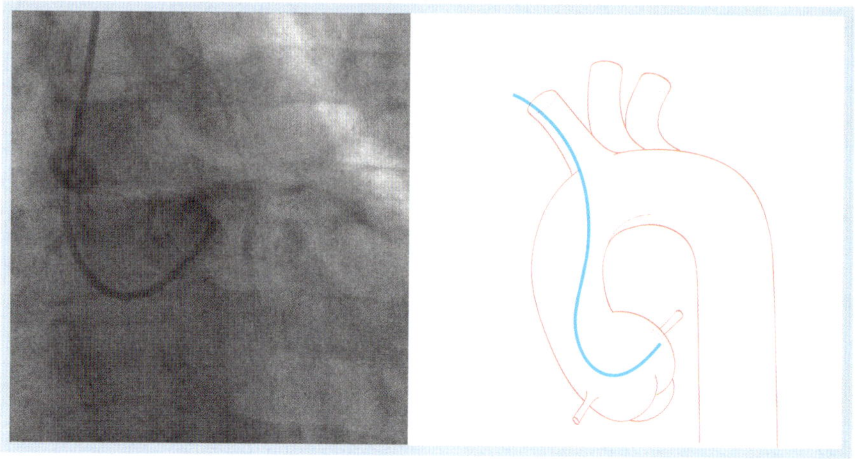

We gradually pushed and rotated the catheter counterclockwise.

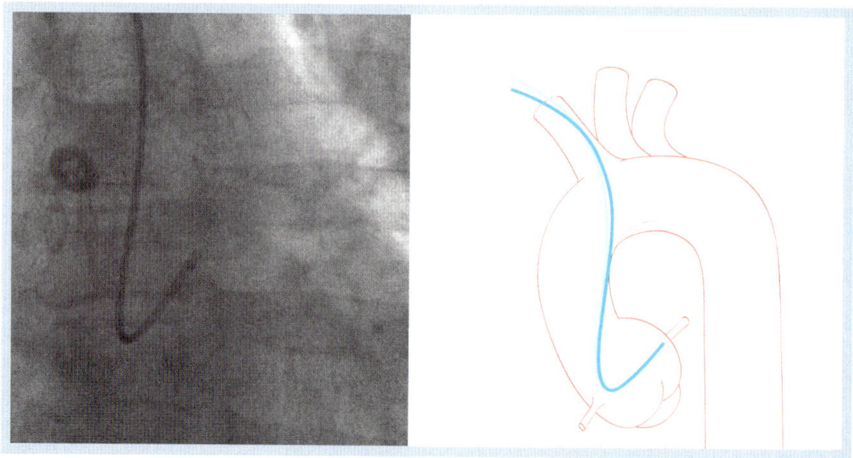

The catheter tip approached the left coronary artery ostium.

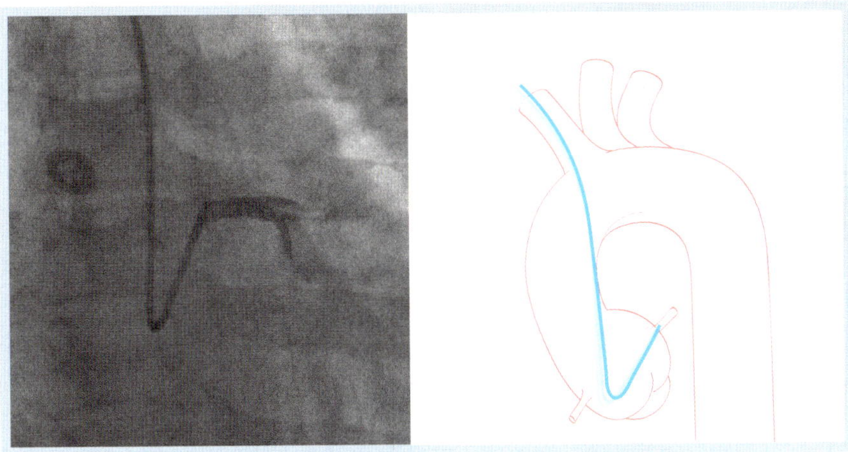

Continuation of the counterclockwise rotation and a gentle push of the catheter resulted in cannulation of the left coronary artery ostium.

Tips

- In most cases, the operator should be able to cannulate the coronary ostium by using the regular curves i.e. Optitorque TIG, Judkins or an EBU curve. In selected cases, special curves may be needed.
- If there is significant tortuosity in the subclavian region, or there are loops due to dilatation and/or distortion of the aorta, or if there is arteria lusoria, normal torque of the catheter is not preserved. Therefore, rather than fussing about clock or counterclockwise rotation, the operator should concentrate on the movement of the catheter's tip to direct it into the coronary ostia. Eye-hand coordination is very important in this situation.
- Rather than using the wrist movements for the torque of the catheter (regularly practiced while working through the femoral route), use the finger movements to cannulate coronary ostia while working through the radial route.

Dealing With Special Situations

❶ At times, while engaging the RCA ostium, a 5 Fr TIG Optitorque catheter tends to cannulate the conal artery selectively. It is identified by a damping of the aortic pressure tracing. Removed the catheter immediately and make a second attempt to engage the RCA ostium. If the phenomenon repeats, the following maneuver should be tried: Take a 0.032-inch or 0.035-inch standard guidewire and introduce the opposite (stiff) end of the guidewire through the catheter lumen. Bring it up to the primary curve of the catheter, not letting it protrude outside the tip. Try to engage the RCA ostium in the regular fashion. Is should engage successfully in most instances.

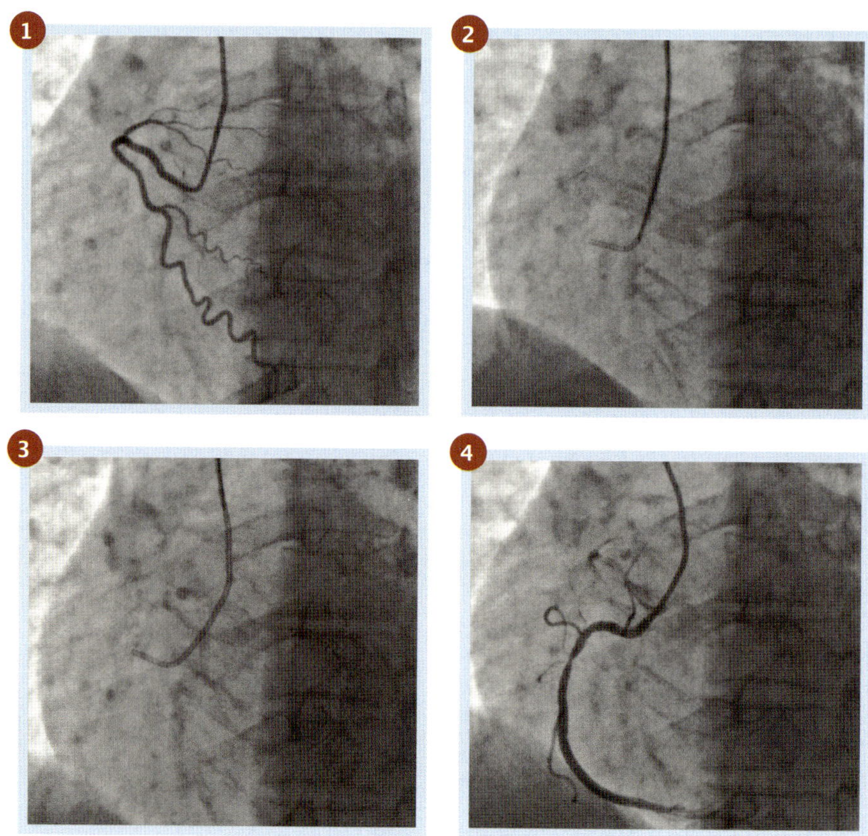

1. While trying selective RCA cannulation using a 5 Fr Optitorque TIG catheter, it tends to selectively cannulate the conal artery.
2. The stiff end of a standard 0.035-inch guidewire was negotiated and brought near the primary curve of the catheter. It transformed this catheter into a right Judkins curve.
3. Successful cannulation of the RCA is done.
4. Right coronary angiogram is done.

❷ At times, a JR guide catheter does not provide an adequate back-up support for RCA intervention. In this situation, a JL 3.5 or JL 4 guide catheter can be tried. It should be carefully rotated in the same fashion to cannulate the RCA ostium. You may also use the stiff end of a 0.032-inch or a 0.035-inch standard guidewire, and the similar technique described previously, to cannulate the RCA ostium. Once it is cannulated using a JL guide catheter, it provides excellent extra back-up support (comparable to the support of an EBU guide catheter for the LCA).

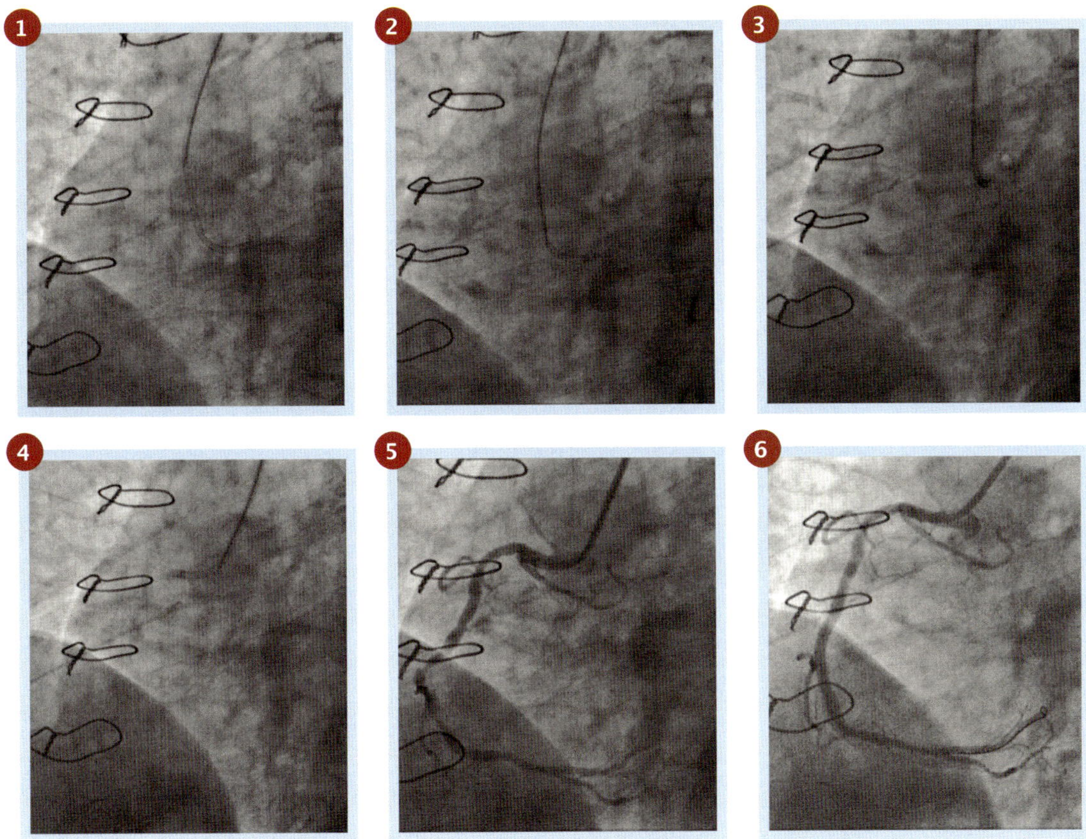

1. After completion of LAD intervention, a 6 Fr JL 3.5 guide catheter was disengaged from LMCA ostium and the opposite end of a 0.035-inch standard guidewire was negotiated.
2. The stiff end of the guidewire was brought near the primary curve, leading to transformation of a JL curve into JR curve.
3. The guide catheter along with the guidewire was rotated in the usual fashion to cannulate the RCA ostium.
4. RCA ostium is cannulated successfully.
5. RCA angiogram reveals a critical mid RCA stenosis.
6. Final result after stenting.

❸ Because an AL guide catheter has a higher chance of damaging or dissecting the RCA ostium, this catheter should be used sparingly to cannulate the RCA through the TRA.

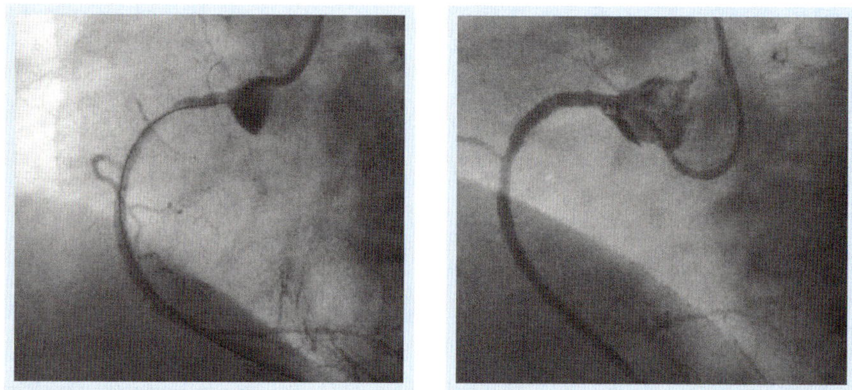

- Aortic dissection in the right coronary cusp was created by the tip of a 6 Fr AL1 guide catheter.

❹ It is possible to use the deep intubation technique through TRA. Although it is an effective technique to tackle difficult distal lesions and to perform thrombosuction, it should be used sparingly and only by very experienced operators.

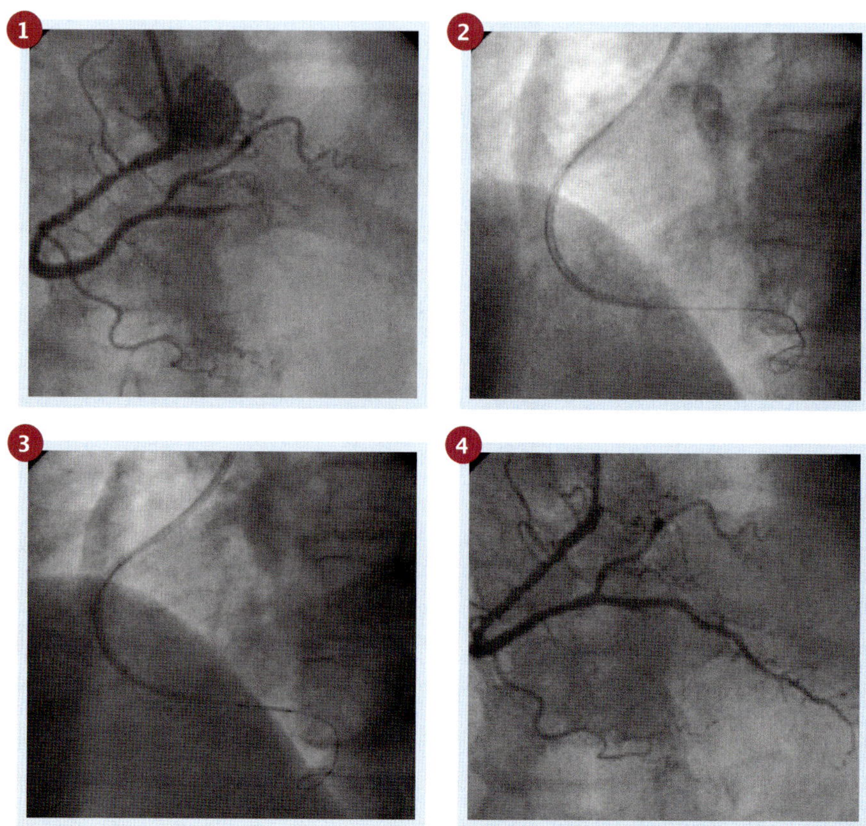

1. RCA injection using a 6F JR4 guide catheter revealed a total occlusion in the PDA.
2. By using a deep intubation technique, the tip of the guide catheter was brought near the bifurcation of RCA.
3. Stenting in progress.
4. Final result.

❺ While performing intervention in an anomalous RCA arising from the left coronary cusp, a JL 3 guide catheter should be the first choice, as it sits coaxially in the RCA ostium and provides good backup.

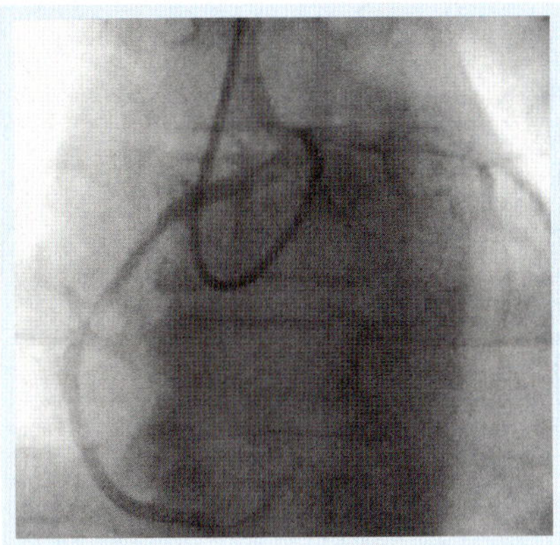

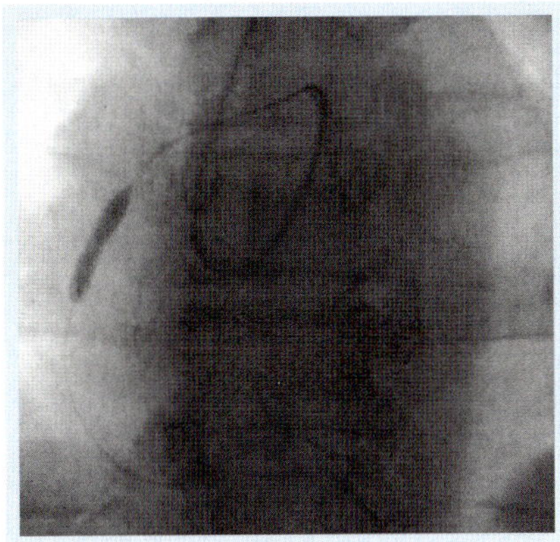

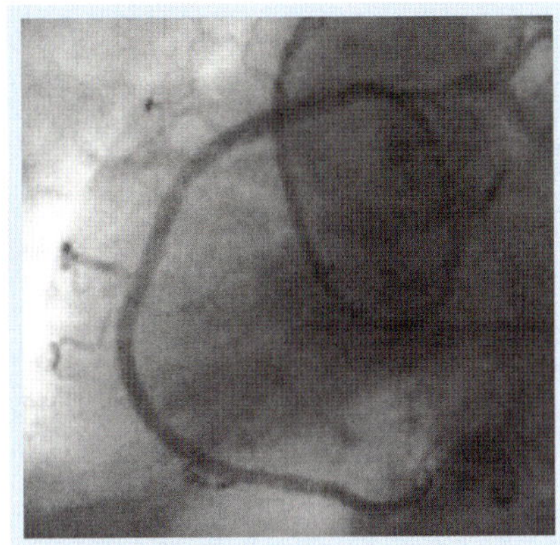

1. A 6 Fr JL 3 guide catheter is used to cannulate an RCA arising anomalously from the left coronary cusp. Selective RCA injection reveals a critical mid-RCA stenosis.
2. Stenting is n progress.
3. In the final result, note the extremely good back-up support provided by the JL 3 guide catheter.

❻ While performing intervention in an anomalous RCA arising high and anteriorly from the ascending aorta, we have used a 6 Fr JR 4 guide catheter. Although we completed intervention successfully, a 6 Fr MP-1 guide catheter would have been a better choice.

1

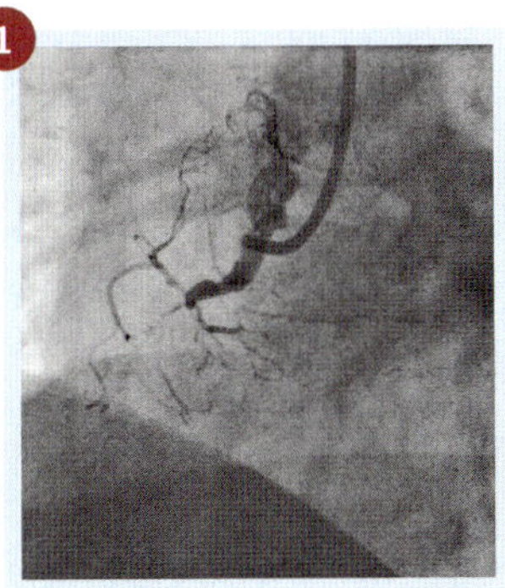

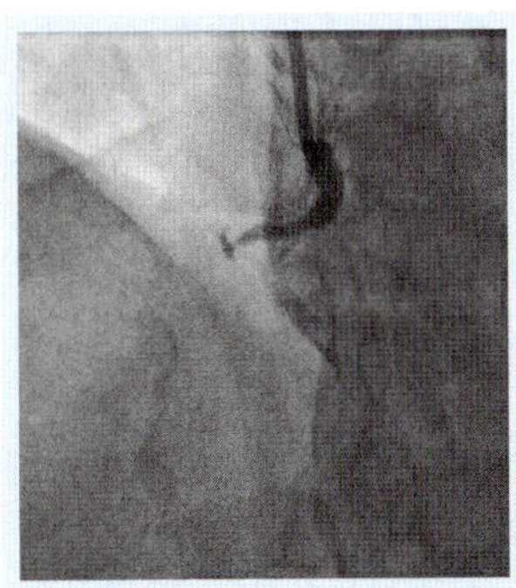

2

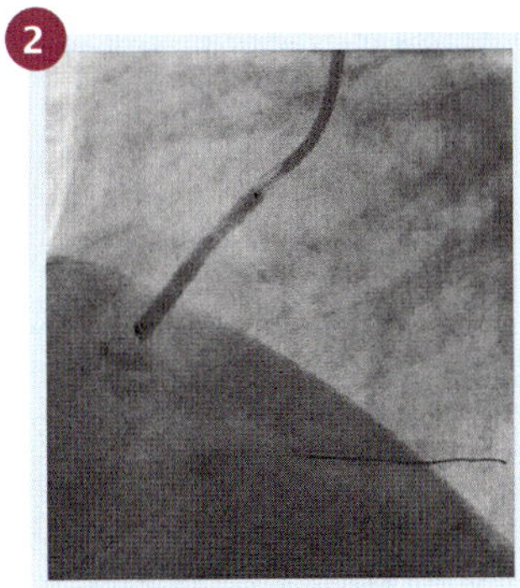

3

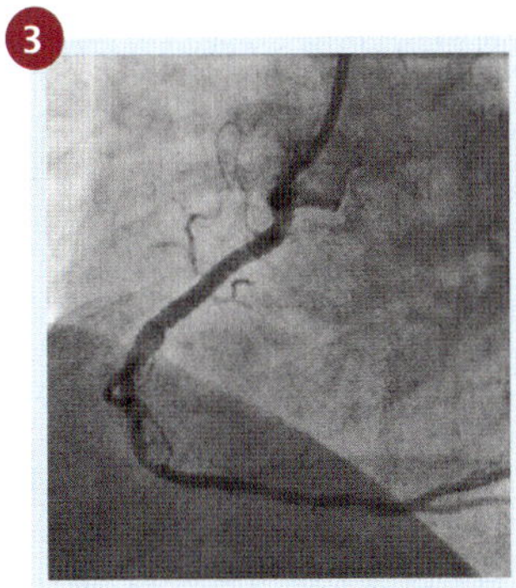

1. A 6 Fr JR 4 guide catheter cannulates an anomalous RCA arising high and anteriorly from the ascending aorta. The RCA is totally occluded after its origin.
2. Stenting is in progress.
3. The final result is pictured.

❼ An example of an anomalous LCX arising from the right coronary cusp and successful intervention of LCX and RCA lesions.

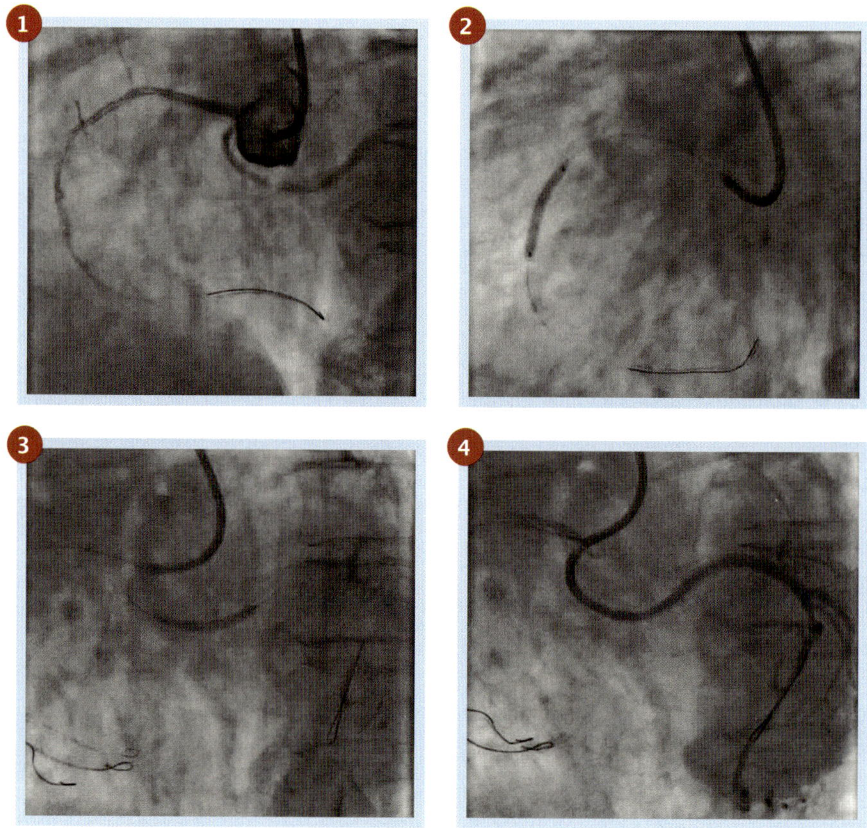

1. A non-selective injection from a 6 Fr JR 4 guide catheter reveals an anomalous origin of the LCX from the right coronary cusp. Note the critical stenosis in mid-RCA and -LCX.
2. RCA stenting is in progress.
3. LCX stenting is in progress.
4. The final result is pictured.

❽ Role of 5 Fr guide catheters

Pros	Cons
• Allows interventions through a 5 Fr introducer sheath. • Offers higher success rate while working through small radials and difficult loops. • Is less traumatic during deep intubation maneuvers.	• Poses higher risk of air trapping and air embolism during PTCA catheter removal. • Has relatively poor visualization of the coronary system compared to 6 Fr or 7 Fr guide catheters. • Kissing balloon technique and use of bulky devices (e.g., rotational atherectomy, distal protection device) is not recommended.

⑨ Role of Sheathless Guide Catheters

(Rajiv Gulati and Charanjit Rihal)

The outer diameter of a standard hydrophilic sheath is approximately 2 Fr sizes larger than the outer diameter of its corresponding guide catheter. Therefore, a sheathless guiding catheter insertion allows for a larger internal lumen without increasing outer diameter size. An 8 Fr sheathless guide, with the same outer diameter as a 6 Fr sheath, will thus enable complex transradial intervention to be undertaken in most radial arteries. A similar strategy allows for 5 Fr and 6 Fr sheathless interventions, equivalent to the use of 3 Fr and 4 Fr sheaths, in patients with small radial arteries or for whom maintenance of radial patency is paramount.

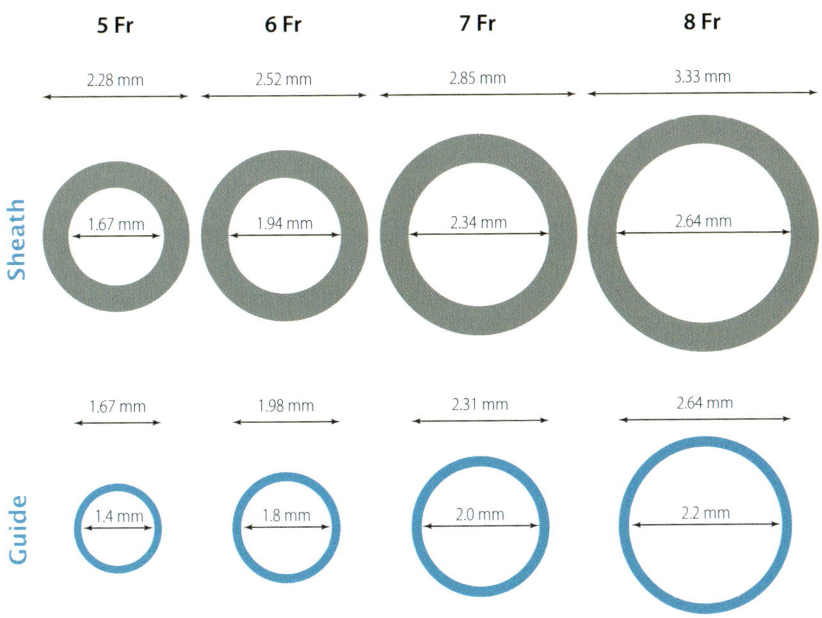

Comparison of inner and outer diameters of introducer sheaths and sheathless guide catheters

Minimizing trauma upon insertion of the sheathless guiding catheter into the radial artery is key to success with such an approach. A custom-made commercial guiding catheter with hydrophilic coating and a long, tapered central dilator are ideal for seamlessly transitioning between wire, dilator and guiding catheter for atraumatic entry into the radial artery. However, these devices are expensive and not universally available. It is also possible to use standard equipment available in all cath labs to fashion an inner dilator for standard guiding catheters. Our approaches are detailed in the following sections.

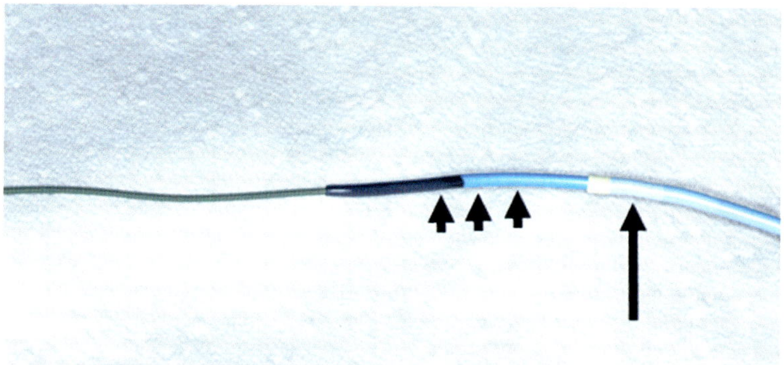

A sheathless guide catheter with dilator and guide wire

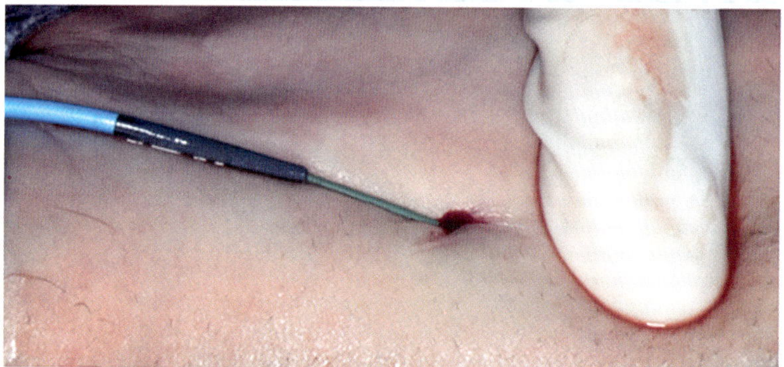

Guide catheter with dilator being advanced over the wire

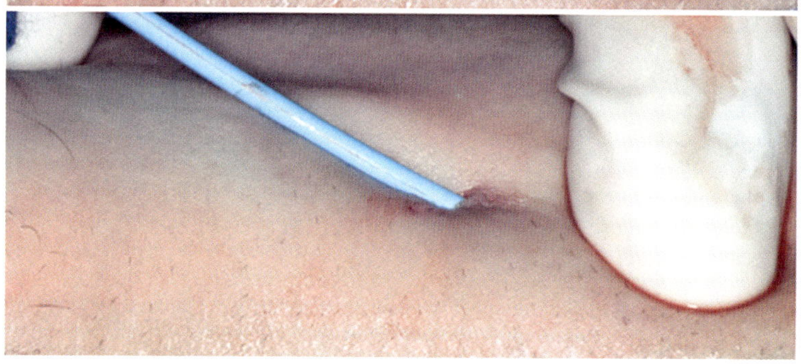

Guide catheter that has entered the radial artery

Larger caliber guides

First, obtain access to the radial artery with a 5 Fr or 6 Fr sheath in a standard manner. The entry-site arteriotomy created by the sheath will facilitate subsequent guide advancement. Next, advance any diagnostic catheter into the aortic root and use this to switch for an exchange-length 0.035-inch stiff wire. A regular wire will also work, but the stiff wire will serve as a stronger rail over which the guide/dilator can be advanced into the radial artery. To create a taper for standard 7 Fr and 8 Fr guides of any configuration, insert a 125 cm 5 Fr or 6 Fr multipurpose diagnostic catheter or a 125 cm 6.5 Fr Shuttle select hydrophilic catheter through the guide. After removing the sheath, advance the guide/dilator over the 0.035-inch wire into the radial artery. It is helpful for the assistant to apply traction on the wire, actually physically pulling it back slowly, as this provides a taut rail which facilitates guide entry. A quick, moderately forceful push may be required to enter the radial, as the transition between wire, dilator and catheter is not perfect. Remember to maintain forward pressure on the dilator at the same time. Once the guide enters the radial, it can be advanced with its dilator, then used to cannulate the coronary in the usual manner. On occasion, there may be minor ooze at the skin-entry site, but this will settle with a minute of gentle compression.

Smaller caliber guides

For 5 Fr and 6 Fr sheathless guide insertion, first access the radial with a micropuncture kit and advance an exchange-length 0.035-inch wire to the aortic root. The dilator associated with the greatest ease of guide-catheter insertion is a 110 cm Cook 4 Fr sheath dilator through a 5 Fr guiding catheter. For a 6 Fr guide, a 5 Fr 125 cm Shuttle Select diagnostic catheter also provides a reasonable transition. Alternatives include a 4 Fr 125 cm multipurpose diagnostic catheter or a 5-in-6 Guideliner, but these require more forward push to get the guide into the radial artery.

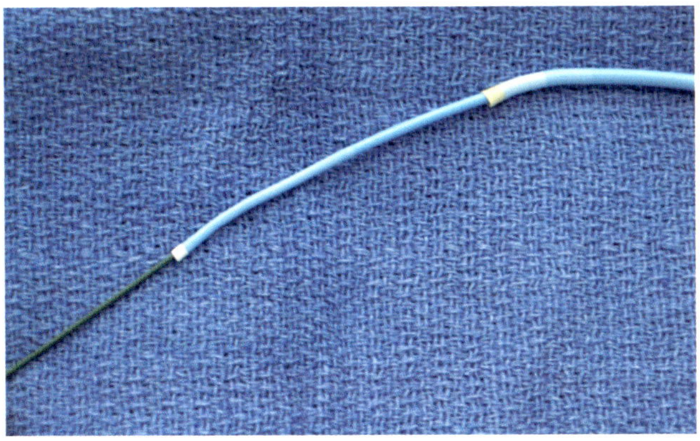

A 7 Fr guide catheter with a 5 Fr diagnostic catheter with a 0.035-inch guide wire.

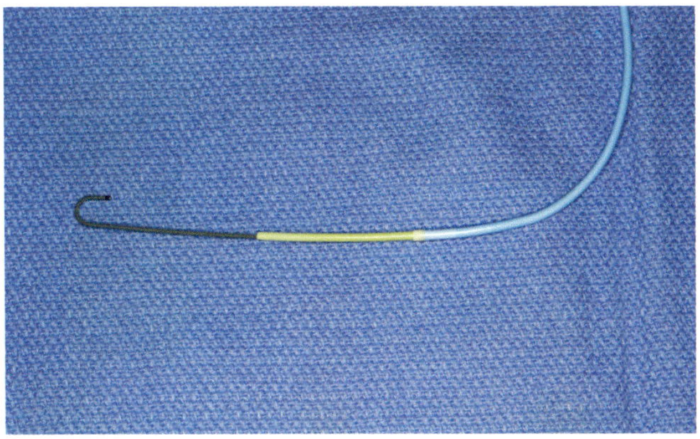

A 5 Fr guide with a 4 Fr Cook sheath dilator and a 0.035-inch guide wire.

Recommended Reading

1. Abhaichand R, Louvard Y, Gobeil J, et al. The problem of arteria lusoria in right transradial coronary angiography and angioplasty. Catheter Cardiovasc Interv. 2001; 54 (2): 196-201.
2. Bhatia G, Ratib K, Lo T, et al. Transradial cardiac procedures and increased radiation exposure: is it a real phenomenon? Heart. 2009; 95 (22): 1879-80.
3. Caputo R, Simons A, Giambartolomei A, et al. Transradial cardiac catheterization in elderly patients. Catheter Cardiovasc Interv. 2000; 51 (3): 287-90.
4. Dehghani P, Mohammad A, Bajaj R, et al. Mechanism and predictors of failed transradial approach for percutaneous coronary interventions. JACC Cardiovasc Interv. 2009; 2 (11): 1057-64.
5. From A, Gulati R, Prasad A, et al. Sheathless transradial intervention using standard guide catheters. Catheter Cardiovasc Interv. 2010; 76 (7): 911-16.
6. Gilchrist I. Transradial technical tips. Catheter Cardiovasc Interv. 2000; 49 (3): 353-54.
7. Ikari Y, Masuda N, Matsukage T, et al. Backup force of guiding catheters for the right coronary artery in transfemoral and transradial interventions. J Invasive Cardiol. 2009; 21 (11): 570-74.
8. Ikari Y, Nagaoka M, Kim J, et al. The physics of guiding catheters for the left coronary artery in transfemoral and transradial interventions. J Invasive Cardiol. 2005; 17 (12): 636-41.
9. Mamas M, D'Souza S, Hendry C, et al. Use of the sheathless guide catheter during routine transradial percutaneous coronary intervention: a feasibility study. Catheter Cardiovasc Interv. 2010; 75 (4): 596-602.
10. Patel T. Right trans-radial approach-working through arteria lusoria. Indian Heart J. 2006; 58 (4): 301.
11. Patel TM, Shah S, Pancholy S. Coronary cannulation through mirror-image right aortic arch during right transradial approach: A rare case report with review of literature. J Invasive Cardiol. 2012, in press.
12. Takeshita S, Saito S. Transradial coronary intervention using a novel 5-Fr sheathless guiding catheter. Catheter Cardiovasc Interv. 2009; 74 (6): 862-65.
13. Valsecchi O, Vassileva A, Musumeci G, et al. Failure of transradial approach during coronary interventions: anatomic considerations. Catheter Cardiovasc Interv. 2006; 67 (6): 870-78.
14. From AM, Bell MR, Rihal CS, Gulati R. Minimally invasive transradial intervention using sheathless standard guiding catheters. Catheter Cardiovasc Interv. 2011; 78: 866-71.

TRA for Addressing Bypass Graft Lesions

Tejas Patel, Sanjay Shah, Tak Kwan and Tejan Patel

8

When TRA was introduced, cannulation of a bypass graft was considered a relative contraindication. In contemporary practice, this is not true. Both right and left radial approaches are equally effective for bypass graft interventions.

Tips

- A 5 Fr Optitorque TIG (Terumo) catheter can be used for cannulating saphenous vein grafts (SVG) and radial artery grafts to the LCA and RCA.
- JR and AR catheters are also effective in cannulating SVGs and radial grafts to the LCA and RCA.
- The multipurpose catheter is useful for cannulating and maintaining co-axiality with the ostium, particularly during intervention of the SVG to RCA.
- An AL catheter is useful to cannulate the SVG to LCA or RCA, particularly when the aortic root is significantly dilated and distorted.
- There is practically no difference in cannulating SVGs and radial grafts working through the right or left TRA.
- A LIMA graft is easy to cannulate through the left TRA using an IMA catheter, although cannulation through the right TRA can be difficult.
- A technique to cannulate the LIMA graft through the right TRA is described later in this chapter. It is important to know this technique because, in many patients whose left radial arteries have already been harvested for use as bypass grafts, right radial access may be the only route.
- For graft interventions through the TRA, 6 Fr guide catheters are usually preferred because it is possible to use practically all distal protection devices through this diameter guide.

Example 1

Diagnostic cannulation of SVG to OM.

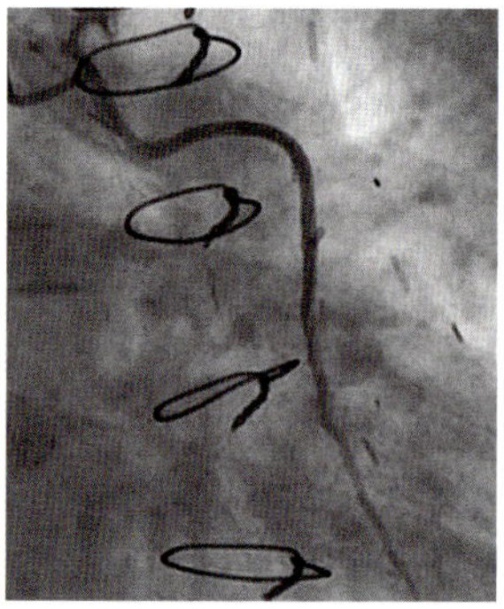

1. Diagnostic cannulation of saphenous vein graft (SVG) to OM artery using an Optitorque TIG catheter.

Example 2

Diagnostic cannulation of SVG to PDA.

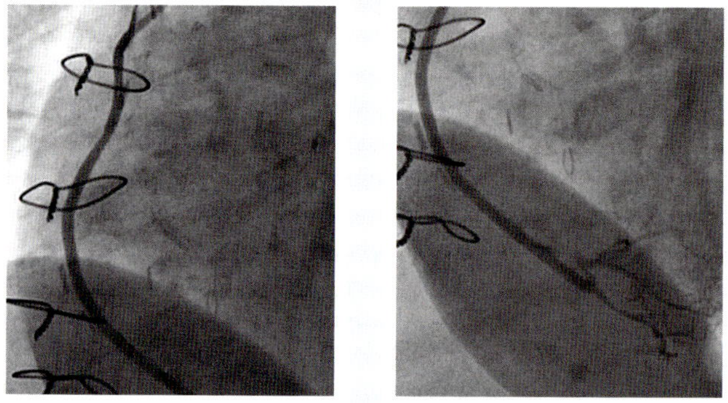

Diagnostic cannulation of SVG to PDA using a JR 4 diagnostic catheter.

Example 3

Intervention of the SVG to OM

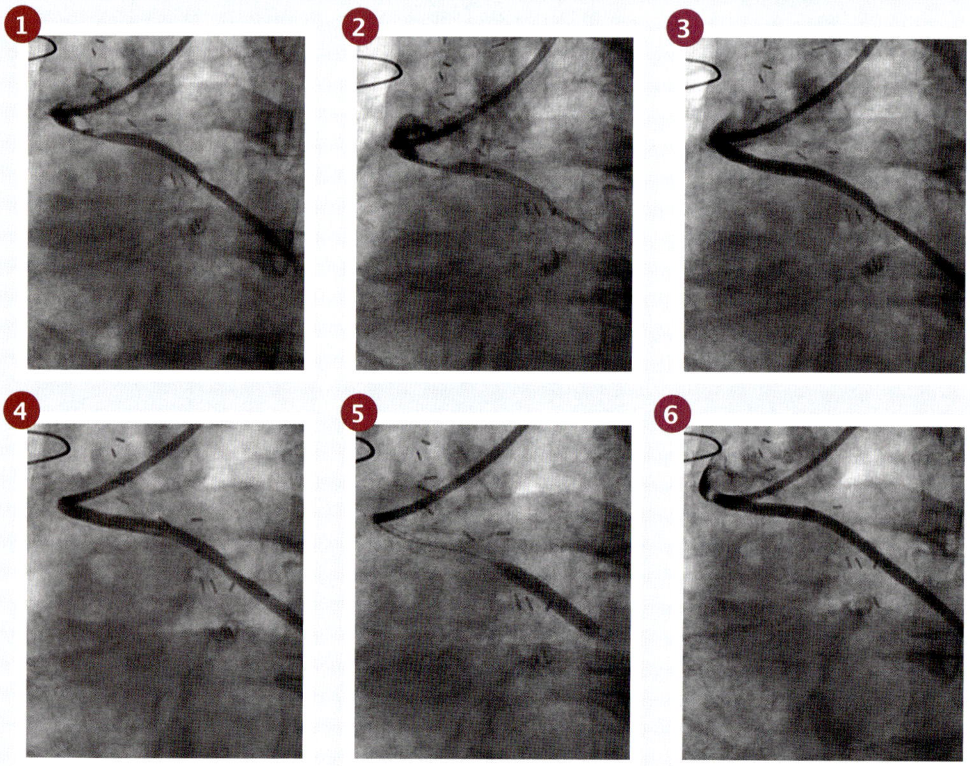

1. Cannulation of the SVG to OM artery using a 6 Fr JR 4 guide catheter showing two tandem lesions in the proximal segment of the graft
2. Stenting of the first lesion in progress
3. Optimal result of the stenting
4. Stenting in progress
5. Stenting of second lesion done
6. Satisfactory end result

Example 4

Intervention of SVG to PDA.

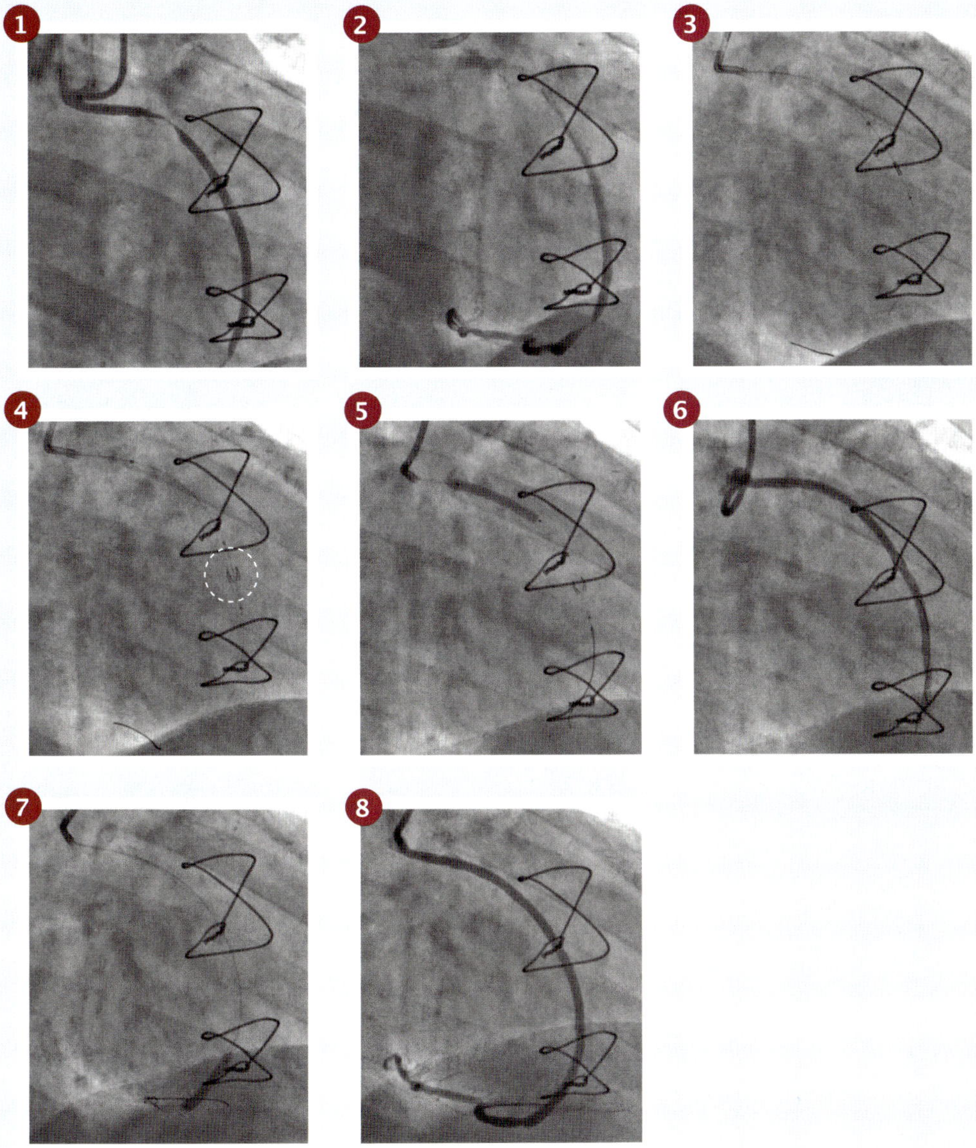

1. Critical lesion in proximal segment of the SVG to PDA
2. Critical lesion in distal segment of SVG to PDA
3. Introducing the distal protection device in the mid-segment
4. Distal protection device is deployed; a white circle denotes the device in place
5. Stenting of the lesion in the proximal segment
6. Optimal result of the stented proximal segment
7. Distal protection device deployed in the distal segment beyond the lesion; lesion stented
8. Optimal result of the stented distal segment

Example 5

LIMA cannulation through left TRA

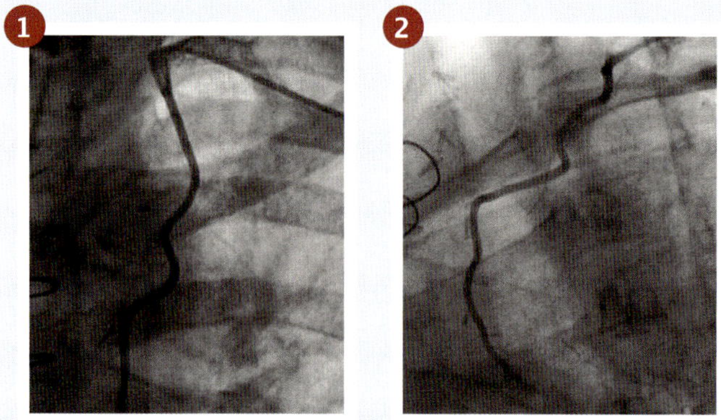

1. LIMA graft cannulation through left transradial approach using an IMA catheter.
2. Normally appearing LIMA graft.

Example 6

LIMA cannulation technique through the right TRA

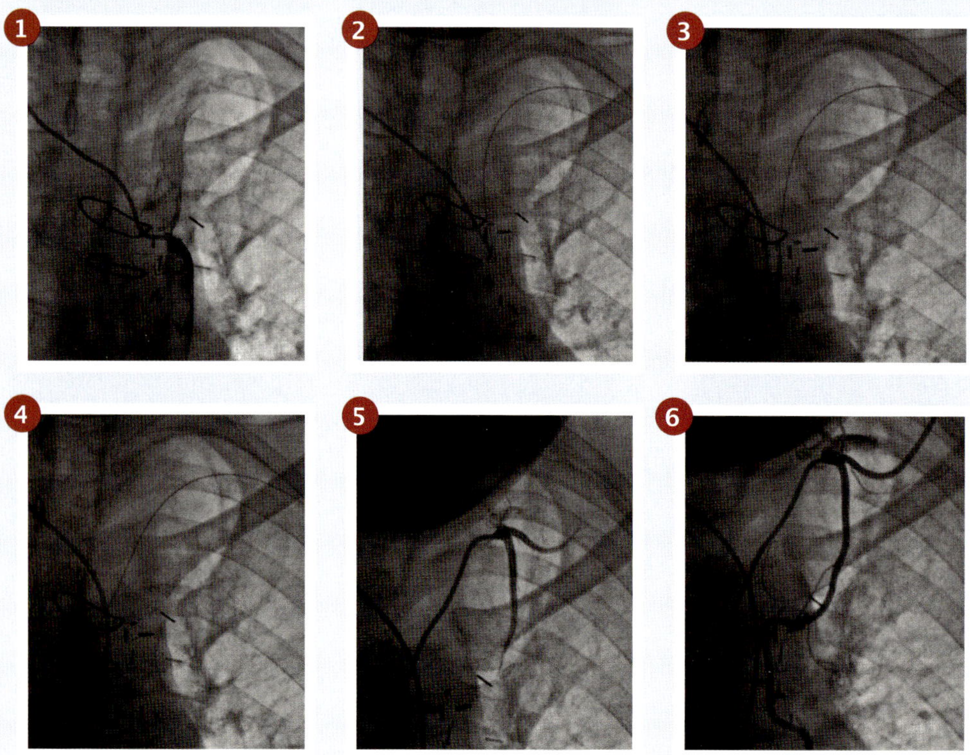

1. LIMA graft cannulation technique through the right transradial approach using an Optitorque TIG catheter
2. Partial cannulation of left subclavian artery with an Optitorque TIG catheter. Then a 0.032-inch hydrophilic wire is negotiated carefully in the subclavian and, subsequently, deep in the brachial artery
3. Negotiating the catheter in the subclavian artery over the wire using a slow jack-hammering technique
4. Further progress of the catheter
5. The tip of the catheter near the ostium of the LIMA; completed selective cannulation of the LIMA
6. LIMA graft angiography

Important tip:

- For better guidewire stability, it can be trapped in the left brachial artery by inflating a BP cuff to 180 mmHg to 200 mmHg, or by complete flexion of the left elbow (provided guidewire is beyond the bifurcation of the brachial artery).

BP-cuff technique

1
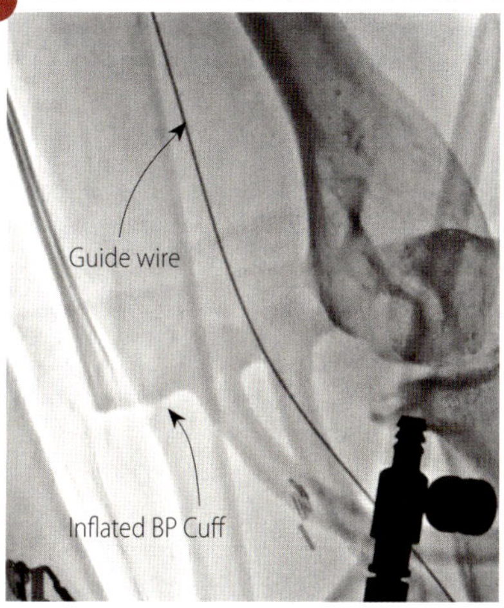

2
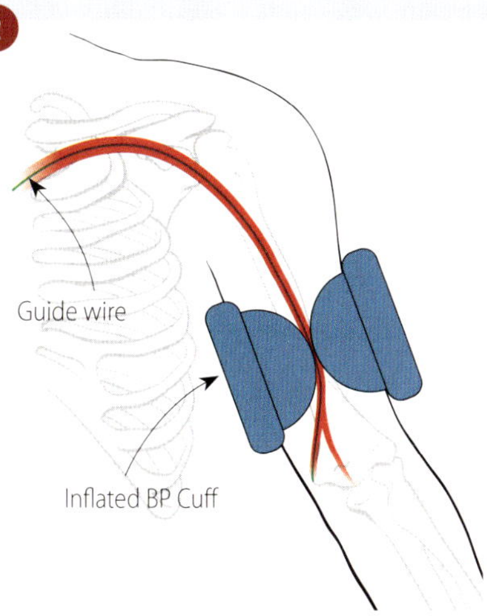

1. Inflated BP-cuff successfully traps the guide wire in left brachial artery
2. Schematic representation of the BP-cuff technique

Elbow-flexion technique

1
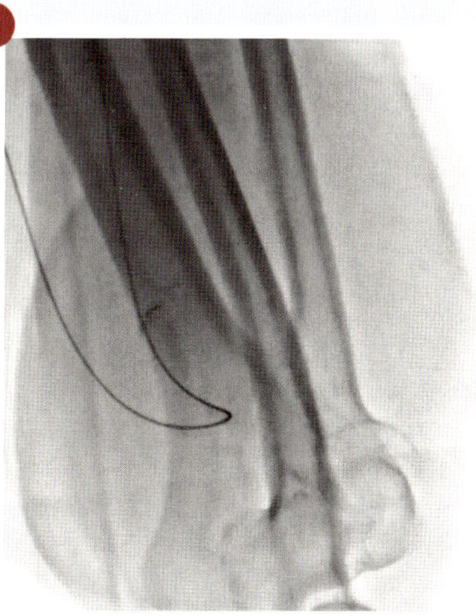

2
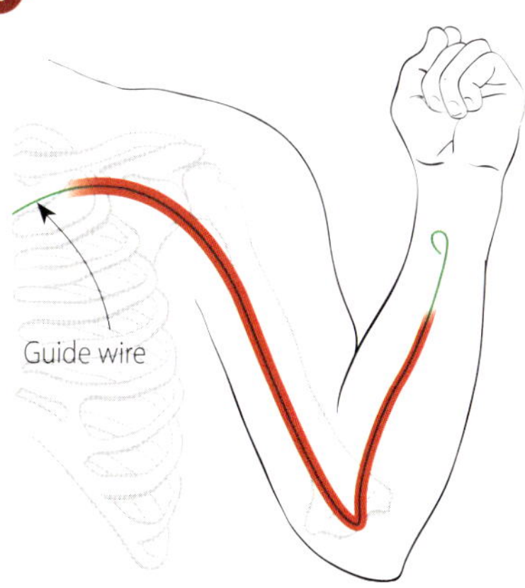

1. Left-elbow flexion traps the guidewire in the left cubital fossa
2. Schematic representation of the elbow-flexion technique

Example 7

LIMA intervention through the right TRA

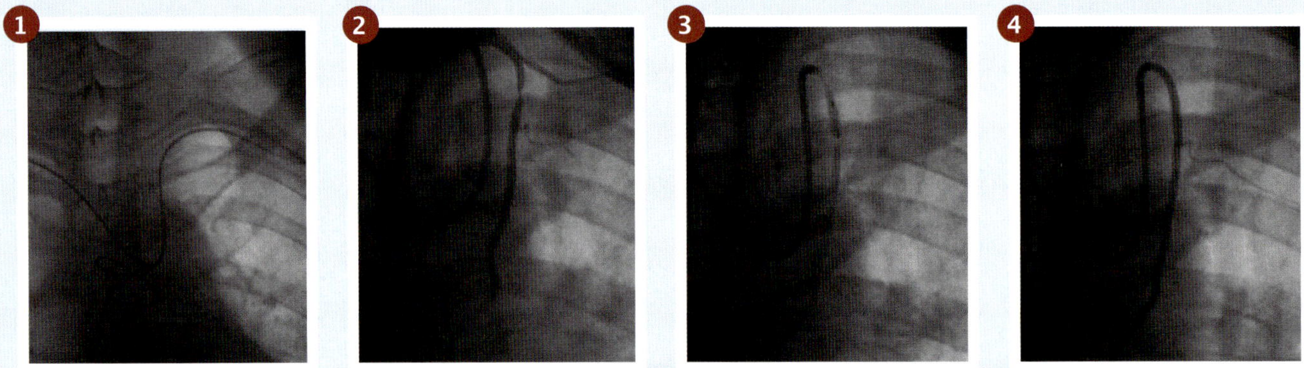

1. Technique of LIMA graft intervention through the right TRA, with a 0.032-inch standard wire negotiated and parked deep into the left subclavian artery using a technique similar to that described in Example 6.
2. The LIMA is cannulated selectively using a 6 Fr JR 4 guide catheter, and the lesion is profiled
3. The stented lesion
4. The satisfactory end result

Recommended Reading

1. Brilakis ES, Lichtenwalter C, de Lemos JA, et al. A randomized controlled trial of a paclitaxel-eluting stent versus a similar bare-metal stent in saphenous vein graft lesions: The SOS (Stenting of Saphenous Vein Grafts) trial. J Am Coll Cardiol. 2009; 53(11):919–28.
2. Burzotta F, Trani C, Hamon M, et al. Transradial approach for coronary angiography and interventions in patients with coronary bypass grafts: Tips and tricks. Catheter Cardiovasc Interv. 2008; 72(2):263–72.
3. Cha K, Kim M. Feasibility and safety of concomitant left internal mammary arteriography at the setting of the right transradial coronary angiography. Catheter Cardiovasc Interv. 2002; 56 (2): 188–95.
4. Kim M, Cha K, Kim H, et al. Bilateral selective internal mammary artery angiography via right radial approach: clinical experience with newly designed Yumiko catheter. Catheter Cardiovasc Interv. 2001; 54 (1): 19–24.
5. Mann T, Cubeddu G, Schneider J, et al. Left internal mammary artery intervention: the left radial approach with a new guide catheter. J Invasive Cardiol. 2000; 12 (6): 298–302.
6. Mann T, Raza J, Whitlock C, et al. Transradial management of saphenous vein bypass graft disease using rheolytic thrombectomy and coronary stenting. J Invasive Cardiol. 2003; 15 (4): 221–23.
7. Patel T, Shah S, Patel T. Cannulating LIMA graft using right transradial approach: Two simple and innovative techniques. Catheter Cardiovasc Interv. 2012 (in press).
8. Pinto B, Rao A, Shah M, et al. Technical tips for transradial approach in post CABG interventions. Indian Heart J. 2008; 60 (1 Suppl A): A38–41.
9. Rathore S, Roberts E, Hakeem A, et al. The feasibility of percutaneous transradial coronary intervention for saphenous vein graft lesions and comparison with transfemoral route. J Interv Cardiol. 2009; 22 (4): 336–40.
10. Sanmartin M, Cuevas D, Moxica J, et al. Transradial cardiac catheterization in patients with coronary bypass grafts: feasibility analysis and comparison with transfemoral approach. Catheter Cardiovasc Interv. 2006; 67 (4): 580–84.

9 TRA for Addressing Bifurcation Lesions

Yves Louvard, Sanjay Shah and Tejas Patel

Bifurcation stenting is a very important subset of coronary intervention. A sizable work history has been done by researchers across the globe, including animal experiments, bench-testing and human studies. As a result, techniques have evolved to address this area. Important techniques include provisional T-stenting, crush technique, reverse-crush technique, culottes technique and simultaneous kissing stent (SKS) technique. It is possible to use all these techniques through TRA. We prefer provisional T-stenting, as it is easily reproducible and offers consistent results. The issue of LMCA bifurcation stenting will be discussed separately in Chapter 10.

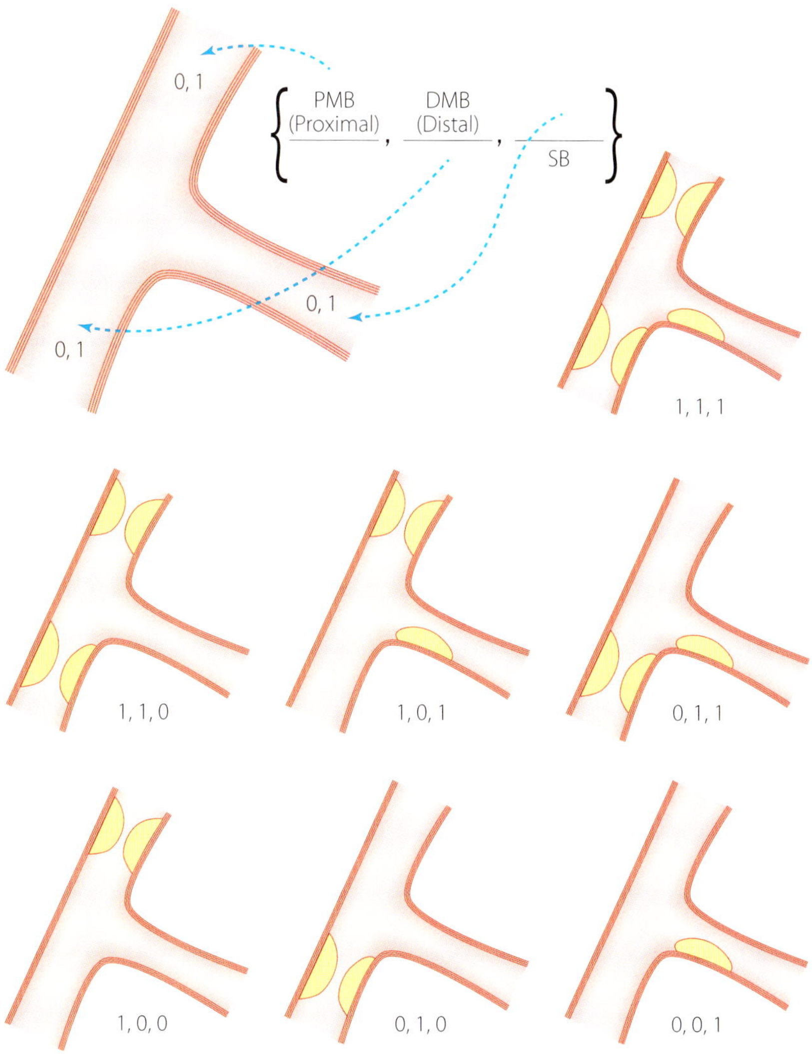

Tips

- 6 Fr EBU guide catheter for LCA and 6 Fr JR catheter for RCA are the preferred catheters.
- If you are addressing a planned bifurcation stenosis, it is reasonable to do a radial angiogram to know the radial anatomy and diameter. If the RA anatomy is favorable and diameter is more than 2 mm, a 7 Fr introducer sheath can be used, and bifurcation stenosis can be addressed comfortably using a 7 Fr guide catheter. In our experience, it is possible in more than 70% of patients.
- The guidewire, PTCA catheter and stents may be selected using the standard protocol of your cath lab.

Example 1

LAD–D1 bifurcation (provisional T-stenting)

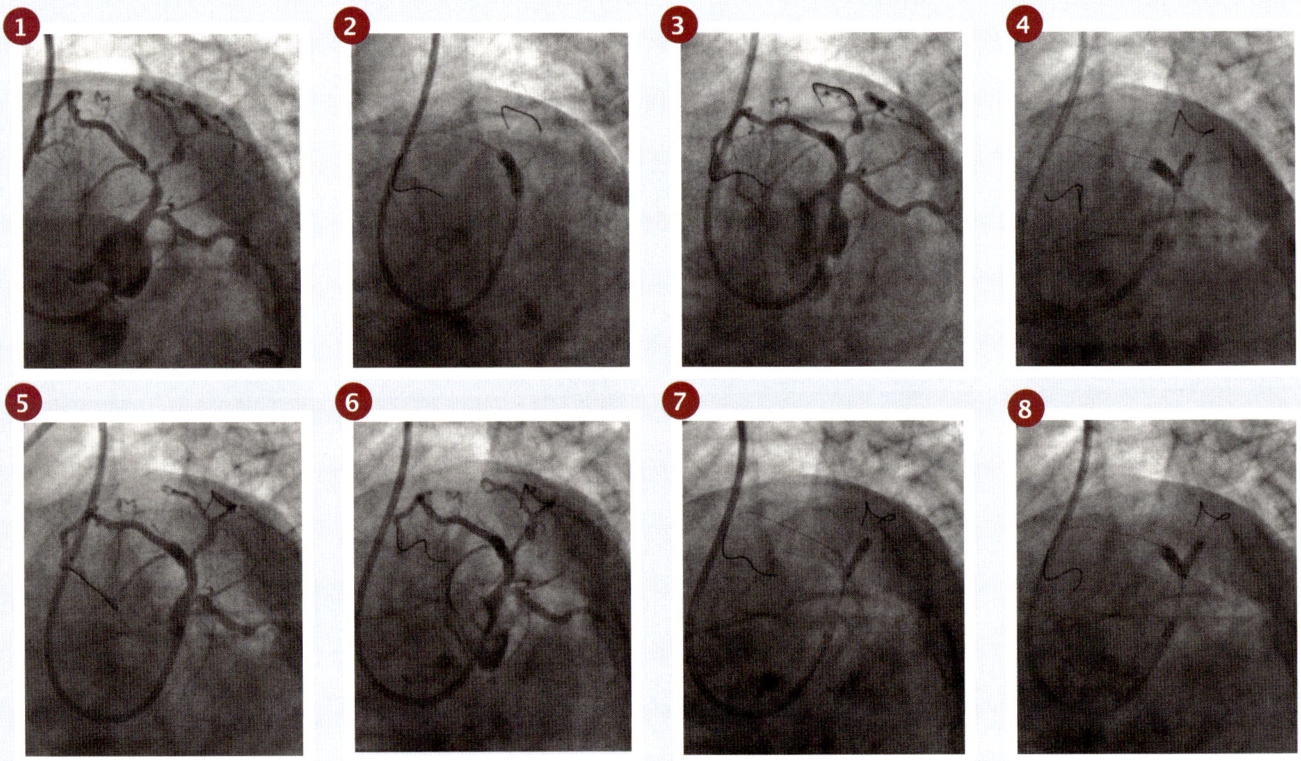

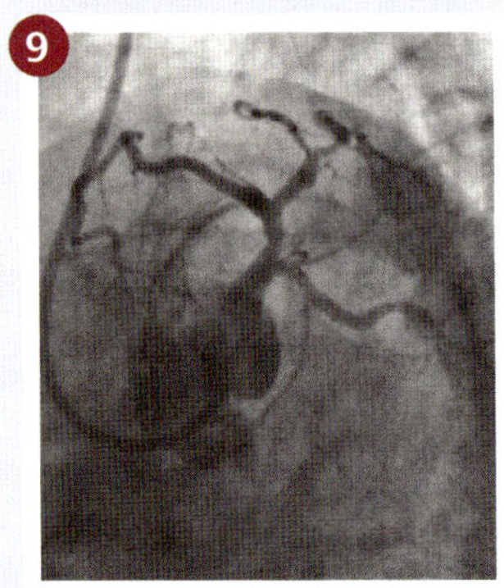

1. This is a case of LAD - D1 bifurcation stenosis (1-1-1).
2. A 6 Fr EBU 3.5 guide catheter is used to cannulate the LMCA, and two 0.014-inch BMW PTCA guidewires have been deployed in the LAD and D1 branches. The LAD lesion is then stented across the D1 branch.
3. The optimal stent result is shown.
4. Use of the kissing balloon technique for LAD and D1 lesions is shown.
5. A suboptimal result of a D1 lesion is seen.
6. A stent is negotiated in the D1 through the struts of the LAD stent.
7. The stent is deployed in the D1.
8. Again, the kissing balloon technique is used.
9. An optimal end result of the provisional T-stenting technique is shown.

Example 2

LAD D1 bifurcation (crush technique)

1
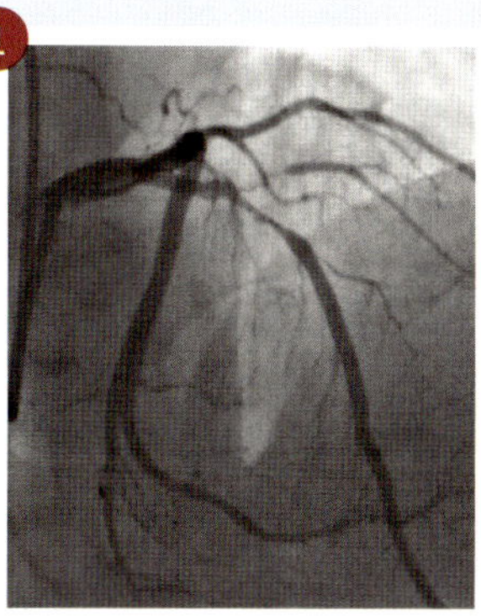

2
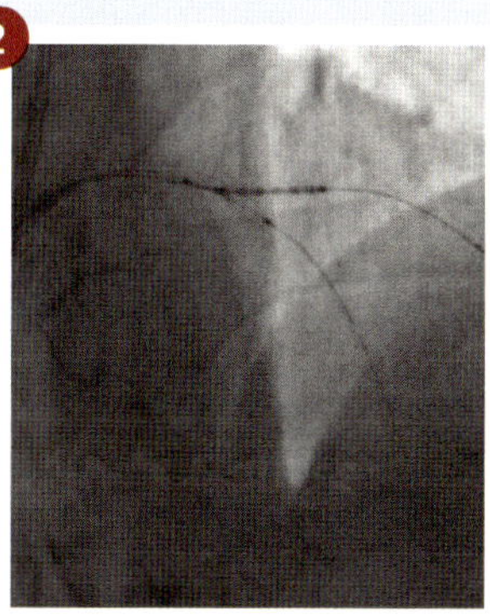

3
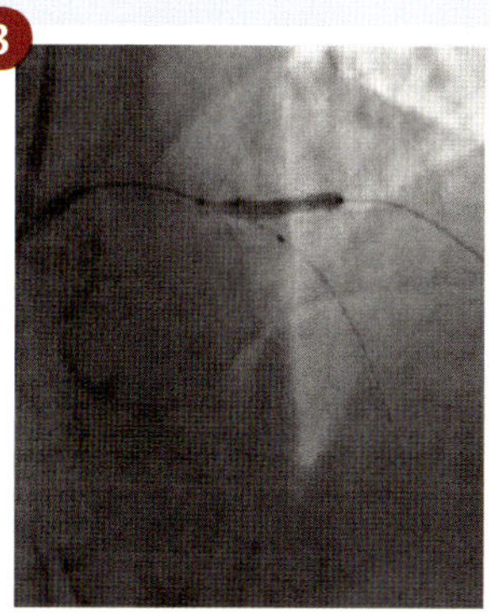

4
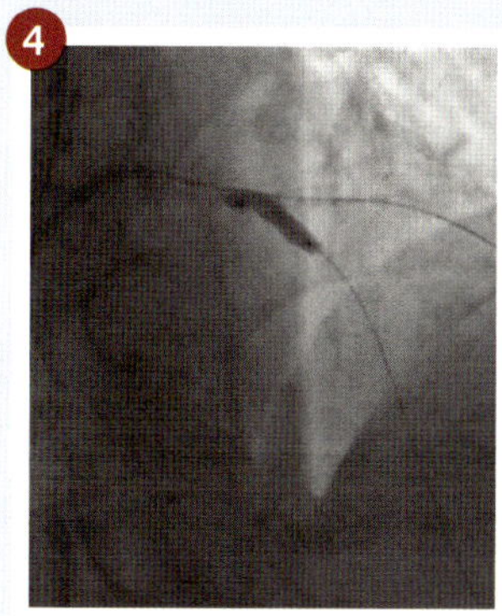

5
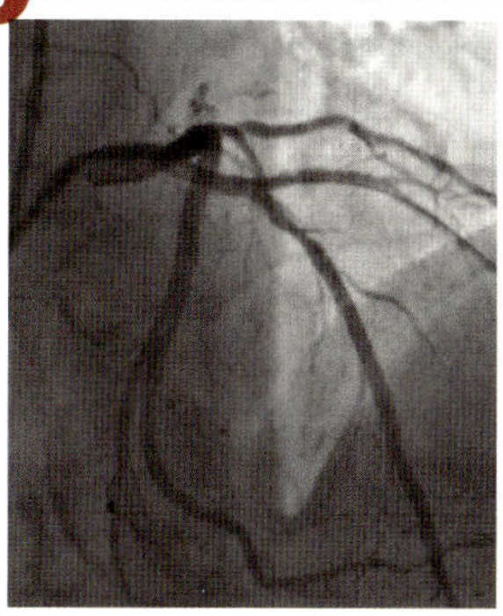

6
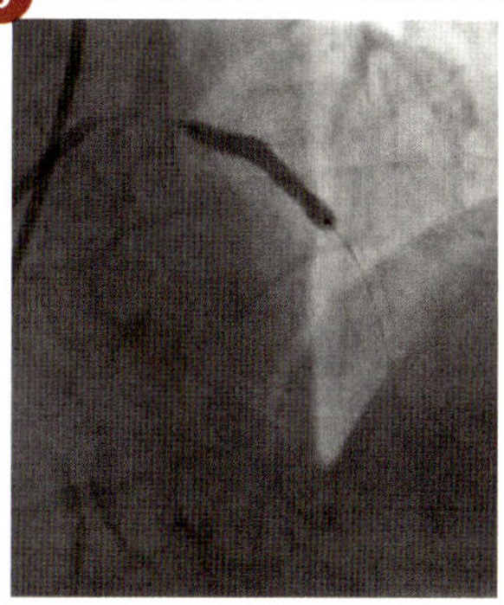

7
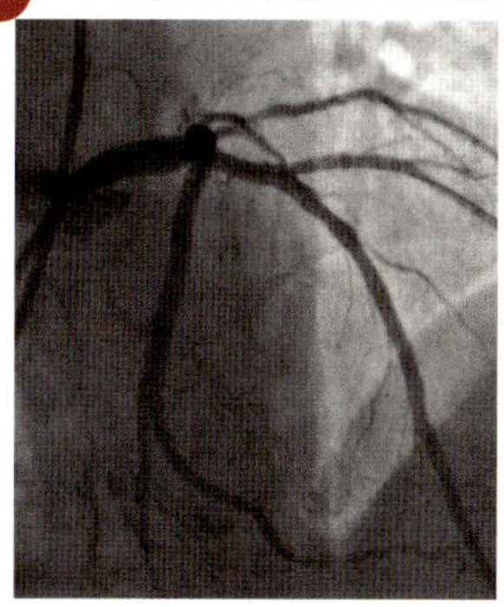

8
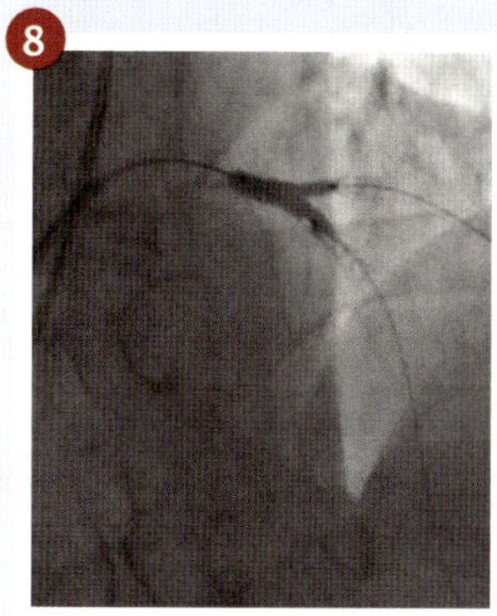

9
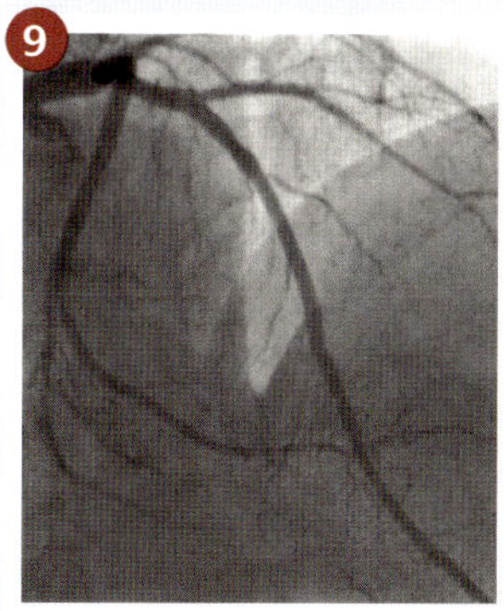

1. This is another case of LAD -D1 bifurcation stenosis (1-1-1).
2. A 7 Fr EBU 3.5 guide catheter is used to cannulate the LMCA, and two 0.014-inch BMW PTCA guidewires are deployed in the LAD and D1 branches. After that, the stent is placed across the D1 lesion, keeping a PTCA balloon across the LAD lesion.
3. The stent is deployed across the D1 lesion. Note that the balloon across the LAD lesion is uninflated.
4. After removing the balloon catheter from the D1, the balloon across the LAD lesion is inflated.
5. The angiogram reveals the stented D1 segment and ballooned LAD segment.
6. The LAD lesion is now stented.
7. An angiogram reveals the stented LAD segment.
8. The kissing balloon technique is used.
9. Successful end result of LAD D1 bifurcation stenting using the crush technique is shown.

Example 3

LCX–OM bifurcation (provisional T-stenting)

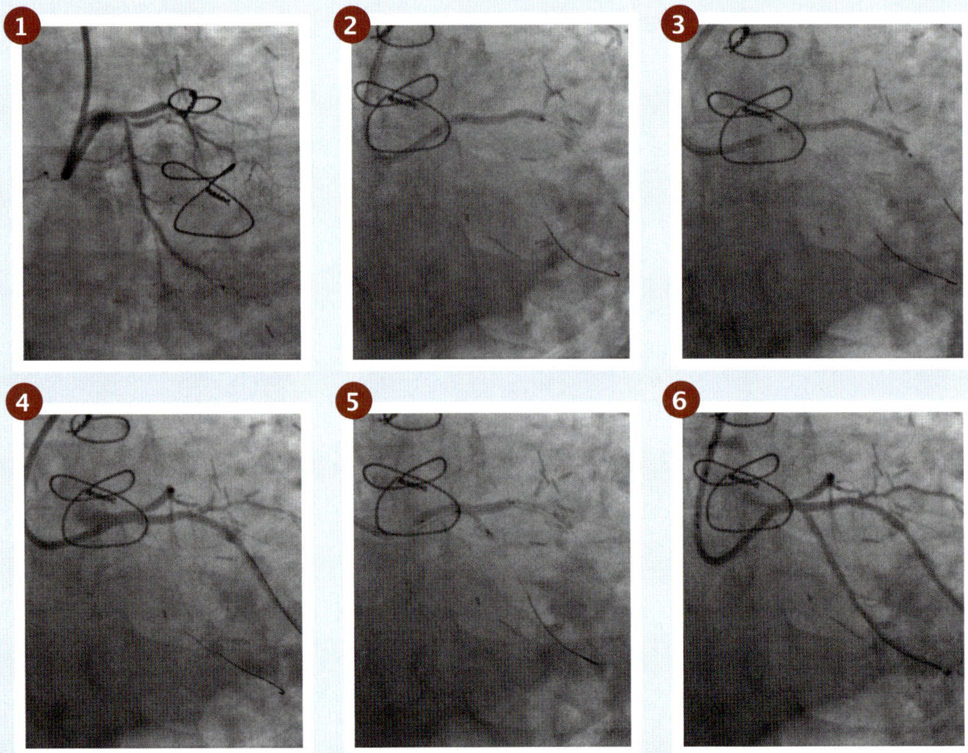

1. This is a case of LCX – OM1 bifurcation stenosis (1-1-1).
2. A 6 Fr EBU 3.5 guide catheter was used to cannulate the LMCA, and two 0.014-inch BMW PTCA guidewires were deployed in the OM and LCX branches. The OM lesion was stented across the LCX.
3. The OM stenting is shown in progress.
4. An angiogram reveals the optimal result of the OM stenting.
5. The kissing balloon technique was used for the LCX and OM lesions.
6. A satisfactory end result is shown.

Example 4

PDA-PLV bifurcation (provisional T-stenting)

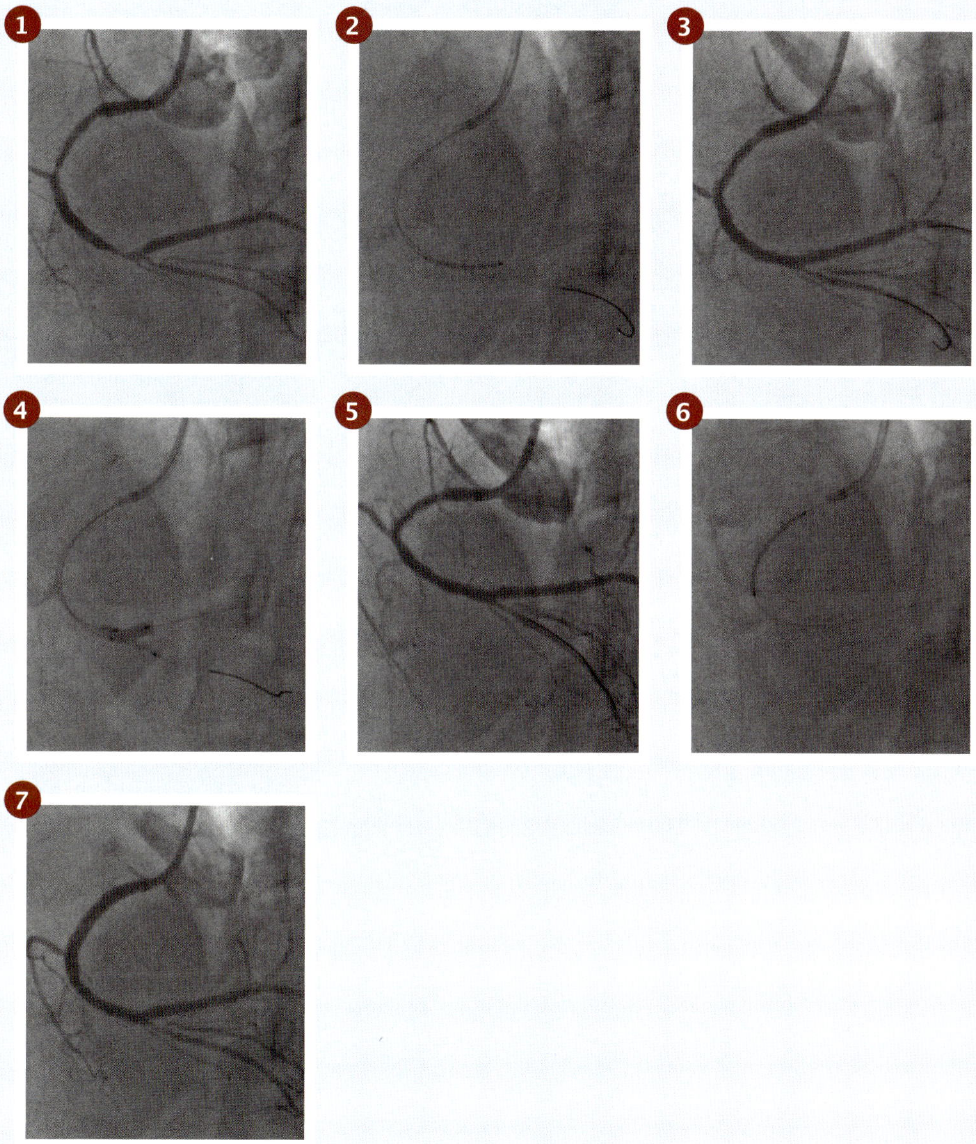

1. A case of PDA-PLV bifurcation stenosis (1-1-1) is shown.
2. A 6 Fr JR 4 guide catheter was used, and two 0.014-inch BMW PTCA guidewires were deployed in the PDA and PLV branches. The stent was deployed across the bifurcation in the PLV branch.
3. The result of stenting is shown.
4. The use of the kissing balloon technique is shown.
5. The optimal end result of the kissing balloon technique is shown.
6. The mid-RCA lesion was then stented.
7. The final result is shown.

Recommended Reading

1. Aziz S, Morris J. Transradial treatment of bifurcation coronary disease using the Multi-Link Frontier bifurcation stent system. J Invasive Cardiol. 2005; 17 (10): E1-3.
2. Ho P. Transradial complex coronary interventions: expanding the comfort zone. J Invasive Cardiol. 2008; 20 (5): 222.
3. Kim WJ, Kim YH, Park DW, et al. Comparison of single-versus two-stent techniques in treatment of unprotected left main coronary bifurcation disease. Catheter Cardiovasc Interv. 2011; 77(6):775-82.
4. Lefèvre T, Louvard Y, Morice MC, et al. Stenting of bifurcation lesions: A rational approach. J Interv Cardiol. 2001; 14(6):573-85.
5. Liang M, Puri A, Linder R. Transradial simultaneous kissing stenting (SKS) with sheathless access. Catheter Cardiovasc Interv. 2010; 75 (2): 222-24.
6. Lim P, Dzavík V. Balloon crush: Treatment of bifurcation lesions using the crush stenting technique as adapted for transradial approach of percutaneous coronary intervention. Catheter Cardiovasc Interv. 2004; 63 (4): 412-16.
7. Lotan C, Hasin Y, Salmoirago E, et al. The Radial Artery: An applicable approach to complex coronary angioplasty. J Invasive Cardiol. 1997; 9 (8): 518-522.
8. Matsukage T, Masuda N, Ikari Y. Simultaneous triple-balloon inflation technique within a 6 Fr guiding catheter for a trifurcation lesion. J Invasive Cardiol. 2008; 20 (7): E210-14.
9. Movahed MR, Stinis CT. A new proposed simplified classification of coronary artery bifurcation lesions and bifurcation interventional techniques. J Invasive Cardiol. 2006; 18(5):199-204.
10. Rizik DG, Klassen KJ, Hermiller JB. Bifurcation coronary artery disease: current techniques and future directions (part 1). J Invasive Cardiol. 2008; 20(2):82-90.
11. Rizik DG, Klassen KJ, Hermiller JB. Bifurcation coronary artery disease: current techniques and future directions (part 2). J Invasive Cardiol. 2008; 20(3):135-41.

TRA for Addressing LMCA Lesions

10

Tejas Patel, Ronald Caputo and Sanjay Shah

Patients with significant LMCA lesions are traditionally considered as surgical candidates. However, in the last several years, several studies have been published on the feasibility, safety and results of LMCA stenting using bare-metal and drug-eluting stents. Although most of the studies have been done through TFA, a few studies have demonstrated effective use of TRA for stenting. LMCA lesions can be broadly classified as ostial, mid-body and bifurcation lesions.

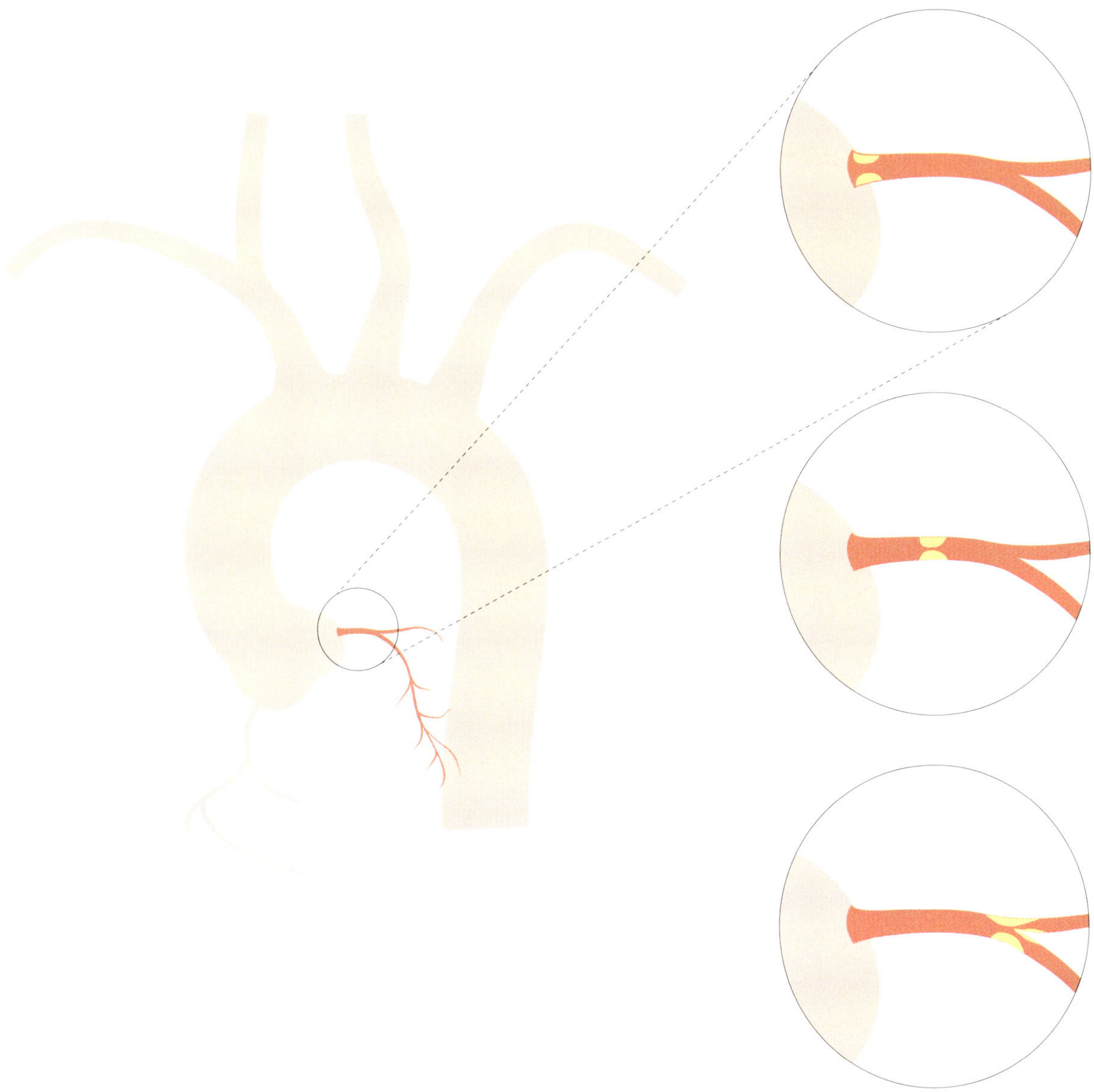

Tips

- This subset should be addressed by experienced radial operators.
- When treatment of bifurcation disease is anticipated, it is reasonable to perform a radial angiogram through an arterial cannula to know the diameter of the RA and other abnormalities. If the diameter is more than 2 mm and RA anatomy is favorable, a 7 Fr introducer sheath should be considered and 7 Fr EBU or left Judkins guide catheter employed for reliable, simultaneous use of two balloons for the kissing technique.
- An experienced radialist can address LMCA stenosis using even a 6 Fr guide catheter. However, it is often difficult to use two non-compliant balloons simultaneously.
- For addressing the ostium in LMCA stenosis, it is important to use a guide catheter with side holes to avoid damping or ventricularization.
- To avoid missing the ostium while addressing ostial LMCA stenosis, 1 or 2 mm of stent segment should be allowed to protrude outside the LMCA and should be separately flared using high pressure.
- For addressing LMCA body stenosis, precision in the stent placement is important, particularly to avoid its protrusion in the LAD or LCX ostium. This can be done by using two PTCA guidewires (one for the LAD and one for the LCX), and their separation should be taken as a road map. Finding the optimal angiographic view also aids in defining the location of the bifurcation (extreme LAO caudal is often used). Pre-dilation with a short balloon will help when determining the proper stent length.
- For LMCA bifurcation stenosis, there are several techniques described in the literature. We recommend provisional T-stenting, as it is easily reproducible and offers consistently good results.
- If there is significant plaque burden and/or calcification, debulking with rotational atherectomy followed by provisional T-stenting is a good option.
- Regardless of the lesion type, IVUS after stent placement in the LM lesion should be considered. Often the LMCA diameter is larger than suspected by angiography, and optimal stent strut apposition is critical for these high-risk lesions.

Example 1

LMCA ostial stenting through the TRA

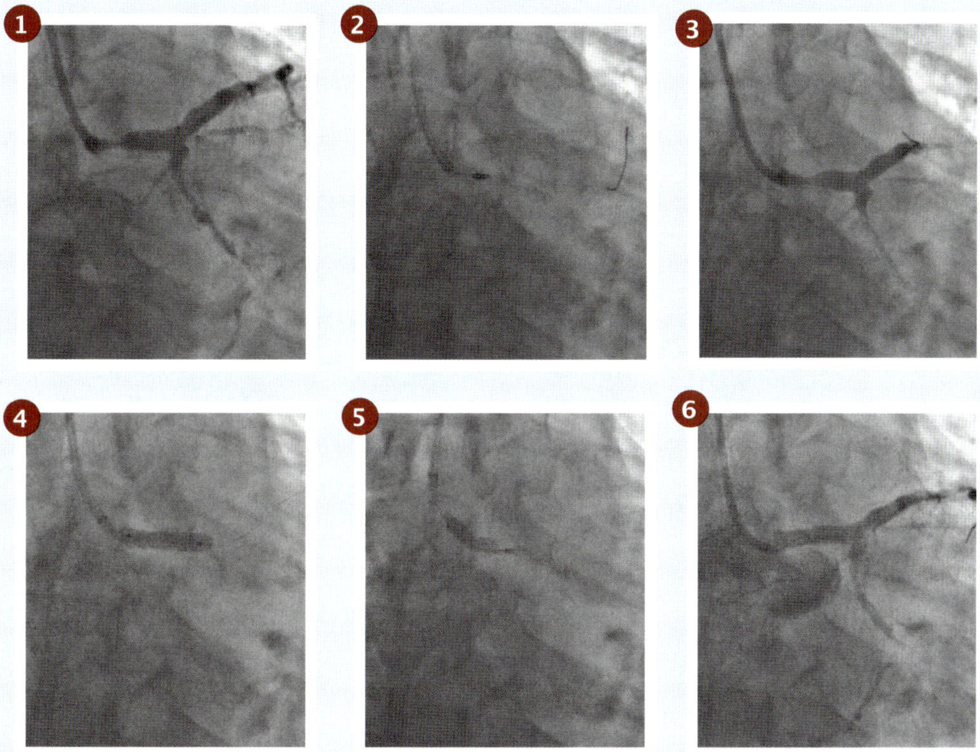

1. A critical LMCA osteal lesion is shown.
2. A 6 Fr JL 4 guide catheter with side holes has been used to cannulate the LMCA, and a 0.014-inch BMW PTCA guidewire is deployed in the LAD artery. After that, rotational atherectomy of the lesion is performed using a 1.5 mm burr.
3. An angiogram reveals satisfactory debulking.
4. Stenting of the ostial LMCA lesion is in progress.
5. Flaring of the stent is done.
6. A satisfactory end result is shown.

Example 2

LMCA body stenting through the TRA

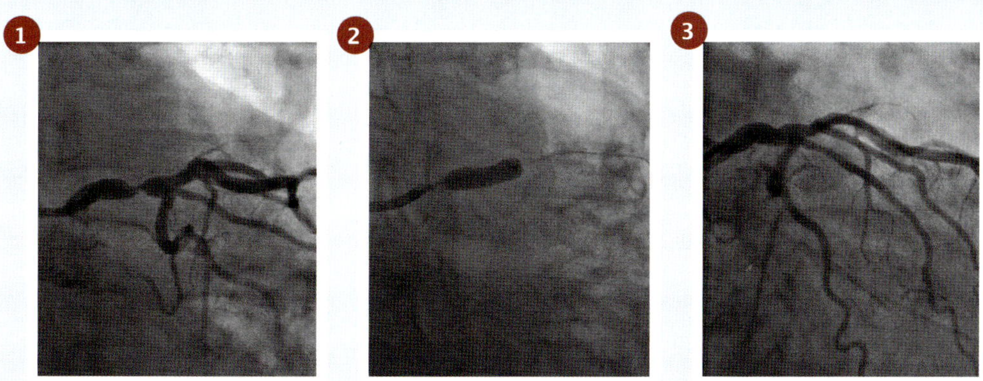

1. An angiogram reveals a critical LMCA body (mid-segment) stenosis.
2. A 6 Fr JL 3.5 guide catheter is used to cannulate the LMCA, and a 0.014-inch BMW PTCA guidewire is deployed in the LAD. Then the stent is deployed.
3. A satisfactory end result is shown.

Example 3

LMCA bifurcation stenting (provisional T-stenting) through the TRA

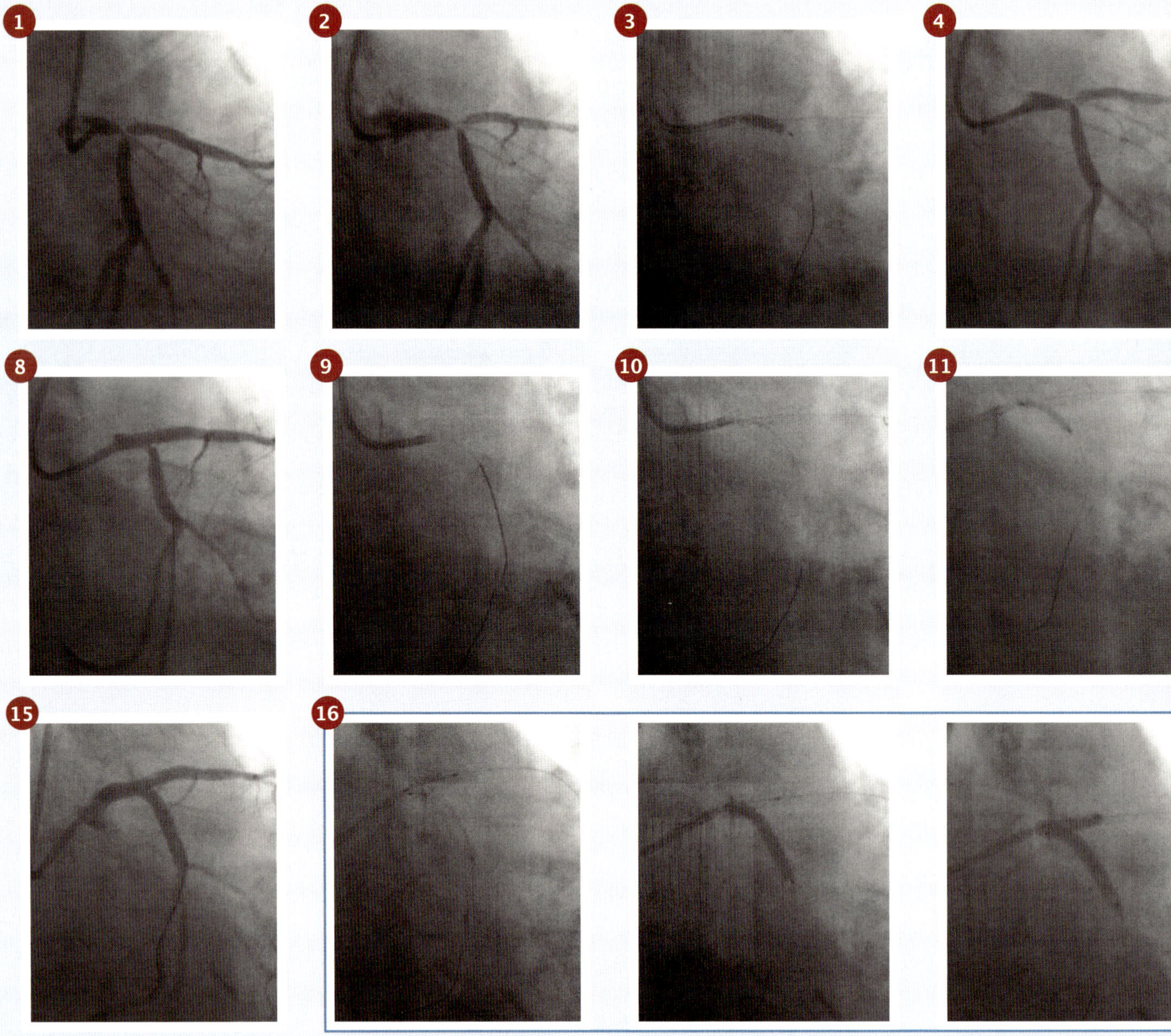

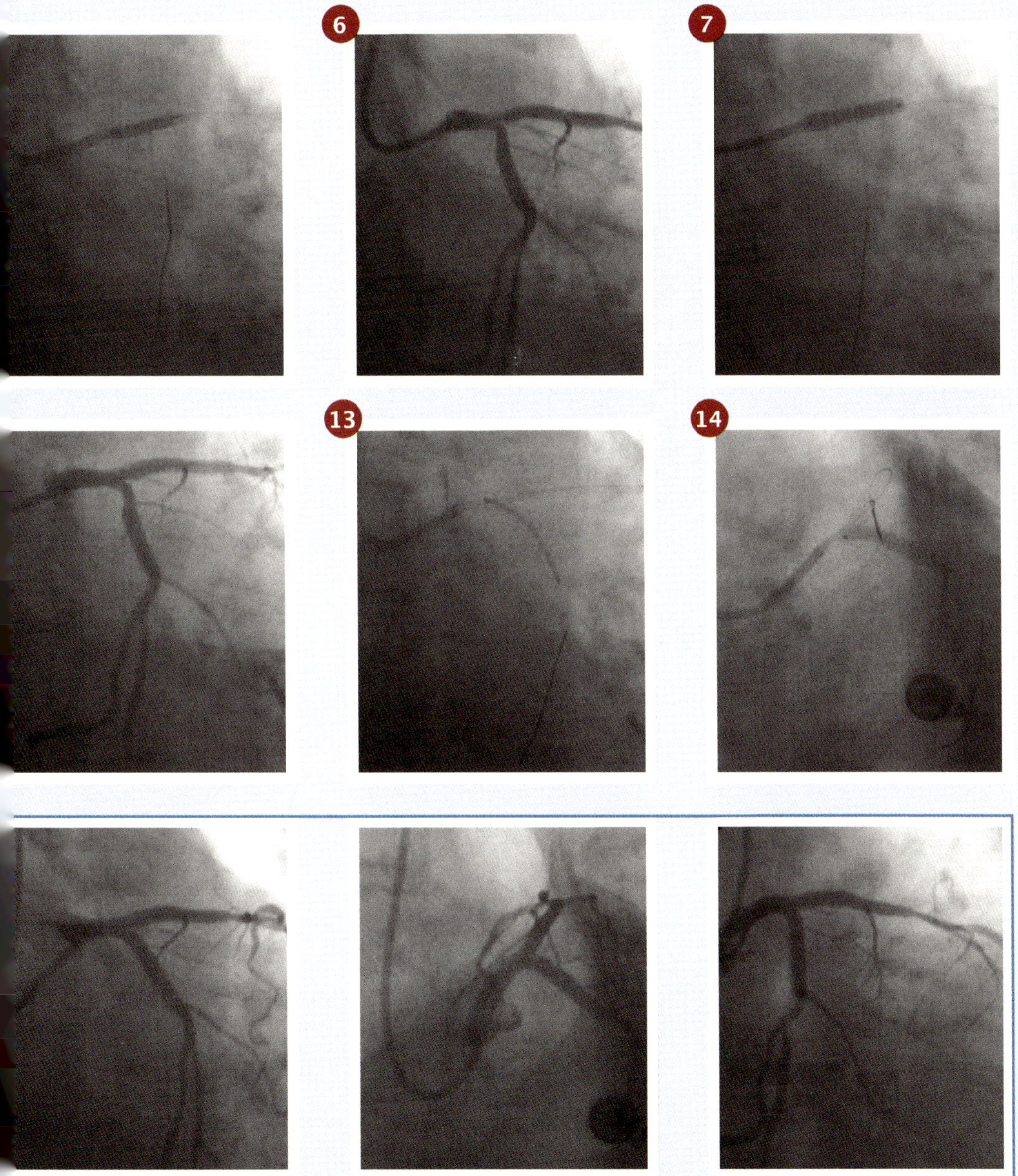

1. An angiogram reveals a critical bifurcation LMCA stenosis (1-1-1).
2. A 7 Fr EBU 3.5 guide catheter is used to cannulate the LMCA ostium, and two 0.014" BMW PTCA guidewires are deployed in the LAD and LCX.
3. The balloon is inflated across the LMCA into the LCX.
4. The balloon result is seen.
5. The balloon inflated across the LMCA into the LAD.
6. The balloon result is seen.
7. A stent is deployed across the bifurcation in the LAD.
8. The stent result is shown.
9. The PTCA guidewire of the LAD is pulled back; the LCX was entered through the struts of the stent with the same wire.
10. The wire from the LCX is pulled back and negotiated through the stent into the LAD.
11. The balloon is inflated across the stent struts in the LCX.
12. The struts are widened.
13. A stent is deployed in the LCX.
14. Stenting is shown in progress.
15. The LCX stent result is seen.
16. The kissing balloon technique is shown.
17. A satisfactory result is shown.

Example 4

LMCA bifurcation rota-stenting through the TRA

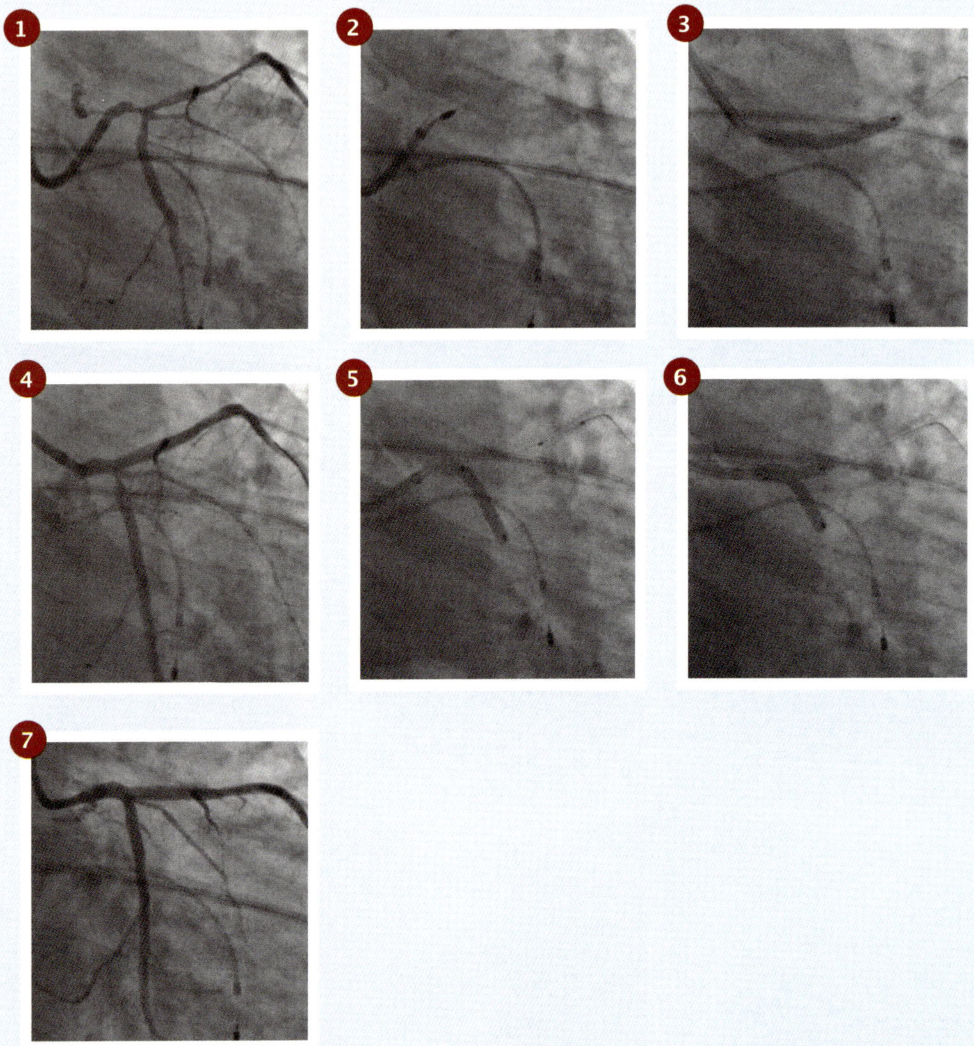

1. Another case of LMCA bifurcation stenosis (1-1-1) is shown.
2. A 7 Fr EBU 3.5 guide catheter was used, and a Rota wire was deployed in the LAD. Rotational atherectomy was done using a 1.5 mm burr.
3. The stent is being deployed.
4. The stent result is shown.
5. Another stent was deployed.
6. Final kissing is shown.
7. The final result is shown.

Recommended Reading

1. Beijk MA, Rittersma SZ, Koch KT, et al. Long-term follow-up after nonurgent percutaneous coronary intervention in unprotected left main coronary arteries. Catheter Cardiovasc Interv. 2010; 75(7):1026-36.
2. Burzotta F, Trani C, Coroleu S. Retrograde recanalization of left main from saphenous vein graft supported by percutaneous Impella Recover LP 2.5 assist device. J Invasive Cardiol. 2009; 21 (8): E147-50.
3. Cheng C, Wu C, Fang C, et al. Feasibility and safety of transradial stenting for unprotected left main coronary artery stenoses. Circ J. 2007; 71 (6): 855-61.
4. Ellis SG. Percutaneous left main invention: An evolving perspective. JACC Cardiovasc Interv. 2010; 3(6): 642-7.
5. Ho P. Transradial complex coronary interventions: expanding the comfort zone. J Invasive Cardiol. 2008; 20 (5): 222.
6. Hussein H, Fang H, Wu C. Transradial complex left main trifurcation intervention. Catheter Cardiovasc Interv. 2010; 76 (5): 679-83.
7. Kim WJ, Kim YH, Park DW, et al. Comparison of single-versus two-stent techniques in treatment of unprotected left main coronary bifurcation disease. Catheter Cardiovasc Interv. 2011; 77(6):775-82.
8. Sunami K, Saito S, Tanaka S. Successful transradial coronary angioplasty and stenting using a self-expandable RADIUS stent to the anomalous left main coronary artery. J Invasive Cardiol. 2003; 15 (1): 46-48.
9. Yang Y, Kandzari D, Gao Z, et al. Transradial versus transfemoral method of percutaneous coronary revascularization for unprotected left main coronary artery disease: comparison of procedural and late-term outcomes. JACC Cardiovasc Interv. 2010; 3 (10): 1035-42.
10. Ziakas A, Klinke P, Mildenberger R, et al. Comparison of the radial and femoral approaches in left main PCI: a retrospective study. J Invasive Cardiol. 2004; 16 (3): 129-32.

11 TRA for Addressing Chronic Total Occlusions

Tejas Patel, Ramon Quesada and Sanjay Shah

Chronic total occlusion (CTO) intervention is a challenging area. The success rate has increased from 60% to almost 90% among experienced operators. This increased success is largely due to the development of procedure-specific hardware, in particular CTO-specific guidewires, balloons, microcatheters and other relevant devices. While TFA is the traditionally preferred approach, in the last decade, many studies have documented feasibility, efficacy and reasonable success rates using TRA. An experienced radialist should be able to achieve an acceptable success rate in practically all subsets of CTO.

Example 1

TRA for CTO of the LAD artery

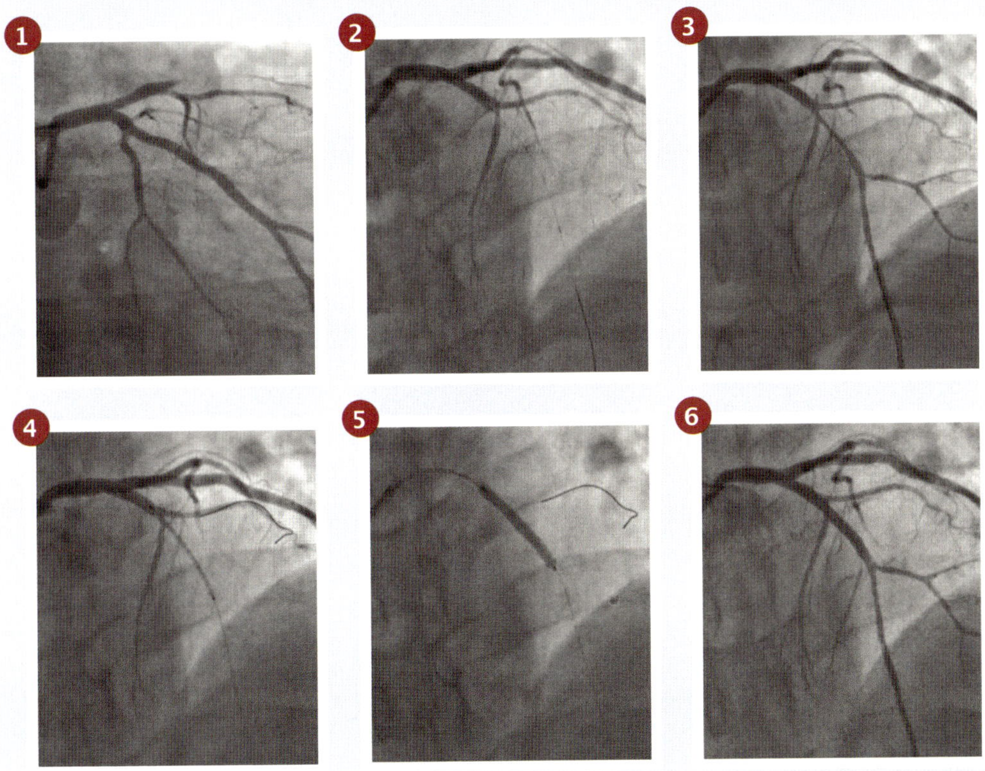

1. An example of CTO of the proximal LAD segment is shown.
2. A 6 Fr EBU 3.5 guide catheter was used, and the lesion was crossed successfully using a Pilot 150 PTCA guidewire.
3. The balloon result is shown.
4. A 0.014-inch BMW PTCA guidewire was deployed in the D1 branch, and the stent was negotiated across the LAD lesion.
5. Stenting is shown in progress.
6. A satisfactory end result is shown.

Example 2

TRA for CTO of the LCX artery

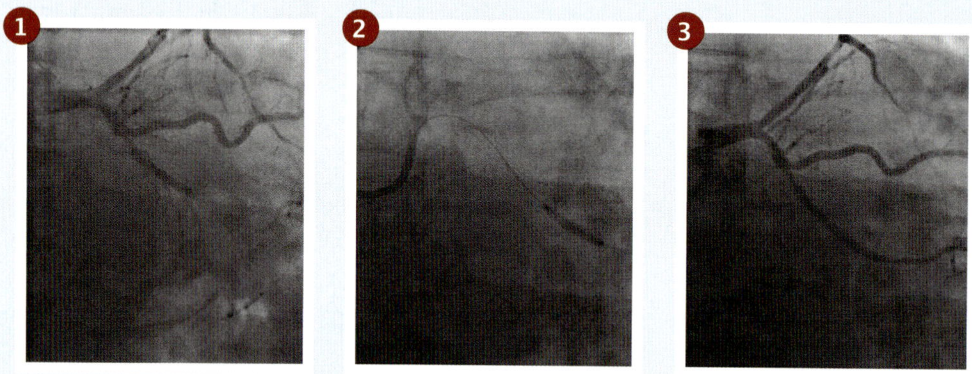

1. An example of CTO of the mid-LCX segment.
2. A 6 Fr EBU 4 guide catheter and a 0.014-inch Pilot 50 guidewire were used. The CTO was crossed and stented successfully.
3. A satisfactory end result is shown.

Example 3

TRA for CTO of RCA

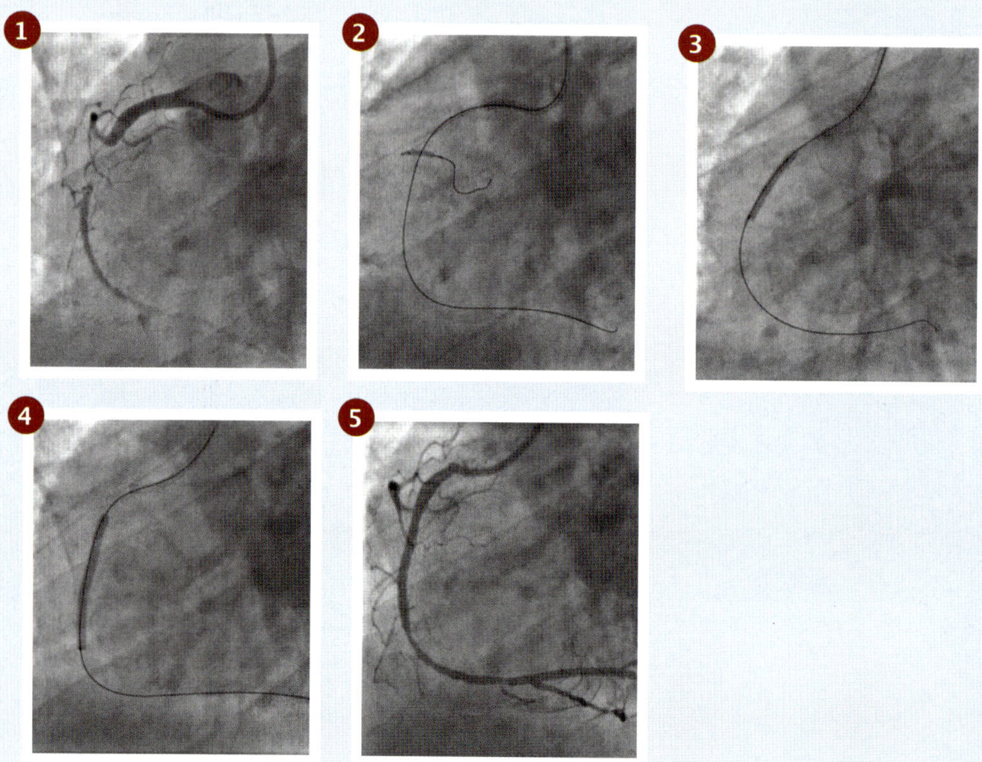

1. An example of CTO of the mid-RCA segment.
2. The RCA was cannulated using a 7 Fr AL 2 guide catheter. The CTO was crossed using a Miracle 4.5 PTCA guidewire. The anchor balloon technique has been demonstrated.
3. Segmental balloon dilation was performed.
4. The lesion was stented.
5. A satisfactory end result is shown.

Example 4

TRA for CTO of the LAD artery (retrograde injection from the RCA)

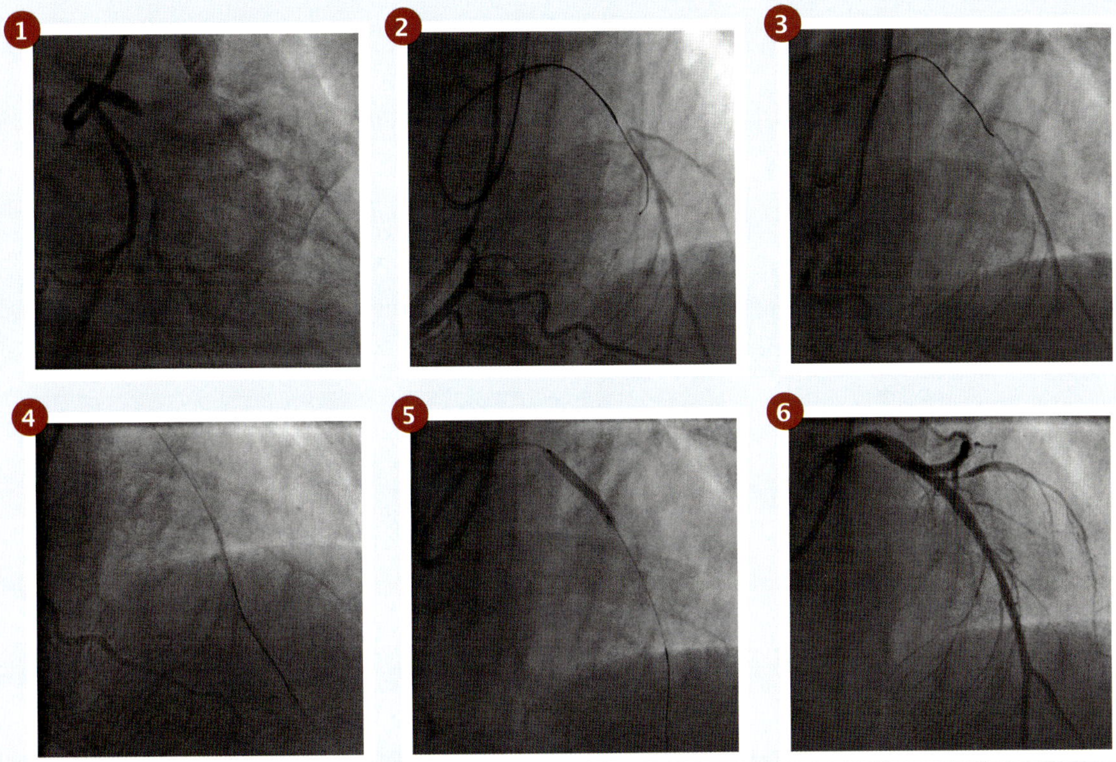

1. The LCA was cannulated using a 7 Fr EBU 3.5 guide catheter. LCA injection revealed CTO of the proximal LAD.
2. A Miracle 4.5 guidewire was negotiated through CTO. Simultaneous RCA injection confirmed its entry in a false channel.
3. Entry to the true channel was tried.
4. Successful entry of the guidewire in the true channel is shown.
5. Stenting is shown in progress.
6. The final result is shown.

Tips

- Radial angiography or vascular ultrasound of the radial artery should be performed to assess the diameter of the RA and the presence of any abnormality.
- If the RA diameter is more than 2 mm and the RA course is relatively straight, a 7 Fr guide catheter should be the first choice.
- If the RA diameter is less than 2 mm, a 6 Fr guide catheter should be the first choice.
- Middle or distal short-segment CTOs with a good nipple — particularly in the LAD or RCA — can be treated with a predictably high success rate through TRA.
- Although an experienced radialist can treat almost any CTO, for a beginning or a medium experience radialist, it is advisable to avoid very proximal and long segment CTOs with flat stumps and the presence of intra-arterial collaterals.

Example 5

TRA for CTO of the RCA (retrograde injection from the LAD)

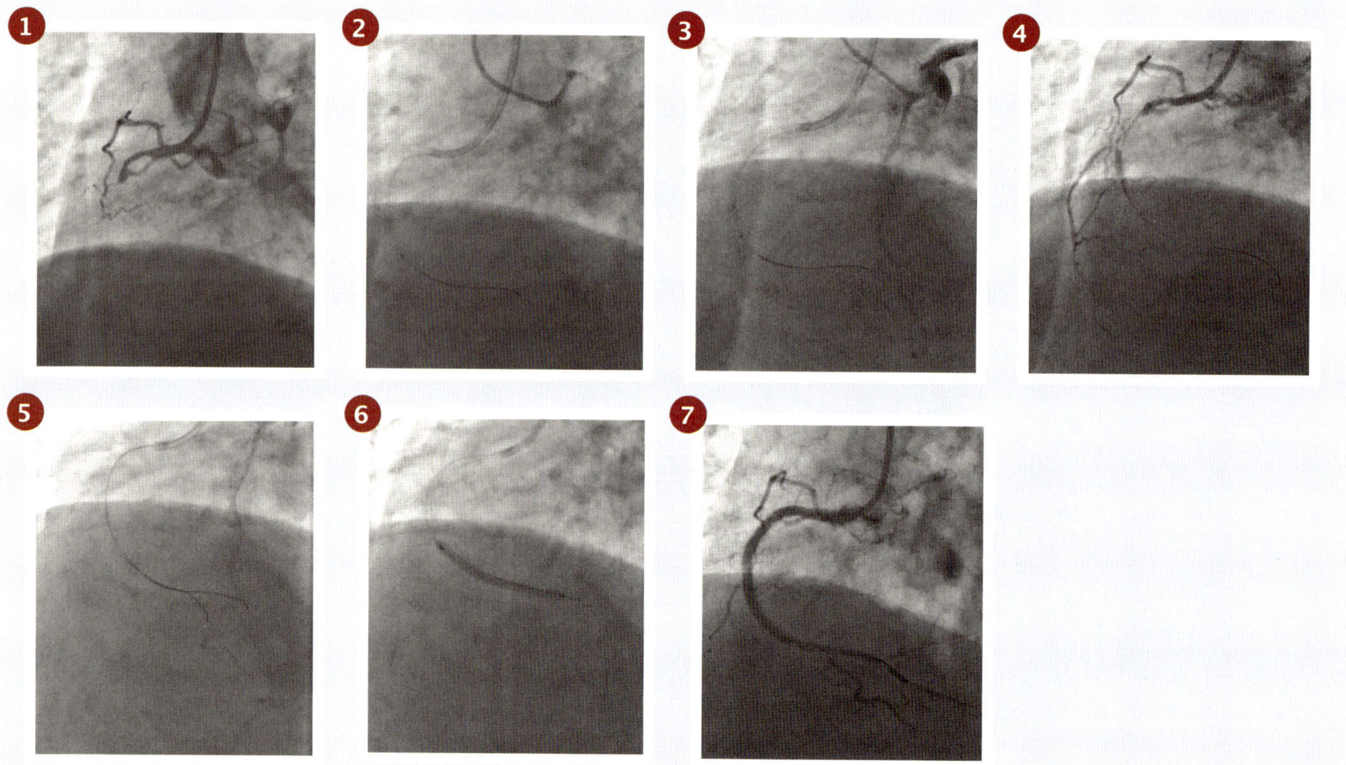

1. An example of CTO of the proximal RCA segment is shown.
2. The RCA was cannulated using a 6 Fr JR 4 guide catheter through the right TRA, and the LCA was cannulated using a 5 Fr JL 4 diagnostic catheter through the left TRA. A 0.014-inch Pilot 150 PTCA guidewire crossed the CTO.
3. An LCA injection revealed the distal RCA segment that was useful to enter. Using the proper branch avoids formation of a false passage.
4. Segmental balloon dilatation was done.
5. An LCA injection helped to negotiate the second PTCA guidewire in the distal RCA.
6. Endoluminal reconstruction of the whole length of the RCA was done using multiple overlapping stents.
7. A satisfactory end result is shown.

Example 6

TRA for CTO of the RCA (retrograde approach from the LAD)

1

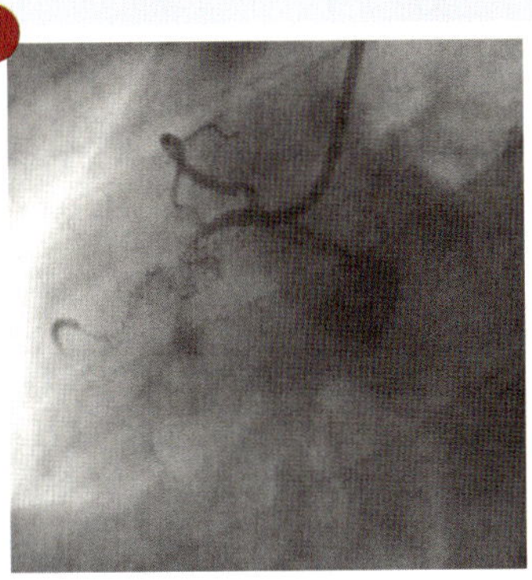

2

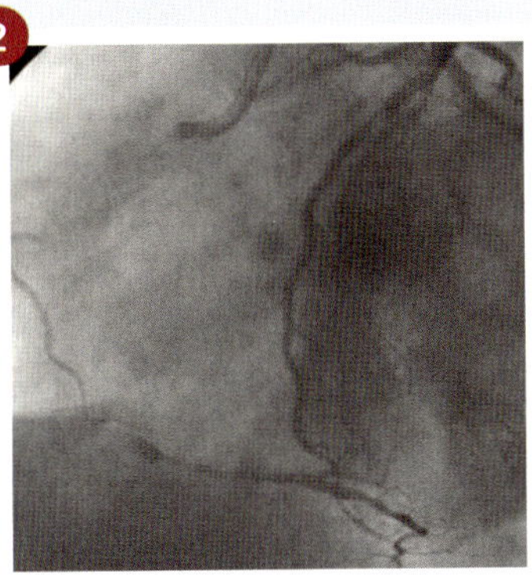

3

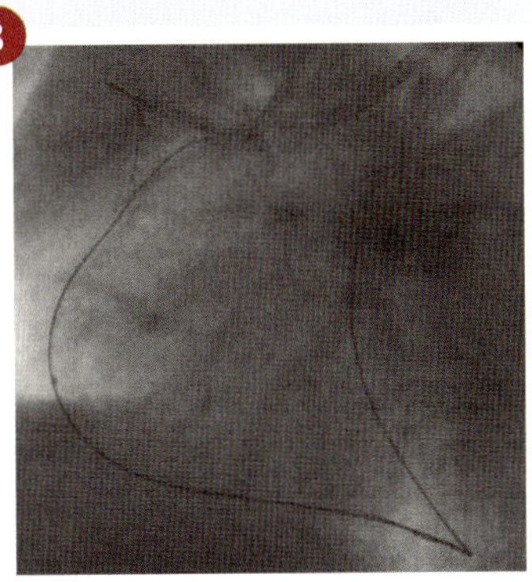

4

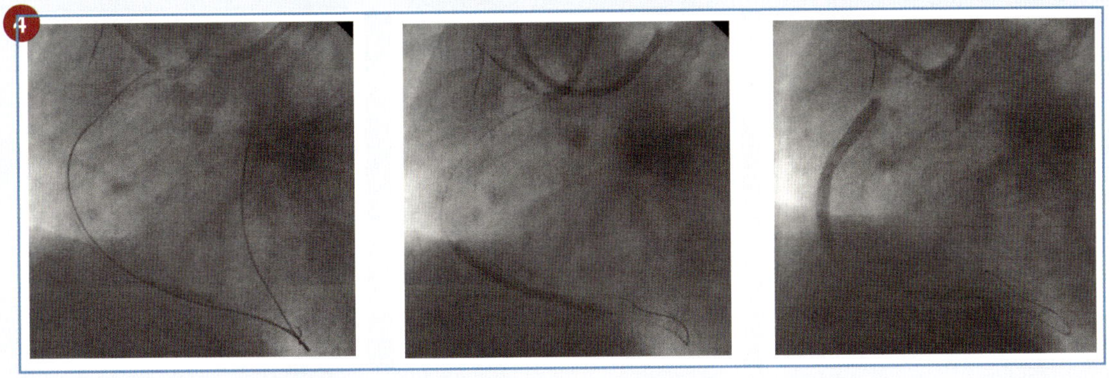

5

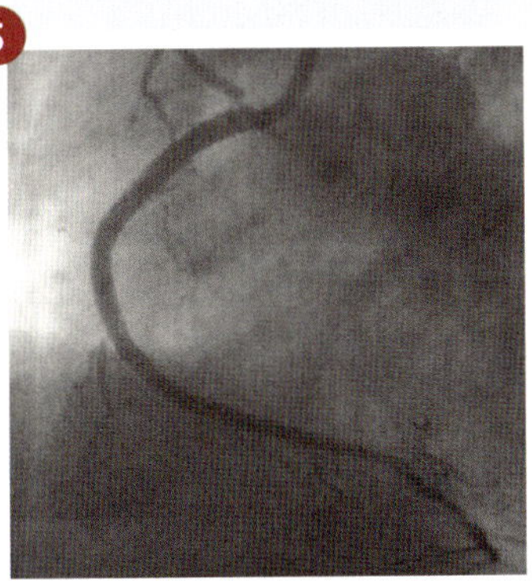

1. A long segment CTO of the RCA is seen.
2. A 7 Fr JR 4 guide catheter was used to cannulate the RCA through the right TRA, and a 6 Fr EBU 3.5 guide catheter was used to cannulate the LCA through left TRA.
3. Demonstration of a retrograde approach and anchor balloon technique is shown.
4. Endoluminal reconstruction of RCA was done using multiple overlapping stents.
5. The excellent end result is shown.

Tips

- It is important to monitor length of procedure and contrast dose to avoid renal complications and minimize radiation exposure for the patient. Rather than continue in these cases, it is advisable to have the patient return for a second attempt.
- EBU guide catheters specifically designed for the LCA should be used; JR or AL guide catheters for the RCA should be used when treating CTOs through the TRA.
- The operator's discretion should govern the choice of guidewires, microcatheters, balloons and relevant devices, along with whether to perform traditional rotational atherectomy or use a Tornus catheter.
- Sheathless guide catheters can accommodate multiple guidewires and balloons, as a 6 Fr sheathless guide catheter has an internal lumen diameter (ILD) of a 7.5 Fr regular guide catheter, and a 7 Fr sheathless guide catheter has an ILD equal to an 8.5 Fr regular guide catheter.
- While addressing very difficult CTOs, the operator should be familiar with the use of the mother-and-child guide catheter technique and the anchor balloon technique for higher success rates.
- Keeping the armboard for the access site parallel and close to femoral position instead of perpendicular should greatly resolve the issue of higher radiation exposure with TRA.

Recommended Reading

1. Godino C, Sharp AS, Carlino M, et al. Crossing CTOs-the tips, tricks, and specialist kit that can mean the difference between success and failure. Catheter Cardiovasc Interv. 2009; 74(7):1019-46.
2. Hayashida K, Louvard Y, Lefèvre T. Transradial complex coronary interventions using a five-in-six system. Catheter Cardiovasc Interv. 2011; 77 (1): 63-68.
3. Ho P. Transradial complex coronary interventions: expanding the comfort zone. J Invasive Cardiol. 2008; 20 (5): 222.
4. Liu W, Wagatsuma K, Toda M, et al. Short- and long-term follow-up of percutaneous coronary intervention for chronic total occlusion through transradial approach: tips for successful procedure from a single-center experience. J Interv Cardiol. 2011; 24 (2): 137-43.
5. Okamura N, Takeshita S, Saito S. Transradial coronary intervention using a four-French child catheter through a six-French guiding catheter. Int J Cardiol. 2011; 151 (3): e93-5.
6. Prasad A, Rihal CS, Lennon RJ, et al. Trends in outcomes after percutaneous coronary intervention for chronic total occlusions: a 25-year experience from the Mayo Clinic. J Am Coll Cardiol. 2007; 49(15):1611-8.
7. Rathore S, Hakeem A, Pauriah M, et al. A comparison of the transradial and the transfemoral approach in chronic total occlusion percutaneous coronary intervention. Catheter Cardiovasc Interv. 2009; 73 (7): 883-87.
8. Saeed B, Kandzari DE, Agostoni P, et al. Use of drug-eluting stents for chronic total occlusions: a systematic review and meta-analysis. Catheter Cardiovasc Interv. 2011; 77(3):315-32.
9. Saito S, Tanaka S, Hiroe Y, et al. Angioplasty for chronic total occlusion by using tapered-tip guidewires. Catheter Cardiovasc Interv. 2003; 59 (3): 305-11.
10. Shah PB. Management of coronary chronic total occlusion. Circulation. 2011; 123 (16): 1780-4.

TRA for Acute Myocardial Infarction (AMI) Interventions

12

Tejas Patel, Christopher Pyne, Sanjay Shah and Samir Pancholy

Interventions in AMI have been performed for nearly two decades. This is the only subset offering mortality benefit. Worldwide, TFA has traditionally been the preferred route. Since 1999, studies have been published documenting feasibility, reproducibility and results of TRA in this subset. It is well known that, compared to TFA, TRA generally reduces bleeding and related complications, and is also more economically efficient. These are additional benefits of TRA for AMI interventions, which carry a higher risk of bleeding due to higher intensity of anticoagulation. A recently completed, large, multicenter randomized clinical trial demonstrated a marked survival advantage for STEMI patients treated with TRA compared to the femoral approach. There are certain problems with TRA in this situation, including a learning curve and additional mental pressure on the operator to reduce door-to-balloon time, however they tend to resolve with experience.

Tips

- Start a TR-AMI program only after achieving adequate experience with TRA. There is no magic number at which one becomes a TR-AMI expert; the more done, the better an operator will get. We recommend performing at least 250 coronary angiograms and 75 PCI through TRA in stable patients before attempting a TR-AMI program. These numbers will let an operator handle an adequate number of anatomical variations in the radio-brachial and subclavian regions, and should result in increased comfort levels while performing interventions in this demanding subset.
- It is important to select at least 25 hemodynamically stable AMI patients in the initial stage of a TR-AMI program, to overcome a learning curve without significantly delaying reperfusion time.
- It is important to prepare the groin and the wrist simultaneously in the cath lab. Although preparation time is slightly prolonged when compared to provisional femoral access, it is typically justified to minimize this activity when femoral access is needed during the procedure (e.g., for femoral crossover or in IABP/hemodynamic support-device placement). Operators who begin with the radial approach in STEMI patients should not hesitate to add hemodynamic support through the femoral approach if indicated. Such crossover is part of the procedure and not a failure of the initial strategy.
- Although it is not a routine practice, we strongly recommend that beginners inject contrast through the puncture cannula to define the vascular anatomy before introducing the sheath. If anatomy is unfavorable or very difficult, immediate switch-over to femoral access will save important time. As experience increases, the number of crossovers will decrease remarkably.
- Avoid working through extreme subclavian tortuousities and arteria lusoria during the initial phase of the program.
- Selection of guide catheter, guidewire, balloon, stent and thrombectomy device should be left to the discretion of an operator. However, we strongly recommend against using a 5 Fr guide catheter in initial stage of the program.
- Operators may wish to consider the left approach in certain STEMI patient populations (e.g., elderly, small stature, previous CABG). Data suggest equivalent success and reperfusion times, and may be particularly helpful for new operators.

Example 1

TRA for primary PCI of an LAD lesion

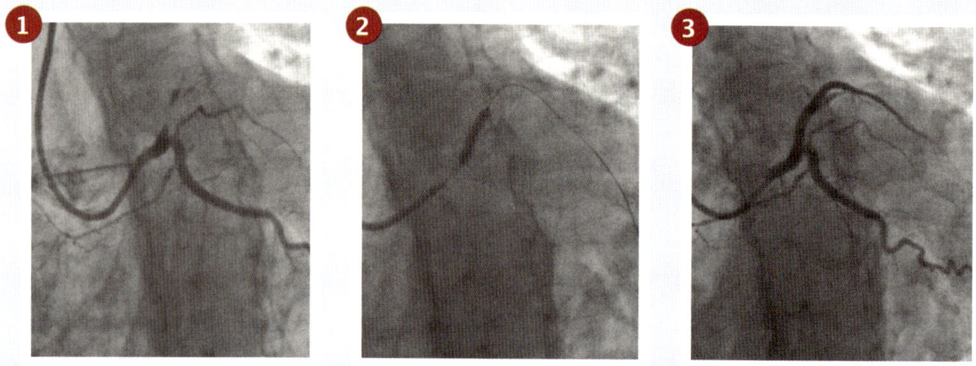

1. The acute anterior wall MI. The LAD is totally occluded after its origin.
2. Stenting is shown in progress.
3. The final result is shown.

Example 2

TRA for primary PCI of an RCA lesion

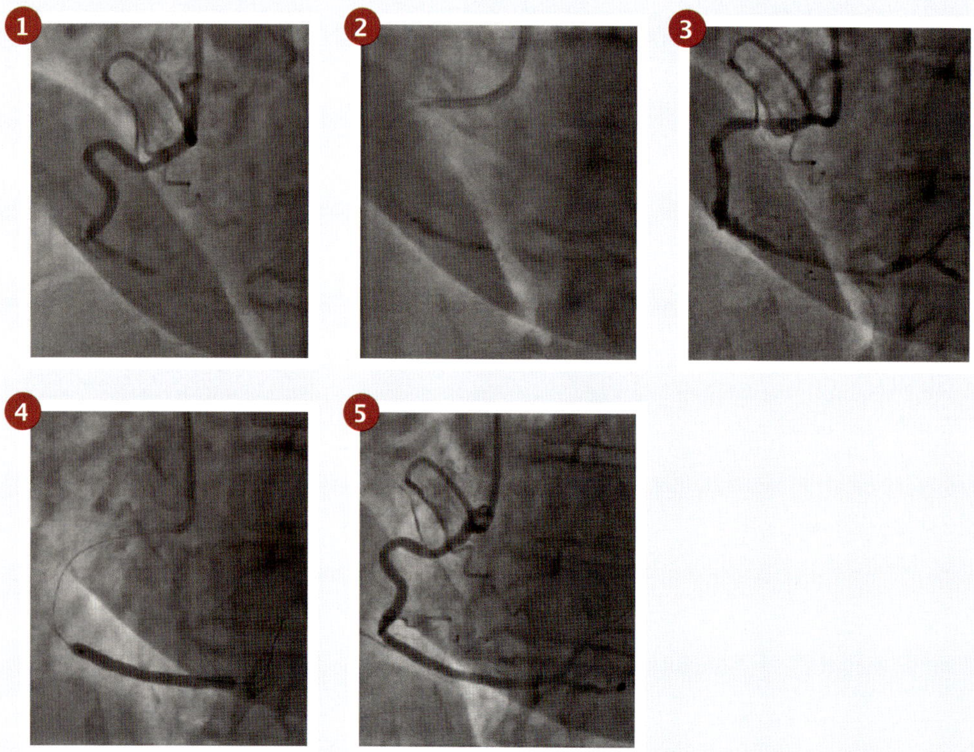

1. Selective RCA injection using a 6 Fr JR 4 catheter reveals total occlusion, with thrombus in the mid-part.
2. The lesion was crossed using a 0.014-inch Whisper guidewire, and PTCA was done.
3. The PTCA result is shown.
4. A long stent was deployed.
5. A satisfactory end result is shown.

Example 3

TRA for primary PCI of an LMCA lesion

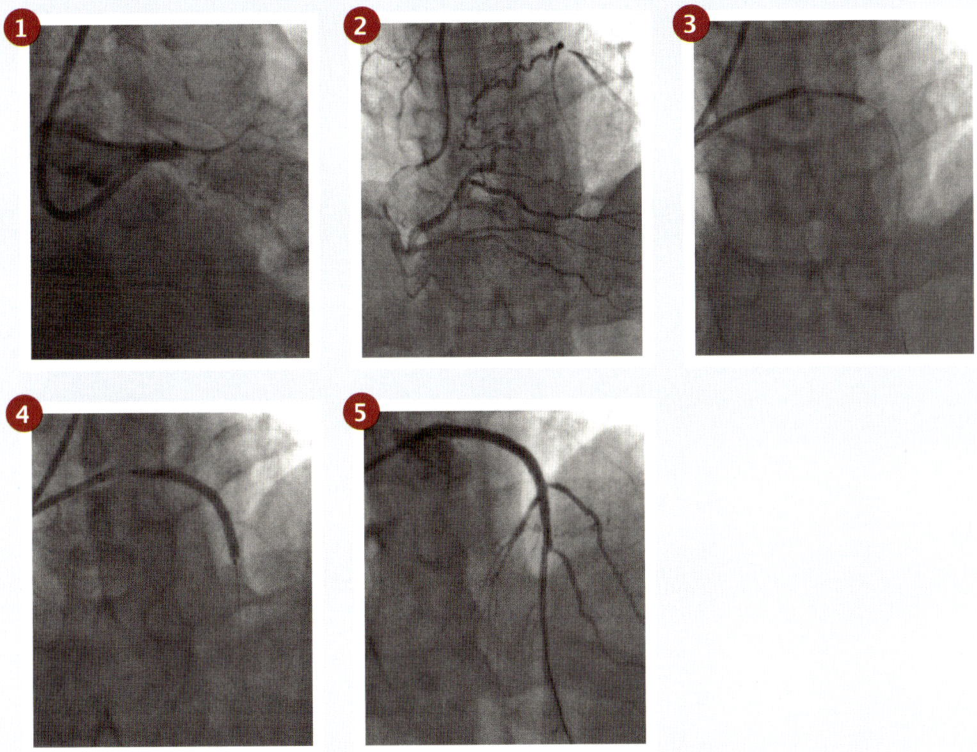

1. Selective LMCA injection through a 6 Fr EBU 3.5 guide catheter reveals a total occlusion of the LMCA, with thrombus.
2. An RCA injection reveals retrograde filling of LCA.
3. 0.014-inch BMW PTCA guidewire was deployed, and PTCA was performed.
4. Stenting was done.
5. Excellent result of primary PCI of the LMCA is shown.

Example 4

TRA for primary PCI of an LMCA lesion

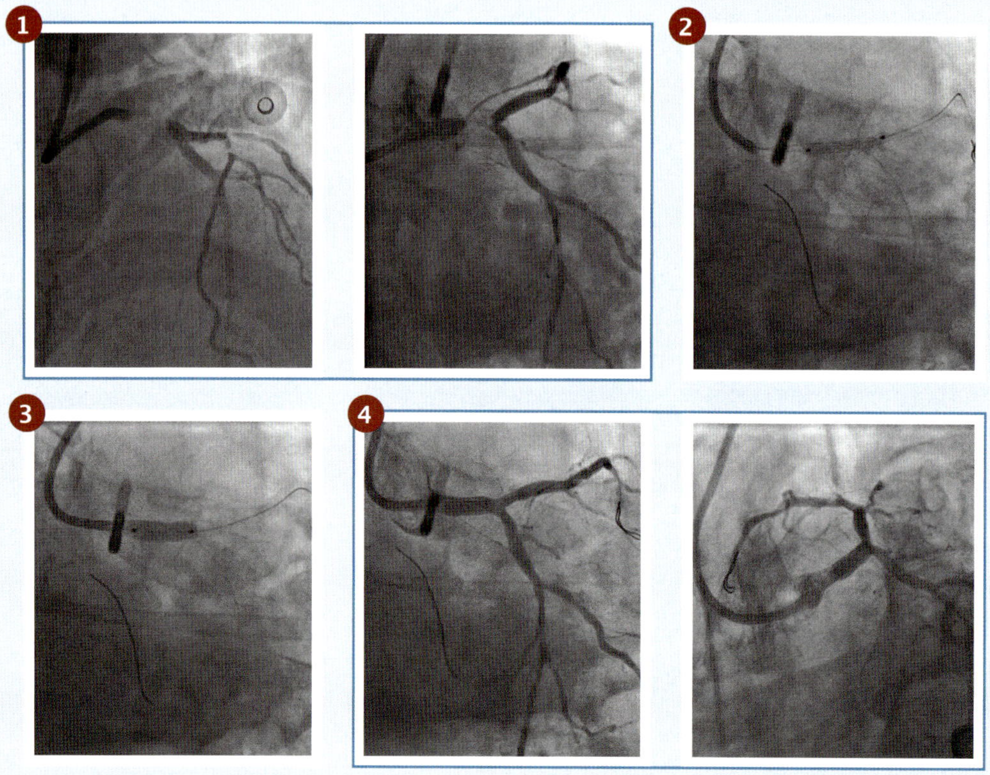

1. An LCA injection using a 6 Fr EBU 3.5 guide catheter reveals a 99% occlusion and a big thrombus in the distal LMCA.
2. Two 0.014-inch BMW PTCA guidewires were deployed in the LAD and LCX, and balloon dilatation was given in the culprit area.
3. The LMCA was stented.
4. An excellent end result is shown.

Example 5

TRA for primary PCI of an RCA lesion (deep intubation technique)

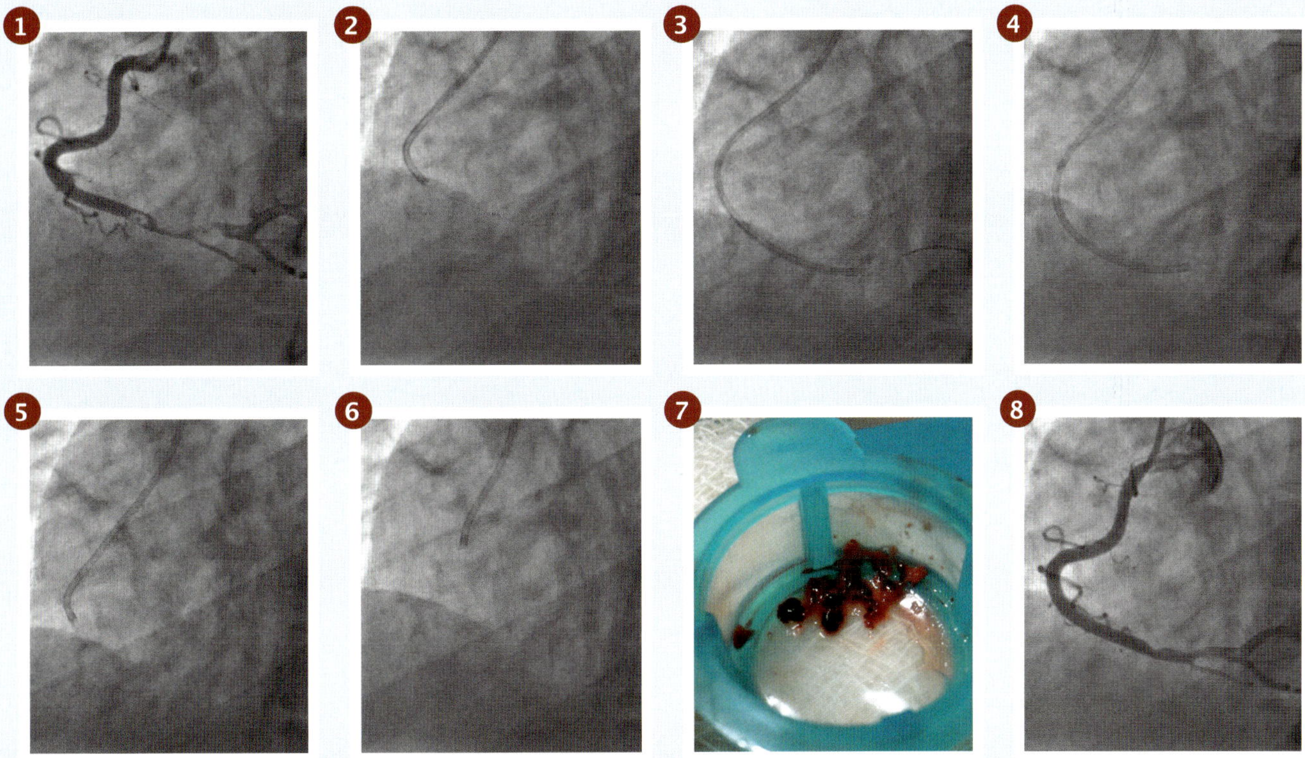

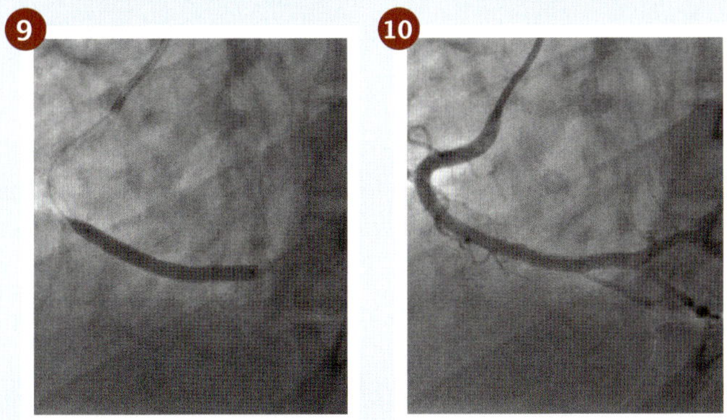

1. An example of acute inferior wall MI and cardiogenic shock that shows a huge thrombus burden in the large RCA.
2. Deep intubation with a 6 Fr JR 4 guide catheter was performed.
3. The distal tip of catheter was placed at the site of thrombus.
4. Thrombosuction was performed through the guide catheter itself.
5. Thrombosuction is in progress.
6. Thrombosuction is in progress.
7. A large amount of thrombus was removed.
8. An RCA angiogram was done after thrombosuction.
9. The affected segment was stented.
10. The final result is shown.

Recommended Reading

1. Amoroso G, Kiemeneij F. Transradial access for primary percutaneous coronary intervention: the next standard of care? Heart. 2010; 96 (17): 1341-44.
2. Bertrand O, Larose E, Costerousse O, et al. Effects of aspiration thrombectomy on necrosis size and ejection fraction after transradial percutaneous coronary intervention in acute ST-elevation myocardial infarction. Catheter Cardiovasc Interv. 2011; 77 (4): 475-82.
3. Bertrand O, Rodés-Cabau J, Larose E, et al. Early Discharge after Transradial Stenting of CoronarY Arteries in Acute Myocardial Infarction (EASY-MI) Study Investigators. Intracoronary compared to intravenous Abciximab and high-dose bolus compared to standard dose in patients with ST-segment elevation myocardial infarction undergoing transradial primary percutaneous coronary intervention: a two-by-two factorial placebo-controlled randomized study. Am J Cardiol. 2010; 105 (11): 1520-27.
4. Cantor W, Puley G, Natarajan M, et al. Radial versus femoral access for emergent percutaneous coronary intervention with adjunct glycoprotein IIb/IIIa inhibition in acute myocardial infarction—the RADIAL-AMI pilot randomized trial. Am Heart J. 2005; 150 (3): 543-49.
5. Kernis SJ, Harjai KJ, Stone GW, et al. The incidence, predictors, and outcomes of early reinfarction after primary angioplasty for acute myocardial infarction. J Am Coll Cardiol. 2003; 42(7): 1173-7.
6. Ochiai M, Isshiki T, Toyoizumi H, et al. Efficacy of transradial primary stenting in patients with acute myocardial infarction. Am J Cardiol. 1999; 15; 83 (6): 966-8, A10.
7. Pancholy S, Patel T, Sanghvi K, et al. Comparison of door-to-balloon times for primary PCI using transradial versus transfemoral approach. Catheter Cardiovasc Interv. 2010; 75 (7): 991-95.
8. Ranjan A, Patel T, Shah S, et al. Transradial primary angioplasty and stenting in Indian patients with acute myocardial infarction: acute results and 6-month follow-up. Indian Heart J. 2005; 57 (6): 681-87.
9. Saito S, Tanaka S, Hiroe Y, et al. Comparative study on transradial approach vs. transfemoral approach in primary stent implantation for patients with acute myocardial infarction: results of the test for myocardial infarction by prospective unicenter randomization for access sites (TEMPURA) trial. Catheter Cardiovasc Interv. 2003; 59 (1): 26-33.
10. Stone GW, Brodie BR, Griffin JJ, et al. Prospective, multicenter study of the safety and feasibility of primary stenting in acute myocardial infarction: in-hospital and 30-day results of the PAMI stent pilot trial. Primary Angioplasty in Myocardial Infarction Stent Pilot Trial Investigators. J Am Coll Cardiol. 1998;31(1):23-30.
11. Weaver A, Henderson R, Gilchrist I, et al. Arterial access and door-to-balloon times for primary percutaneous coronary intervention in patients presenting with acute ST-elevation myocardial infarction. Catheter Cardiovasc Interv. 2010; 75 (5): 695-99.
12. Yip H, Chen M, Chang H, et al. Transradial application of PercuSurge GuardWire device during primary percutaneous intervention of infarct-related artery with high-burden thrombus formation. Catheter Cardiovasc Interv. 2004; 61 (4): 503-11.
13. Jolly SS, Yusuf S, Cairns J et al. Radial versus femoral access for coronary angiography and intervention in patients with acute coronary syndromes (RIVAL): a randomised, parallel group, multicentre trial. Lancet. 2011; 377 (9775): 1409-20.
14. Larsen P, Shah S, Pyne C et al. Comparison of procedural times, success rates and safety. between left vs. right radial access in primary percutaneous intervention for acute ST-elevation acute myocardial infarction. Catheter Cardiovasc Interv. 2011; 78 (1): 45-6.

TRA for Addressing Internal Carotid Artery (ICA) Stenosis

13

Tejas Patel, Tift Mann, Sanjay Shah and Alok Ranjan

Carotid artery stenting (CAS) has become an accepted treatment modality for revascularizing the internal carotid artery (ICA). TFA has already been widely accepted. Small feasibility studies of CAS through ipsilateral TRA have already been published. We have recently published a technique for CAS using contralateral TRA. Although CAS through TRA is more challenging, it is important to know this technique, as it provides a useful alternative approach in patients with severe aortoiliac disease and/or anatomical variations of the aortic arch.

CAS Using Contralateral TRA

Example 1

Right ICA stenting using the left TRA

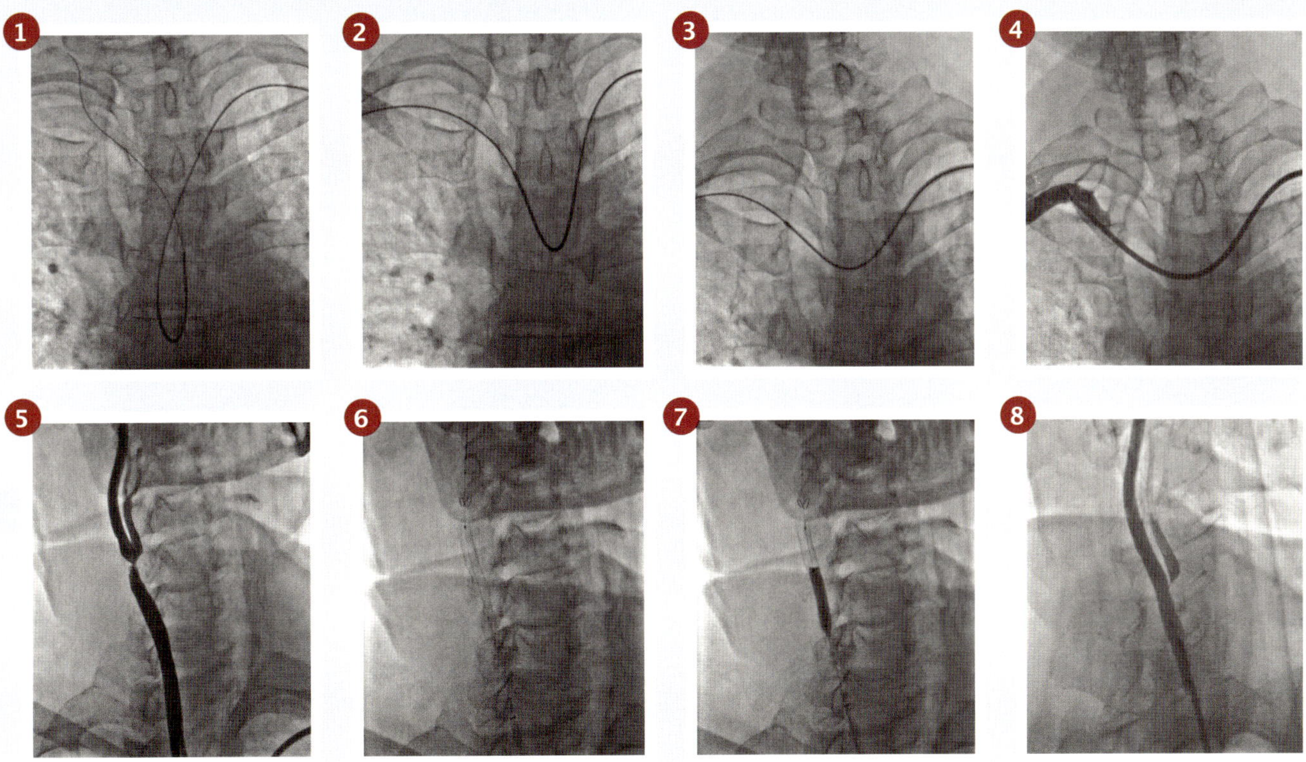

1. An example of right ICA stenting using the left TR approach. A 5 Fr Simmons-1 catheter was used, and a 0.032-inch hydrophilic wire was negotiated into the innominate artery.
2. The guidewire was directed into the right subclavian and, subsequently, the axillary artery.
3. The 6 Fr Pinnacle sheath was negotiated using the telescopic technique over a Simmons-1 catheter.
4. The tip of the Pinnacle sheath was placed in the right subclavian artery.
5. Gentle pullback led to selective cannulation of the right CCA and demonstration of the culprit lesion.
6. The distal protection device was deployed and the lesion was stented.
7. In-stent balloon dilatation was given.
8. A satisfactory end result is seen.

Example 2

Left ICA stenting using the right TRA

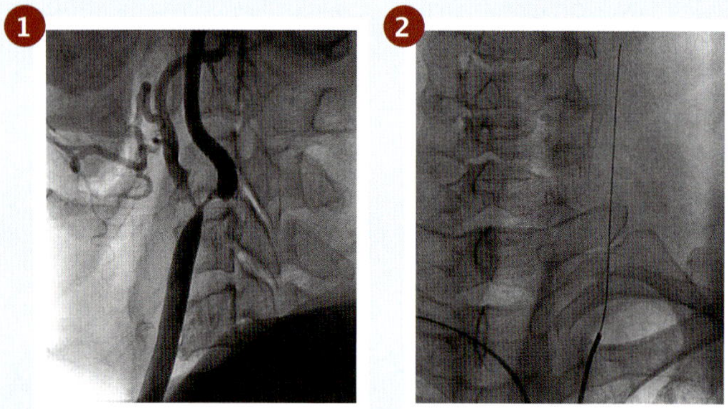

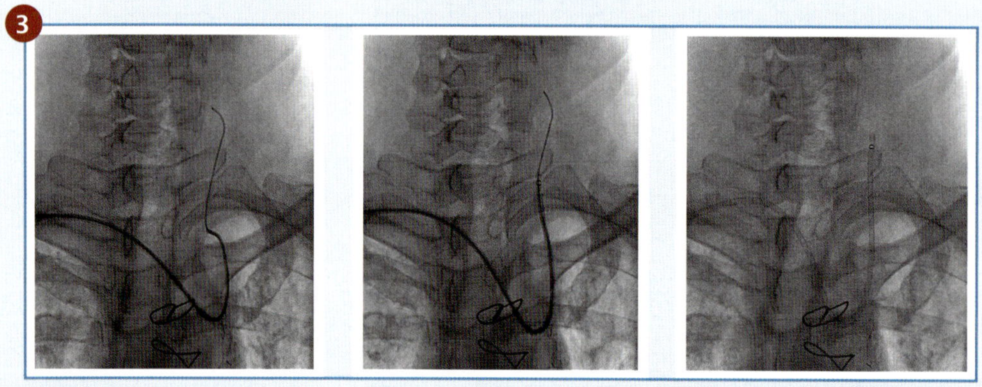

1. Left ICA stenting using the right TR approach is shown. The lesion was profiled.
2. A 5 Fr Simmons-1 diagnostic catheter was used to cannulate the left CCA, and a 0.032-inch standard wire was negotiated through the CCA into the ECA.
3. A Simmons-1 catheter was replaced by a 5 Fr JL 4 diagnostic catheter, and a 6 Fr Pinnacle sheath (90 cm long) was negotiated into the left CCA using the telescopic technique.
4. A distal protection device was deployed, and PTA of the culprit lesion was performed.
5. A self-expanding stent was deployed.
6. In-stent balloon dilatation was performed.
7. The final result is shown.

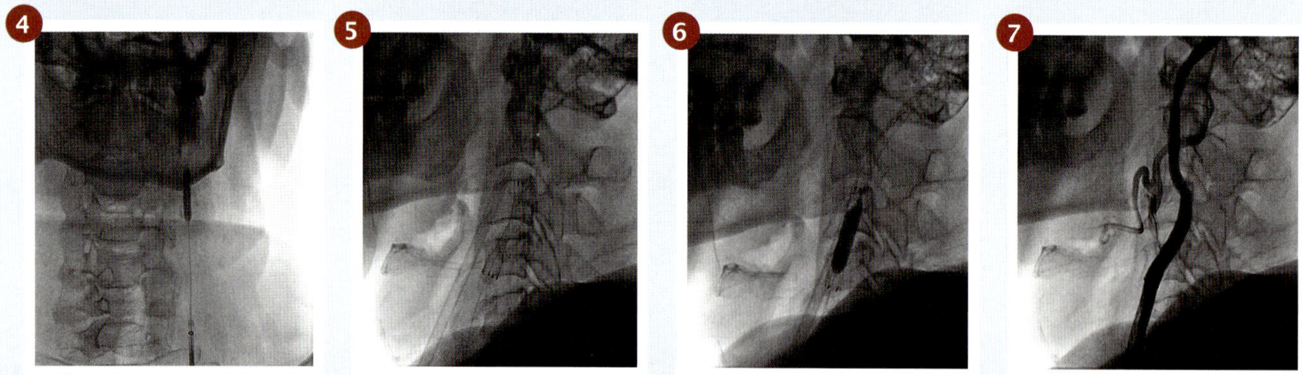

Tips

- We strongly recommend performing a radial angiogram through the arterial puncture cannula to define vascular anatomy before introducing the sheath. In cases of an RA diameter less than 2 mm, severe RA tortuosity and difficult radio-brachial loops, TRA should be avoided.
- For contralateral TRA, the target carotid artery is usually cannulated with a 5 Fr Simmons-1 or a 5 Fr TIG Optitorque catheter.
- A 0.025-inch or 0.032-inch hydrophilic guidewire is then parked at optimal position in the external carotid artery (ECA).
- The catheter is then advanced into the ECA using a corkscrew movement or slow jack-hammering technique.
- Once the catheter is parked in the ECA, the hydrophilic guidewire is removed and replaced by a 0.035-inch super-stiff guide wire.
- The diagnostic catheter and introducer sheath are removed, and a 90 cm long 6 Fr sheath (with introducer) is then slowly negotiated over the super-stiff wire to position it coaxially in the contralateral CCA, just below its bifurcation.
- To enter the contralateral CCA, telescoping is performed. While pushing the sheath from the angle of aortic arch into the subclavian artery, the dilator of the sheath is simultaneously pulled back by gentle maneuvering.
- At times, as an alternative approach, the sheath is kept in the aortic arch, the dilator is removed and a 5 Fr JR diagnostic catheter is replaced. The JR catheter is then advanced into the contralateral CCA, and the sheath is slowly negotiated over it to enter the CCA.
- Once the sheath is deployed coaxially to the CCA, CAS is performed using the standard technique.
- The choice of 90 cm long sheath, stent, filter device and balloon is left to the discretion of the operator.
- Addressing right ICA stenosis using the left TRA is relatively easy because of the favorable angle of the right CCA.

CAS Using Ipsilateral TRA (Tift Mann)

The RAO subclavian arteriogram is useful when selecting the appropriate diagnostic catheter for the right CCA.

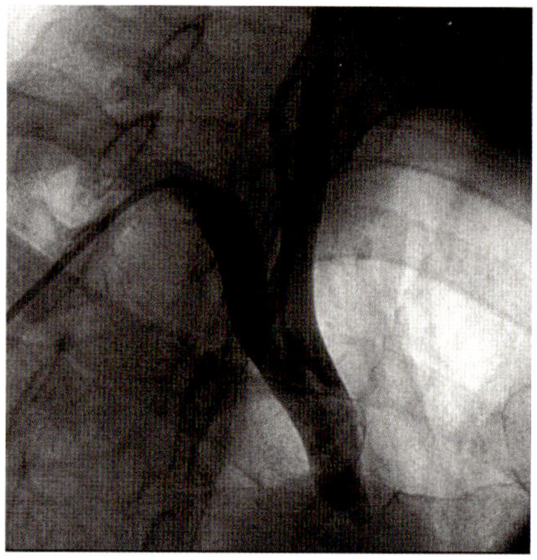

Simmons-1 for vertical takeoff

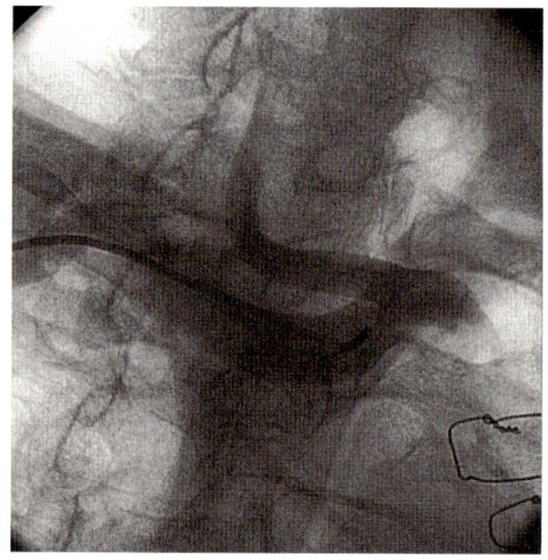

TIG for horizontal takeoff

Bovine aortic arch

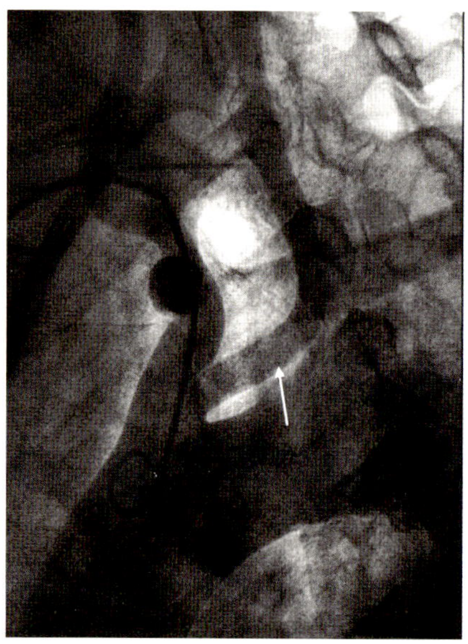

Amplatz R2 for horizontal takeoff

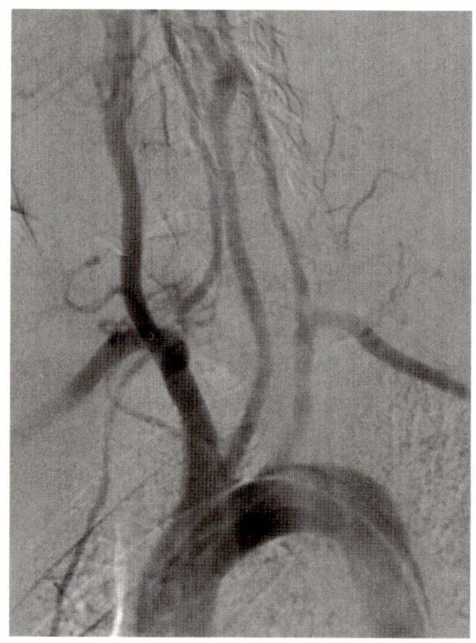

Simmons-1 or -2 for vertical takeoff

Example 1

Right ICA stenting using the right TRA

1

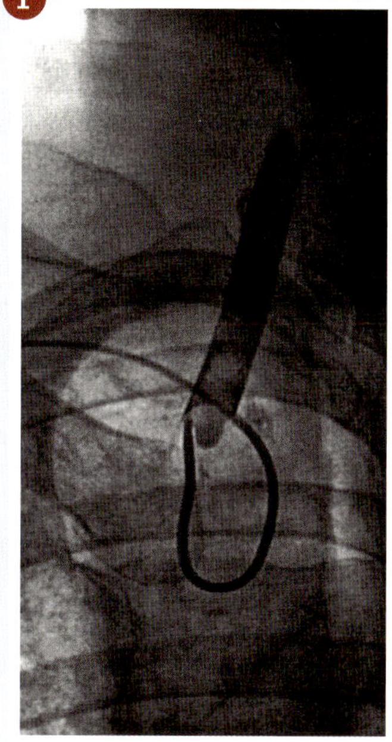

2

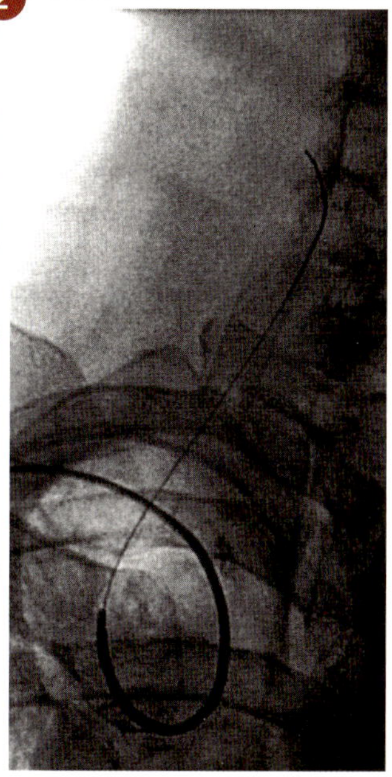

3

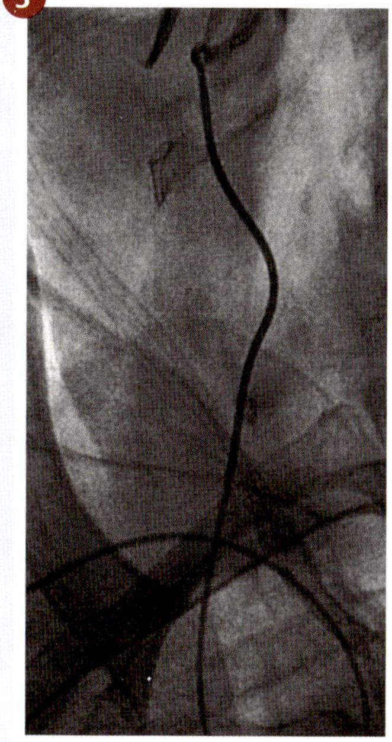

4

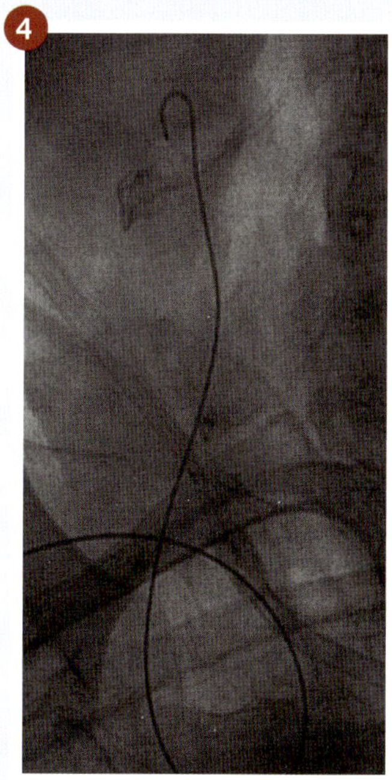

5

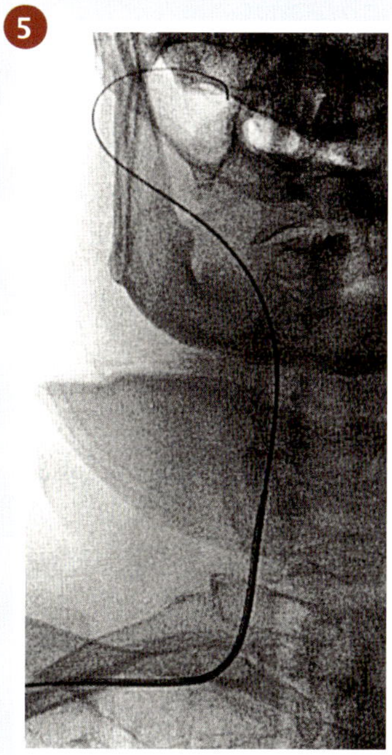

1. The right CCA was cannulated using a Simmons-1 catheter.
2. A 0.014-inch extra support coronary guidewire (Mailman, Boston Scientific) was introduced and parked in the right ECA.
3. The catheter was advanced over the wire into the right ECA.
4. A 0.035-inch exchange length J wire was used to exchange the diagnostic catheter for the Shuttle sheath.
5. A tapered, exchange-length .036″ guidewire (TAD II, Covidien) was advanced through a Simmons-1 catheter directly into the external carotid. The Shuttle sheath can be exchanged over this wire, thus skipping steps 2-3.

Example 2

Left ICA stenting using right TRA

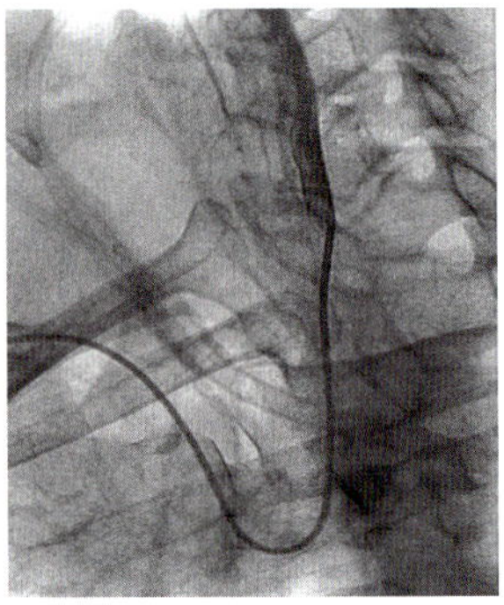

A Simmons-2 catheter is shown in the LICA.

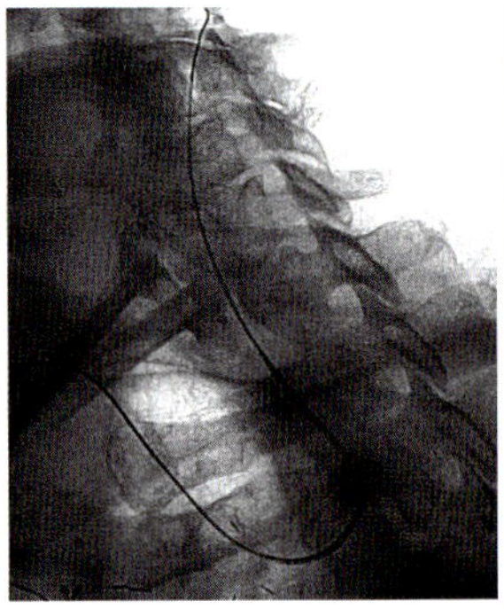

The TAD II guidewire is anchored in the external carotid.

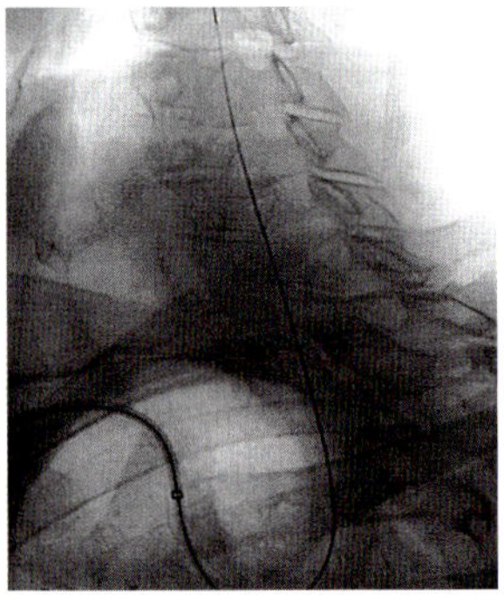

The Shuttle sheath is advanced over the TAD II wire into the LCCA. In patients with extreme angles, it may be necessary to substitute an Amplatz super-stiff guidewire and/or telescope Shuttle sheath over a Simmons-2.

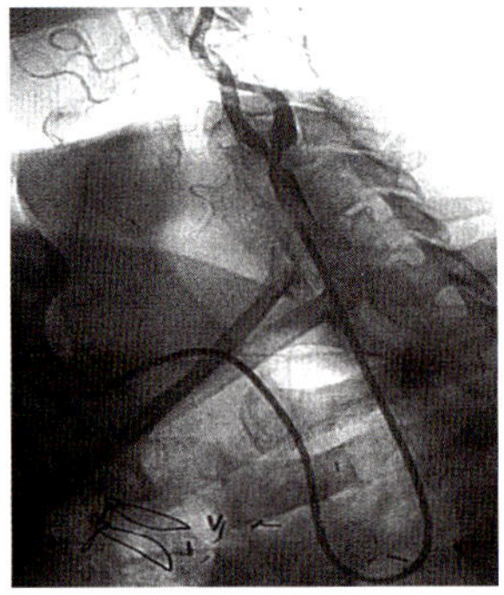

The Shuttle sheath is positioned beneath the bifurcation for deployment of an embolic protection device and carotid stent.

Claret technique

With the Claret technique, carotid stents are deployed through a 7 Fr Kimny guide catheter supported on the right coronary cusp.

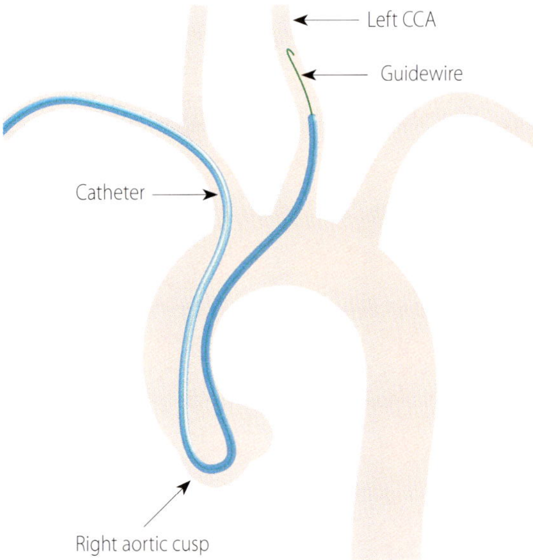

Tips

- The right ipsilateral approach is indicated for right ICA stenting in the presence of a hostile aortic arch or other situations in which femoral access is best avoided.
- For transradial right carotid angiography, catheter selection is based on an initial RAO subclavian arteriogram, which shows the angle of takeoff of the right CCA. A Simmons-1 catheter is used for a vertical origin of the right CCA, and a TIG catheter is used for a more horizontal origin and less acute angles.
- When selecting the right ipsilateral ECA, a 0.014-inch extra support coronary guidewire is an alternative to the standard 0.035-inch angled Glidewire when the angle of takeoff of the right CCA is acute. The diagnostic catheter is then advanced over this wire into the right ECA.
- A 0.035-inch exchange-length J wire is used to exchange the diagnostic catheter for the Shuttle sheath. Stiffer guidewires such as the Amplatz Super Stiff Guidewire are not used from the ipsilateral approach because they create excessive tension due to the acute angle at the origin of the CCA. If the ECA is occluded or cannot be accessed for other reasons, the exchange is carefully made in the CCA.
- Bovine left carotid arteries present a unique situation in which right transradial access may be the preferred strategy for stenting. The bovine left carotid artery can usually be selected from the right arm with an AR2 or Simmons catheter. After baseline angiography, the Shuttle sheath is exchanged for the diagnostic catheter over a 0.035-inch J wire positioned beneath the bifurcation.
- All currently available carotid stents can be delivered through a 6 Fr Shuttle sheath. However, caution must be observed during delivery, because air can be introduced to the system during delivery, creating the risk of air embolization. Allow extra time to bleed back air or deploy the stent using roadmap fluoroscopy mode for positioning.
- The 8 mm by 21 mm Carotid Wallstent, when deployed, covers most lesions. It is a particularly useful option in women with smaller radial arteries, as it can be delivered through a 5 Fr sheath.

Recommended Reading

1. Fang H, Chung S, Sun C et al. Transradial and transbrachial arterial approach for simultaneous carotid angiographic examination and stenting using catheter looping and retrograde technique. Ann Vasc Surg. 2010; 24(5): 670-679
2. Folmar J, Sachar R, Mann T. Transradial approach for carotid artery stenting: a feasibility study. Catheter Cardiovasc Interv. 2007; 69(3):355-361.
3. Gan H, Bhasin A, Wu C. Transradial carotid stenting in a patient with bovine arch anatomy. Catheter Cardiovasc Interv. 2010; 75(4): 540-543.
4. Patel T, Shah S, Ranjan A, et al. Contralateral transradial approach for carotid artery stenting: a feasibility study. Catheter Cardiovasc Interv. 2010; 75 (2): 268-275.
5. Trani C, Burzotta F, Coroleu S. Transradial carotid artery stenting with proximal embolic protection. Catheter Cardiovasc Interv. 2009; 74 (2): 267-72.
6. Wu C, Cheng C, Hung W, et al. Feasibility and safety of transbrachial approach for patients with severe carotid artery stenosis undergoing stenting. Catheter Cardiovasc Interv. 2006; 67 (6): 967-271.
7. Wu C, Hung W, Chen S, et al. Feasibility and safety of transradial artery approach for selective cerebral angiography. Catheter Cardiovasc Interv. 2005; 66 (1): 21-26.
8. Yamashita T, Imai S, Tamada T, et al. Transradial approach for noncoronary angiography and interventions. Catheter Cardiovasc Interv. 2007; 70 (2): 303-308.

14 TRA for Addressing Vertebrobasilar Stenosis

Tejas Patel, Sanjay Shah, Rajnikant Radadiya and Leena Shah

Endovascular intervention for vertebrobasilar stenosis is a relatively new but viable alternative modality of management supported by a few case reports and observational studies. TFA has been the preferred approach in most studies. Our recently published study has documented feasibility and reproducibility of TRA in chronic and acute occlusions of the vertebrobasilar system.

Example 1

Left vertebral ostial stenting using the left TRA

1

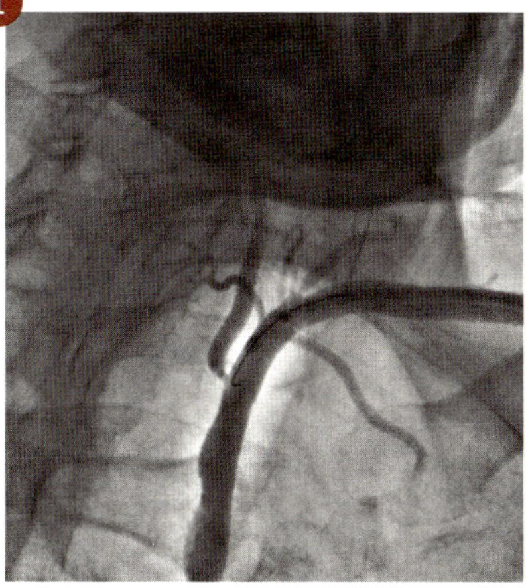

2

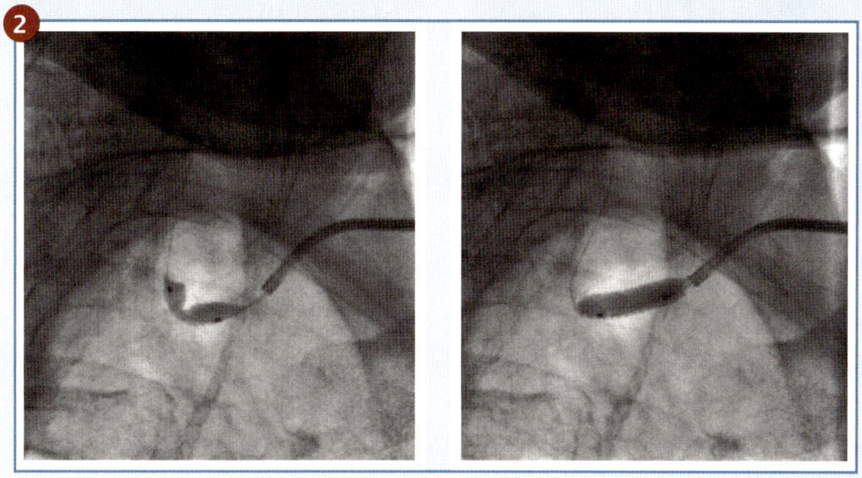

3

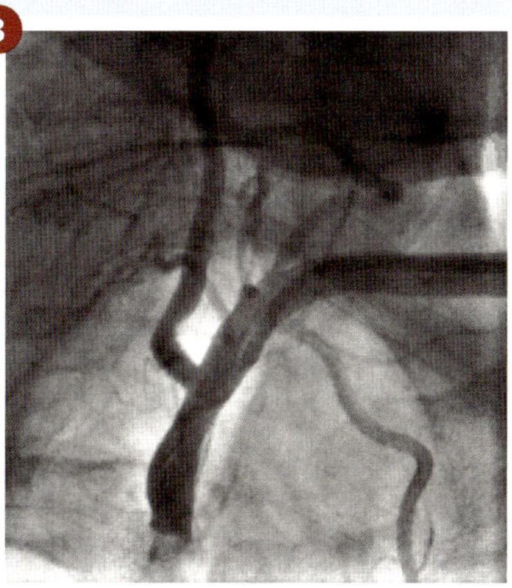

1. A tight left vertebral ostial stenosis was addressed using the left TR approach.
2. A 6 Fr JR-4 catheter was used, and a 0.014-inch BMW PTCA guidewire was negotiated into the vertebral artery. Stenting was completed.
3. A satisfactory end result is shown.

Example 2

Stenting of a chronic left vertebral intracranial stenosis using the left TRA

1

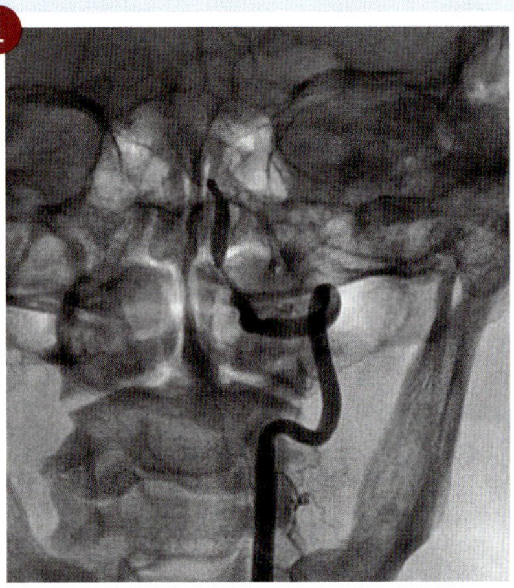

2

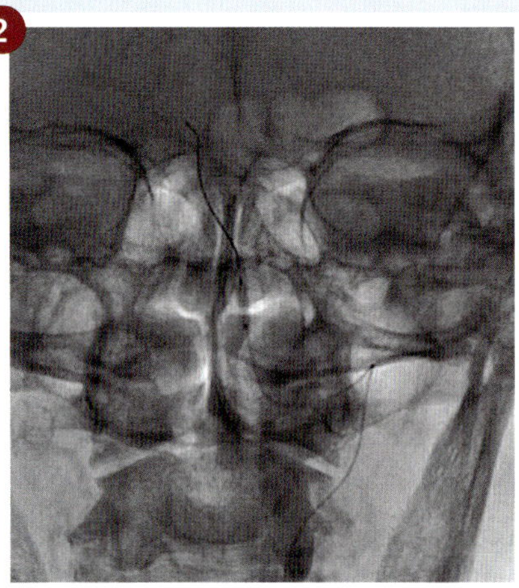

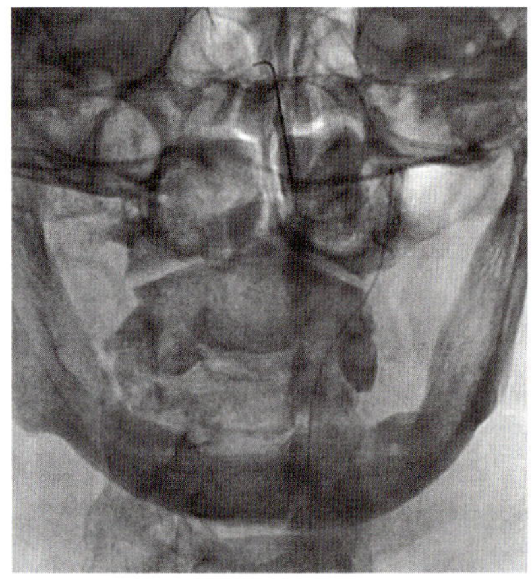

3

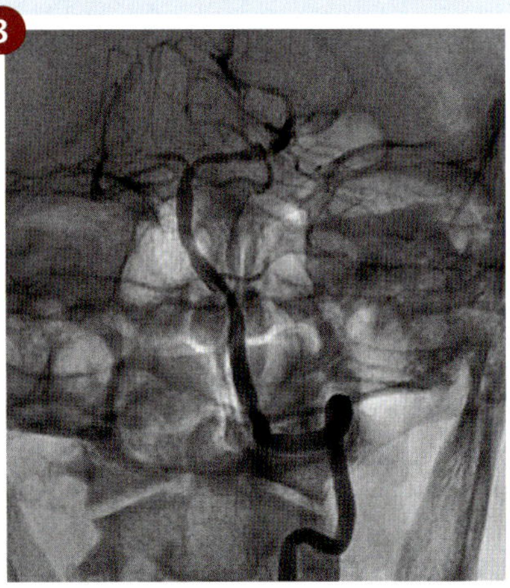

1. Stenting of a chronic intracranial left vertebral artery stenosis using the left TRA is shown. The lesion was profiled.
2. The ostium of the left vertebral artery was cannulated using a 6 Fr IMA guide catheter, and PTA, followed by stenting. This was done in the usual fashion.
3. The final result is shown.

Example 3

Stenting of an acute basilar artery occlusion using the left TRA

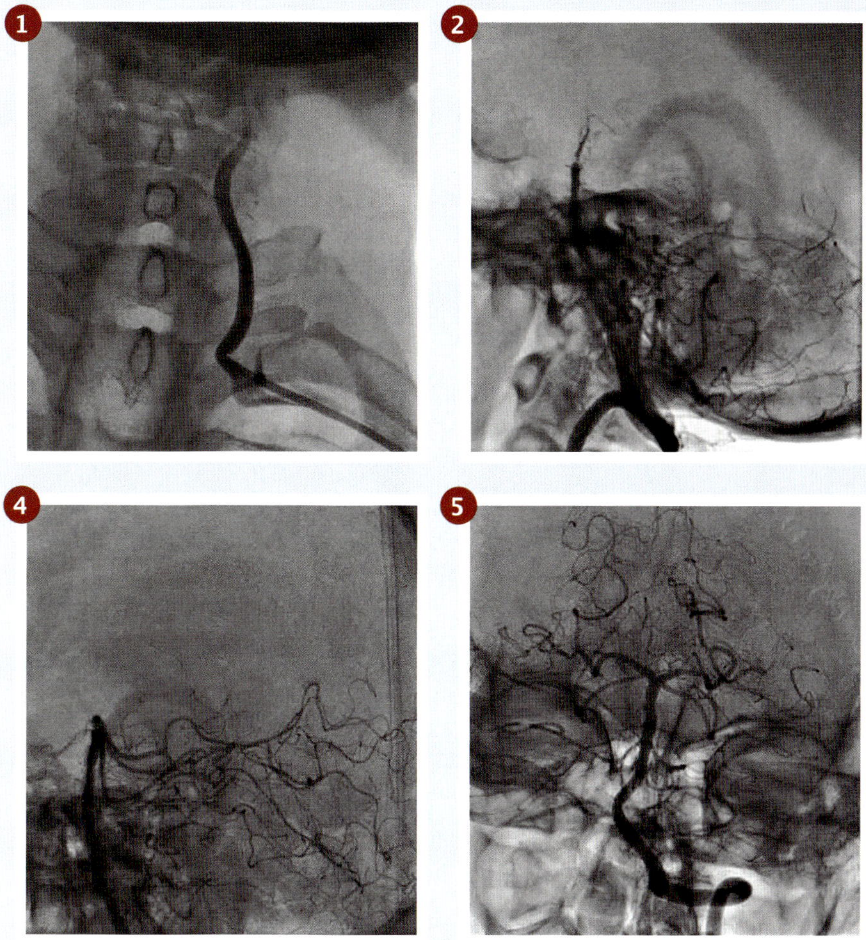

1. Stenting of an acute basilar artery occlusion using the left TRA is shown. The left vertebral artery was cannulated using a 6 Fr IMA catheter.
2. The occlusion was profiled.
3. PTA was done using a 2 mm PTCA catheter at low pressure (4 bars).
4. The distal flow was established and the patient was shifted to the ICU.
5. The next day, the lesion was stented in the usual fashion. The final result was optimal.

This two-stage approach was used to avoid hyperperfusion brain injury.

Example 4

Stenting of a chronic basilar artery occlusion using the right TRA

1
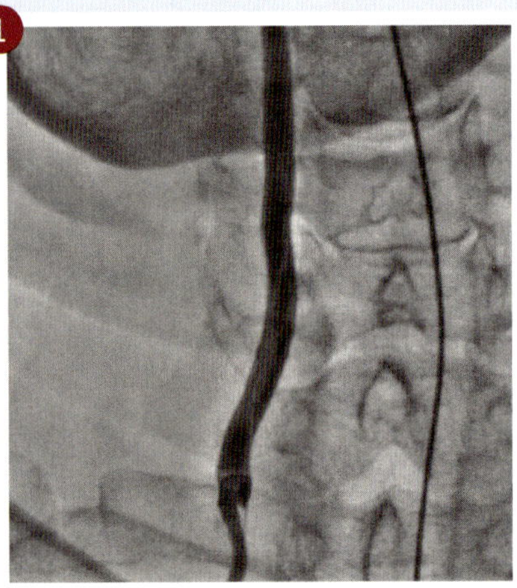

2
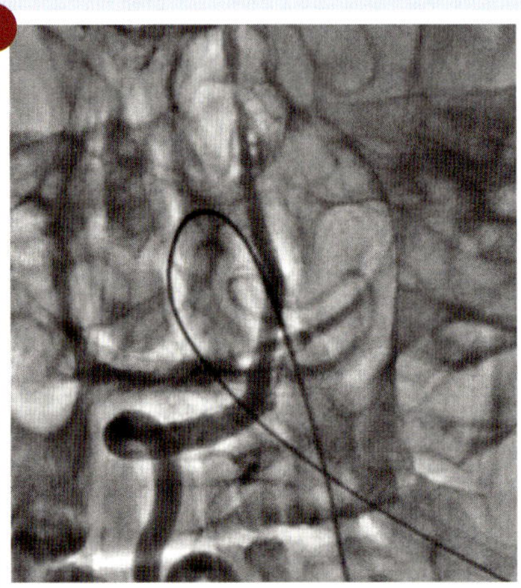

3
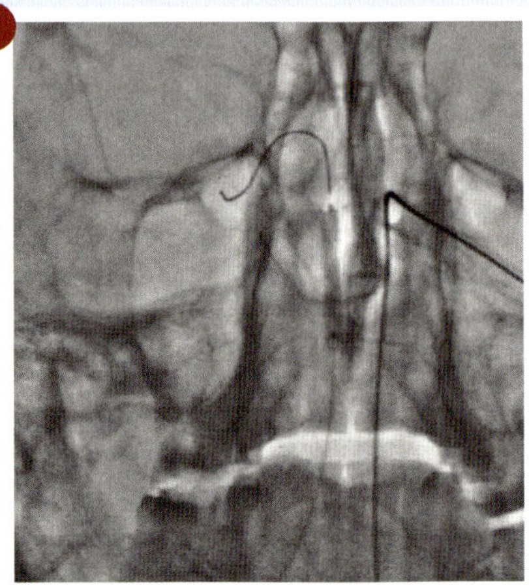

4
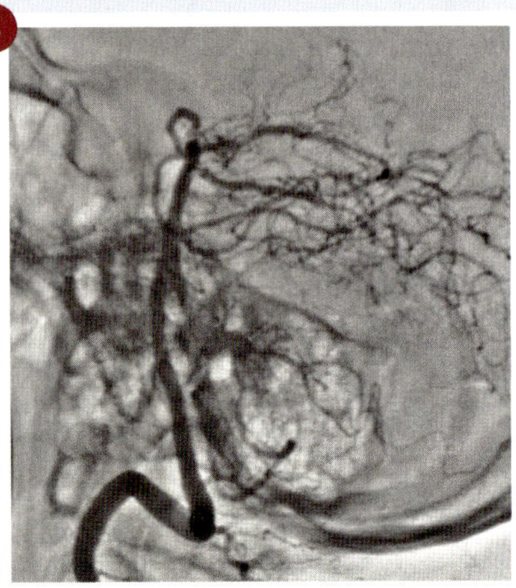

1. Stenting of a chronic basilar artery stenosis using the right TRA is shown. The right vertebral artery was cannulated using a 6 Fr JR 4 guide catheter.
2. The lesion was profiled.
3. The procedure was completed in the usual fashion.
4. The final result is shown.

Tips

- A 6 Fr internal mammary artery guide catheter through the ipsilateral TRA easily cannulates the ostium of the vertebral artery (VA). For addressing ostial VA stenosis, the same guide catheter, with side holes, should be used.
- Regular 0.014-inch floppy PTCA guide wires, balloon catheters and coronary stents should be used.
- Pre-dilation of the lesion should be done with low pressure (between 4 and 6 atmospheres of pressure).
- The stent should be deployed at relatively low pressure (8 to 10 atmospheres of pressure).
- For acute intracranial vertebral or basilar artery occlusions, the procedure should be done in two stages. In the first stage, the lesion should be dilated using a 1.5, 2 x 10 or 12 mm PTCA catheter at 4 to 6 atmospheres to establish the distal flow. In the second stage, the patient should be brought to the cath lab after 24 hours, and the lesion should be stented using a bare-metal coronary stent at 8 to 10 atmospheres. This two-stage approach is recommended to prevent hyperperfusion brain injury.

Recommended Reading

1. Bendok B, Przybylo J, Parkinson R, et al. Neuroendovascular interventions for intracranial posterior circulation disease via the transradial approach: technical case report. Neurosurgery. 2005; 56 (3): E626; discussion E626.
2. Kim J, Park Y, Chung C, et al. Feasibility and utility of transradial cerebral angiography: experience during the learning period. Korean J Radiol. 2006; 7 (1): 7-13.
3. Nohara A, Kallmes D. Transradial cerebral angiography: technique and outcomes. Am J Neuroradiol. 2003; 24 (6): 1247-50.
4. Patel T, Shah S, Malhotra H, Radadia R, Shah L, Shah S. Transradial approach for stenting of vertebrobasilar stenosis: a feasibility study. Catheter. Cardiovasc Interv. 2009; 74 (6): 925-31.
5. Sharma G, Louvard Y, Morice M, et al. Noncoronary transradial angioplasty with coronary equipment: a less invasive technique. Catheter Cardiovasc Interv. 2002; 55 (2): 197-205.
6. Yamashita T, Imai S, Tamada T, et al. Transradial approach for noncoronary angiography and interventions. Catheter Cardiovasc Interv. 2007; 70 (2): 303-8.
7. Yip H, Youssef A, Chang W, et al. Feasibility and safety of transradial arterial approach for simultaneous right and left vertebral artery angiographic studies and stenting. Cardiovasc Intervent Radiol. 2007; 30 (5): 840-46.

TRA for Addressing Subclavian and Innominate Artery Lesions

15

Tejas Patel, Kintur Sanghvi and Sanjay Shah

Occlusive lesions of the innominate and subclavian arteries might cause serious morbidity and should be treated if symptomatic. Endovascular treatment is recommended because it has a lower complication rate compared with surgical treatment. Most studies have used TFA; however, some have used brachial and axillary approaches. We recommend ipsilateral TRA, an easy and reproducible approach.

Example 1

Left subclavian artery stenting using the left TRA

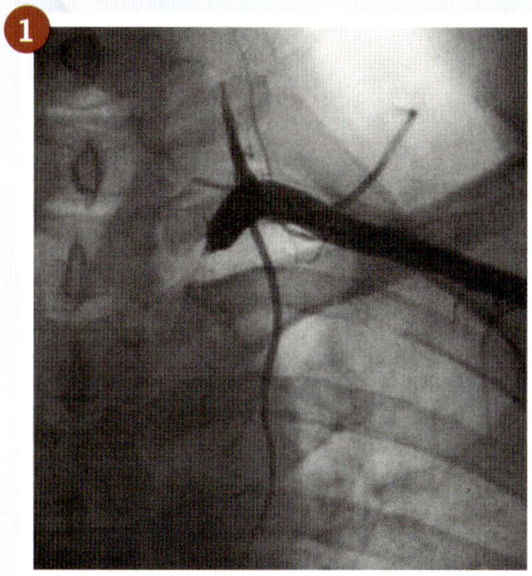

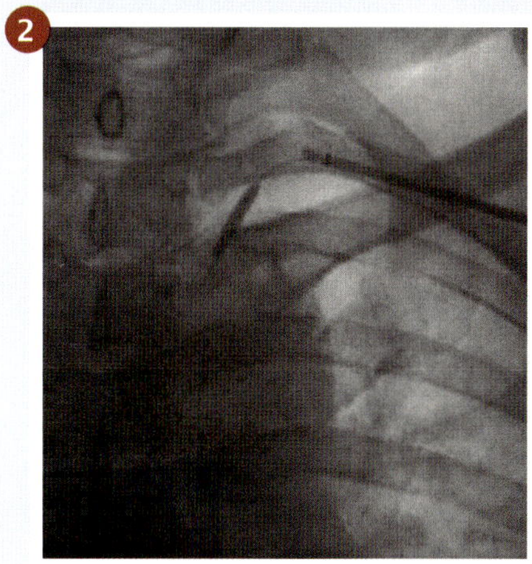

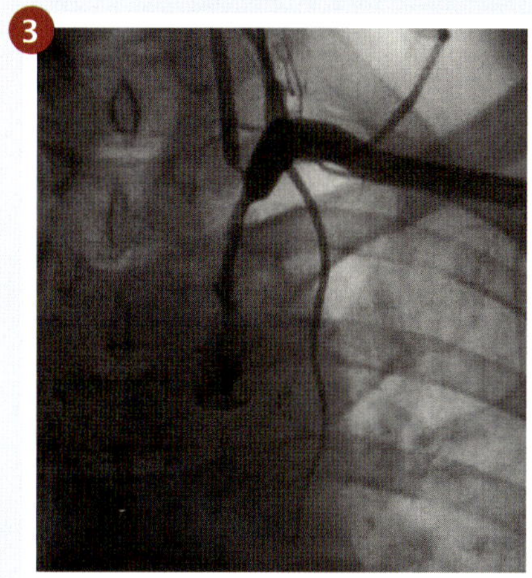

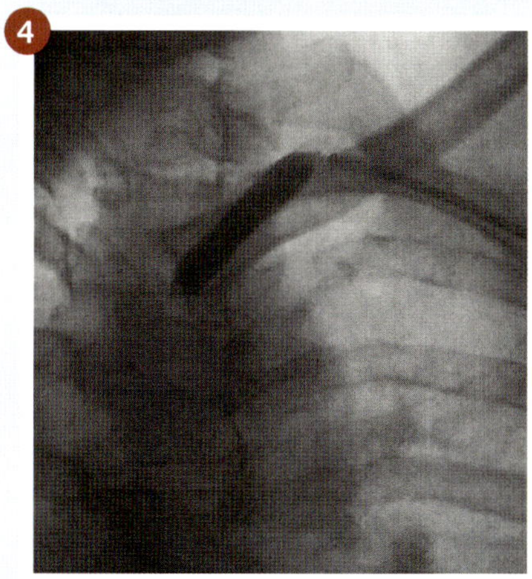

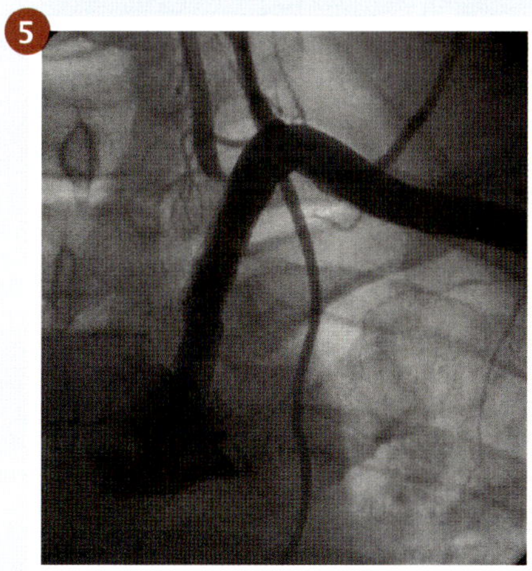

1. Left subclavian artery stenting using the left TRA is shown. A tight left subclavian artery stenosis was seen.
2. A 6 Fr Pinnacle sheath (45 cm long) was deployed near the lesion. The lesion was crossed using a 0.014-inch BMW PTCA guidewire, and PTA was performed.
3. The result of PTA is shown.
4. A balloon-expandable stent was deployed.
5. The final result is seen.

Example 2

Right subclavian artery stenting using the right TRA

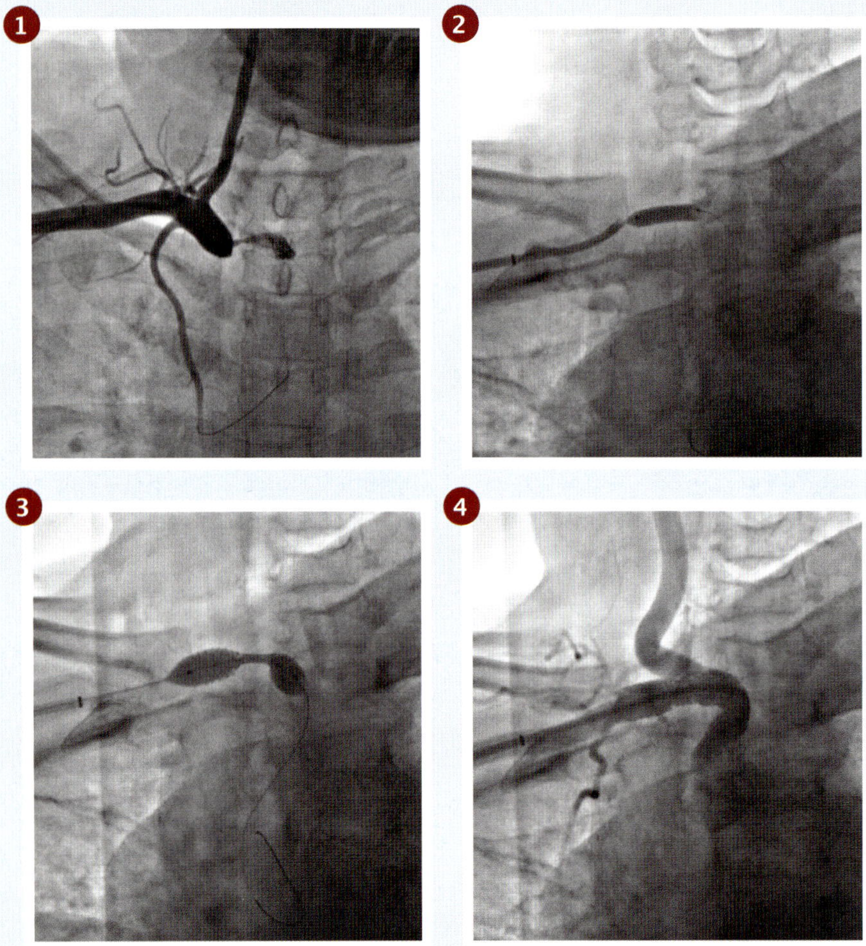

1. Right subclavian stenting using the right TRA is shown. The lesion was profiled.
2. A 6 Fr Pinnacle sheath (45 cm long) was deployed near the lesion, and PTA was performed.
3. After that, the lesion was stented.
4. The final result is seen.

Note that the right CCA origin is not compromised.

Example 3

Subclavian steal phenomenon; left subclavian artery stenting using the left TRA.

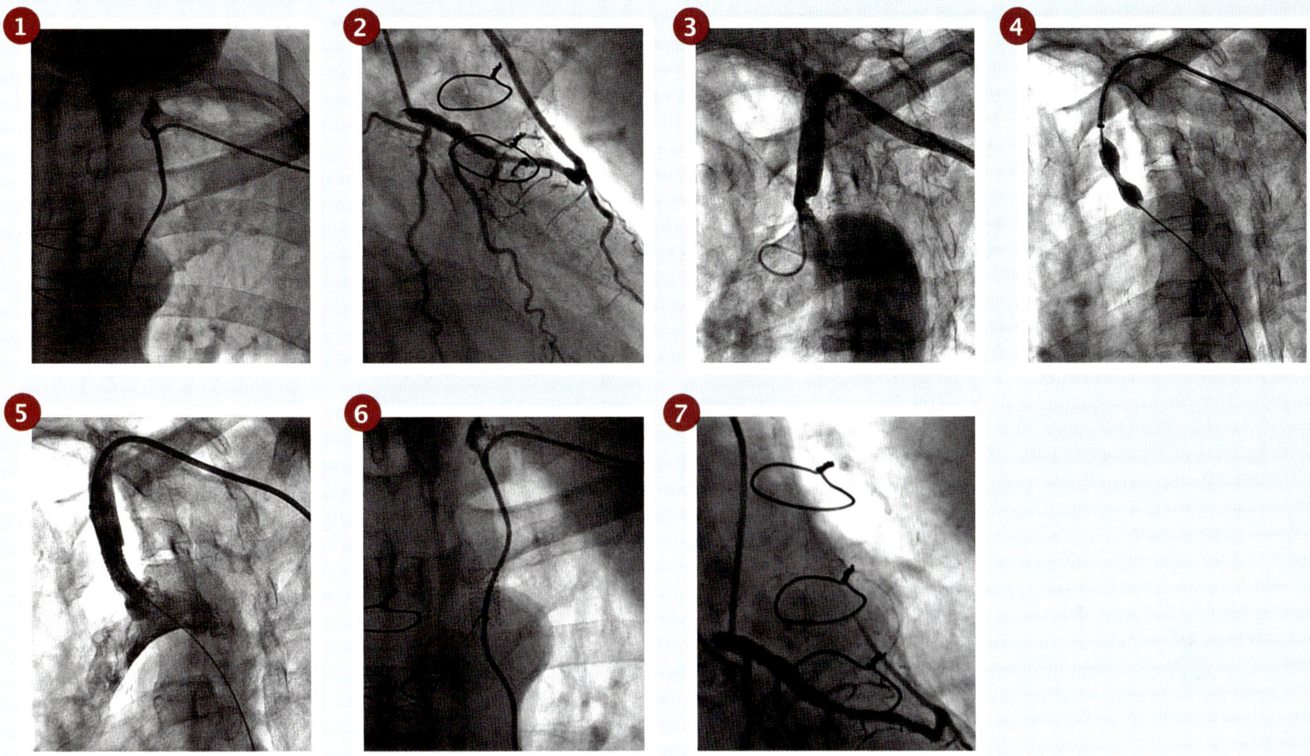

1. Left subclavian artery stenting is done using the left TRA to revert the subclavian–steel phenomenon. Selective LIMA injection revealed sluggish flow.
2. An LCA injection revealed retrograde filling of the LIMA graft from the LAD.
3. A tight left subclavian stenosis was profiled.
4. Stenting was done in the usual fashion.
5. A satisfactory end result is shown.
6. Brisk antegrade LIMA flow is demonstrated.
7. Very slow retrograde LIMA flow is demonstrated.

Tips

- A 45 cm long 6 Fr/7 Fr introducer sheath is preferred through the ipsilateral TRA. The distal tip should be kept 5 mm to 10 mm from the lesion.
- Avoid stent deployment across the vertebral artery (VA) origin, as it could increase the likelihood of VA occlusion and/or brain embolization.
- Avoid stent deployment across the origin of the IMA.
- While addressing innominate artery stenosis, a careful stent deployment is recommended to avoid significant protrusion into the aorta or the orifice of the right CCA.
- For bovine arch variation, care should be taken not to stent across the origin of the left CCA.

Recommended Reading

1. Sharma G, Louvard Y, Morice M, et al. Noncoronary transradial angioplasty with coronary equipment: a less invasive technique. Catheter Cardiovasc Interv. 2002; 55 (2): 197-205.
2. Walker C. Will the transradial approach become the preferred approach in subclavian artery stenting? J Invasive Cardiol. 2010; 22 (5): 207-208.
3. Wood F, Mann J 3rd, Jobe R, et al. Transradial subclavian and coronary stenting in a single procedure. J Invasive Cardiol. 2004; 16 (10): 596-598.
4. Yamashita T, Imai S, Tamada T, et al. Transradial approach for noncoronary angiography and interventions. Catheter Cardiovasc Interv. 2007; 70 (2): 303-308.
5. Yu J, Korabathina R, Coppola J, et al. Transradial approach to subclavian artery stenting. J Invasive Cardiol. 2010; 22 (5): 204-206.

16 TRA for Addressing Renal Artery Stenosis

Tejas Patel, Josef Ludwig and Sanjay Shah

Renal artery stenting (RAS) technique once required the use of large, 8 Fr sheaths or guide catheters to allow the passage of bulky stent systems over 0.035-inch guidewires. It has evolved and, now, contemporary 6 Fr-compatible devices are used over 0.014-inch PTCA guidewires. This revolution in hardware has actually increased the safety and efficacy of RAS, leading to its performance in coronary-like fashion, and to the development of TRA as an effective alternative approach for TFA.

Example 1

Right renal artery ostial stenting using the left TRA

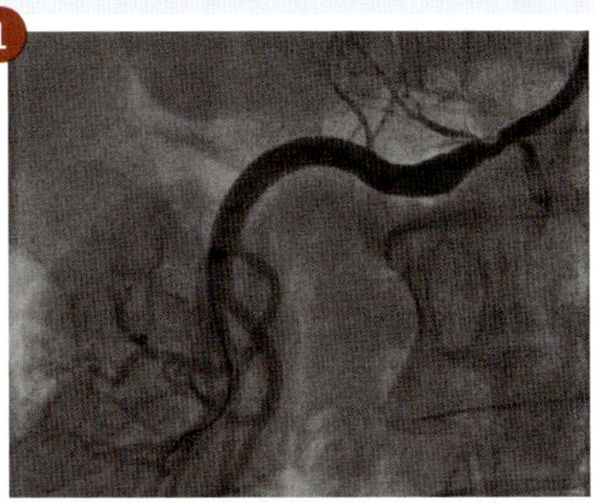

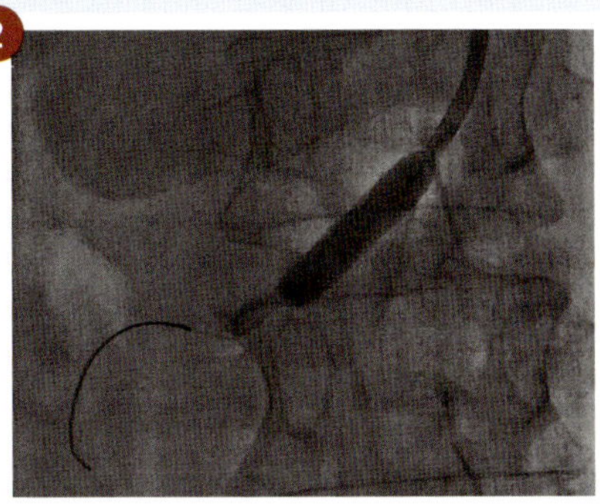

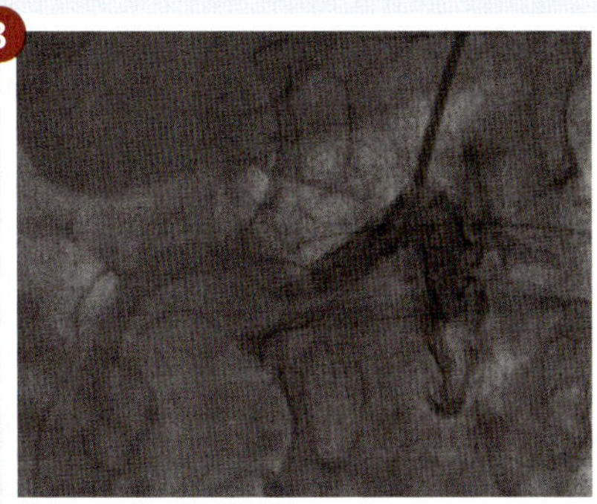

1. The renal artery ostium was cannulated using a 6 Fr JR 4 guide catheter; the lesion was profiled.
2. The lesion was stented in the usual fashion.
3. The final result is shown.

Example 2

Right renal artery mid-segment stenting using the right TRA

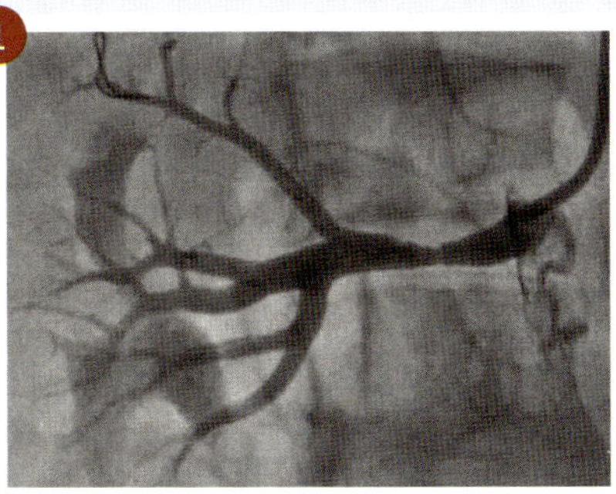

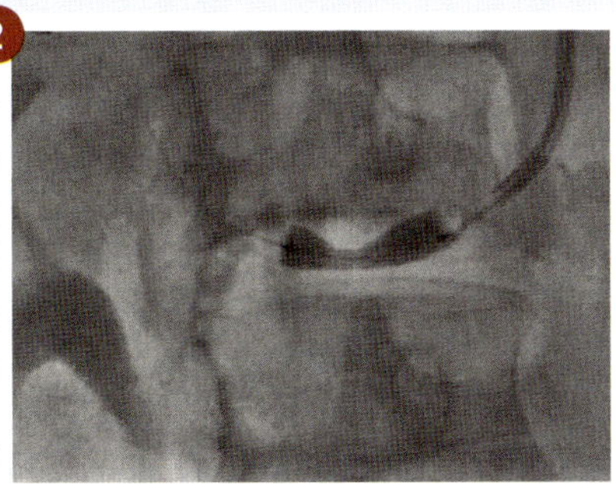

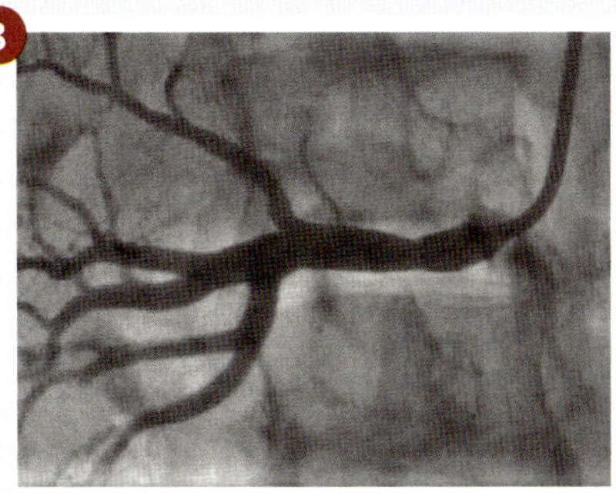

1. The lesion was profiled.
2. Stenting was done in the usual fashion.
3. The final result is shown.

Tips

- For RAS, the left TRA should be considered the first choice, because the distance from access to renals is shorter and less catheter manipulation is required, as there is no need to traverse the aortic arch. Thus, by using regular-length multipurpose (MP) or JR guide catheters, nearly all RAS can be performed.
- However, by using 125 cm 6 Fr/7 Fr MP or JR guide catheters, RAS can be effectively and safely performed in tall patients, even by using the right TRA.

Specific Benefits

- Typically, after the origin, the renal artery points downward; as such, TRA offers more coaxial and less traumatic guide catheter cannulation as compared to TFA.
- Usually, the diameter of the renal artery ranges from 4 mm to 7 mm. 6 Fr- or, sometimes, 7 Fr-catheter-compatible balloons and stents can be comfortably used through the TRA.
- Many patients undergoing RAS have uncontrolled hypertension, despite high doses of antihypertensive medications. TRA is likely to reduce access site-related bleeding complications in this subset.

Recommended Reading

1. Abdou S, Wu C. Successful use of the five-in-six system with IVUS guided transradial renal artery stenting. Catheter Cardiovasc Interv. 2011; 77 (5): 750-3.
2. Braunlich S, Ludwig J, Scheinert D. Transradial renal artery angioplasty and stening. J Invasive Cardiol. 2002; 14 (3): 147-149.
3. Coppola J, Kurian D, Staniloae C. Transradial peripheral vascular interventions. Indian Heart J. 2010; 62 (3): 197-201.
4. Galli M, Tarantino F, Mameli S, et al. Transradial approach for renal percutaneous transluminal angioplasty and stenting: a feasibility pilot study. J Invasive Cardiol. 2002; 14 (7): 386-390.
5. Scheinert D, Bräunlich S, Nonnast-Daniel B, et al. Transradial approach for renal artery stenting. Catheter Cardiovasc Interv. 2001; 54 (4): 442-447.
6. Sharma G, Louvard Y, Morice M, et al. Noncoronary transradial angioplasty with coronary equipment: a less invasive technique. Catheter Cardiovasc Interv. 2002; 55 (2): 197-205.
7. Shuck J, Khan A, Cavros N, et al. Transradial renal angioplasty: initial experience. Catheter Cardiovasc Interv. 2001; 54 (3): 346-349.
8. Trani C, Tommasino A, Burzotta F. Transradial renal stenting: why and how. Catheter Cardiovasc Interv. 2009 15; 74 (6): 951-956.
9. Yamashita T, Imai S, Tamada T, et al. Transradial approach for noncoronary angiography and interventions. Catheter Cardiovasc Interv. 2007; 70 (2): 303-308.

17 TRA for Addressing Iliac Artery Lesions

Tejas Patel, John Coppola, Kintur Sanghvi and Sanjay Shah

Approximately one-third of obstructive lesions in lower-extremity peripheral arterial disease affects the aortoiliac segment. Percutaneous intervention with angioplasty and stenting is less invasive and associated with lower morbidity. PCI is as effective as surgery, with very good long-term outcomes. Although TFA is the most common approach, TRA is evolving as a good alternative approach.

Example 1

Right common Iliac artery stenting using the left TRA

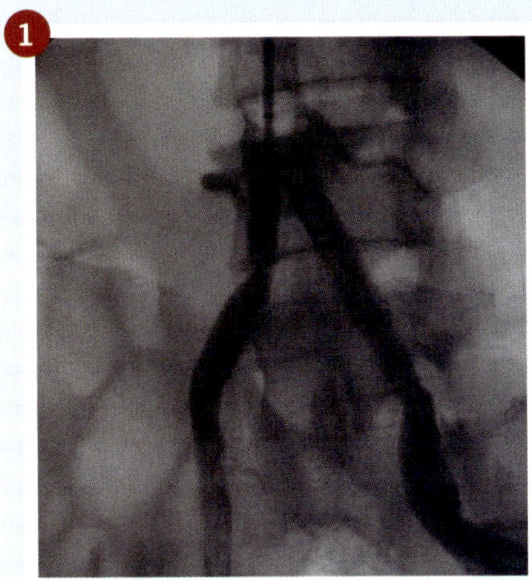

1. A 90 cm long 6 Fr Pinnacle sheath was deployed at the bifurcation, and the lesion was profiled.

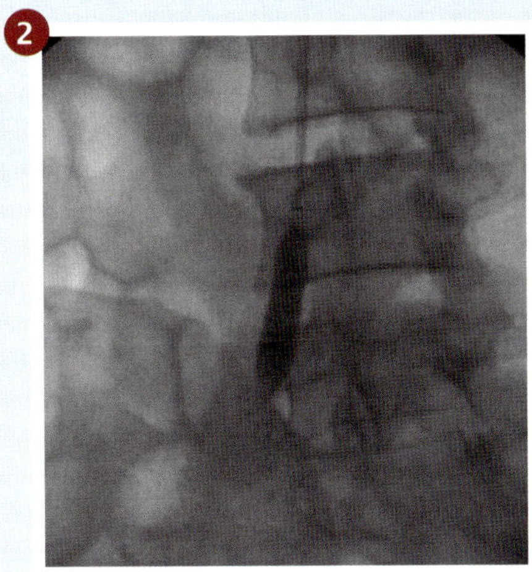

2. A balloon-expandable stent was deployed.

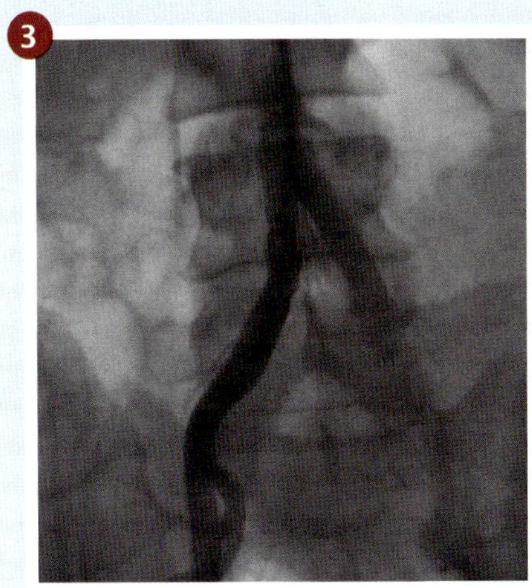

3. The final result is shown.

Example 2

Right common iliac artery stenting using the right TRA.

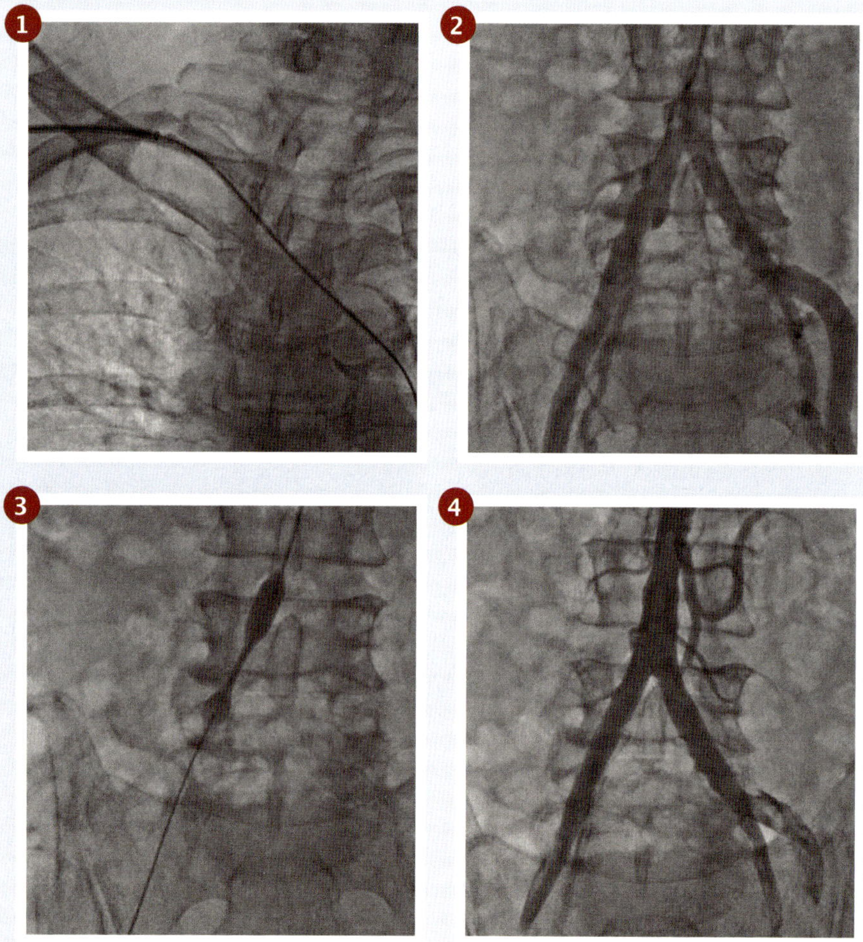

1. A 90 cm long Pinnacle sheath was negotiated from the arch into the descending aorta and kept above the bifurcation.
2. The lesion was profiled.
3. Stenting was done.
4. The final result is shown.

Tips

- Left TRA is a preferred approach because it eliminates the extra length and tortuosity of the aortic arch, allowing relatively easy tracking and deployment of a 100 cm or 110 cm long 6 Fr sheath to the abdominal aorta.
- A patient can be positioned with the head on the caudal end of the cath lab table, leaving the left radial artery approachable from the right side of the table. This can reduce the operator radiation exposure when working on iliacs or the lower extremity. After left radial access is obtained with a 5 Fr short introducer sheath, an IMA, JR 4 or multipurpose catheter is advanced over a long (300 cm) 0.035-inch standard guide wire into the descending aorta. The entire system is then exchanged for a long (90 cm or 110 cm) 6 Fr introducer sheath. The tip of the sheath is positioned at the ostium of the culprit common iliac artery or in the abdominal aorta, just above the bifurcation. The procedure is performed in the usual fashion.
- In difficult cases, the LAO view at 30 to 45 degrees may help in entering the descending aorta along with the use of an angled, hydrophilic, 0.035-inch guide wire.
- Severe tortuosity may make it difficult to advance the long sheath into the descending aorta from the left subclavian artery, and the whole assembly may prolapse in to the ascending aorta. Telescoping over a smaller size multipurpose catheter or exchanging the guidewire for a stiff wire may help in this situation. Selection of a balloon-expandable or self-expandable stent is lesion-specific and left to the discretion of the operator. The shaft length of the stent must be long enough to reach the lesion. In many labs, only short, 80 cm shaft length stents are kept, because TFA is the routine. Availability of the proper equipment should be ensured before starting the procedure.
- If the 110 cm sheath does not reach the ostial Iliac, a 7 Fr multipurpose 125 cm guide through a short (10 cm) 7 Fr sheath can be used in some patients. This will avoid access-contrast use with selective injections of the unilateral extremity and allow better visualization. Equipment accommodated by a 6 Fr introducer sheath can be accommodated by a 7 Fr guide catheter.

Specific Limitations

- Deployment of a long sheath in the descending aorta through the right TRA is more difficult and cumbersome due to aortic arch curvature.
- A 9 mm or larger balloon-expandable stent will not go through a 6 Fr sheath. The longest shaft length on a balloon-expandable stent is 150 cm. Self-expanding stents up to 14 mm can be delivered through a 6 Fr sheath.
- A covered stent up to only 6 mm can be delivered through a 6 Fr sheath. In the case of iliac or external iliac artery perforation, an oversized balloon can be deployed at low pressure to tamponade the artery while anticoagulation is reversed and alternate access is achieved for deploying a larger-size covered stent.

Recommended Reading

1. Flachskampf F, Wolf T, Daniel W, et al. Transradial stenting of the iliac artery: a case report. Catheter Cardiovasc Interv. 2005; 65 (2): 193–195.
2. Pitta S, Barsness G, Lerman A, et al. Transradial iliac artery intervention with dual downstream embolic protection. J Vasc Surg. 2011; 53 (3): 808–810.
3. Sharma G, Louvard Y, Morice M, et al. Noncoronary transradial angioplasty with coronary equipment: a less invasive technique. Catheter Cardiovasc Interv. 2002; 55 (2): 197–205.
4. Staniloae C, Korabathina R, Yu J, et al. Safety and efficacy of transradial aortoiliac interventions. Catheter Cardiovasc Interv. 2010; 75 (5): 659–662.
5. Staniloae C, Kurian D, Coppola J. Transradial bilateral iliac stenting. J Invasive Cardiol. 2006; 18 (10): E256–E257.
6. Yamashita T, Imai S, Tamada T, et al. Transradial approach for noncoronary angiography and interventions. Catheter Cardiovasc Interv. 2007; 70 (2): 303–308.

TRA for Addressing Mesenteric, Celiac and Superficial Femoral Artery Lesions 18

Tejas Patel, John Coppola and Sanjay Shah

Endovascular management of celiac, mesenteric and superficial femoral arterial systems is described in the literature. The TRA is an emerging approach for addressing vascular lesions of these systems, as evidenced by a few case reports and small observational studies.

Example 1

Acute superior mesenteric artery dissection, stenting done through the left TRA

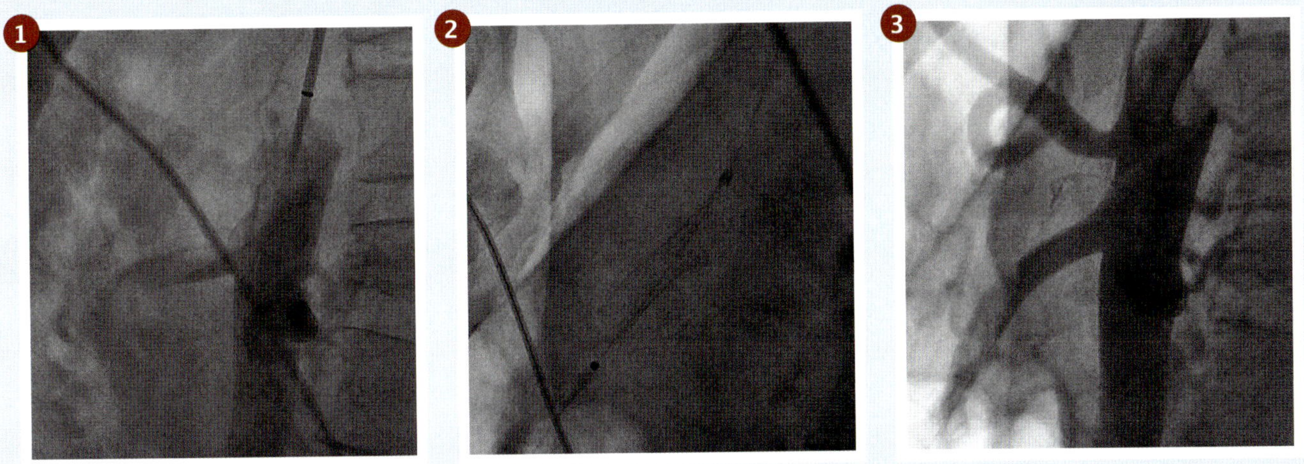

1. A 90 cm long 6 Fr Pinnacle sheath was deployed, and the dissection was profiled.
2. A 0.014-inch BMW PTCA guidewire was negotiated through the true lumen, and a self-expandable stent was deployed.
3. The final result is shown.

Example 2

Left superficial femoral artery PTA done through the left TRA

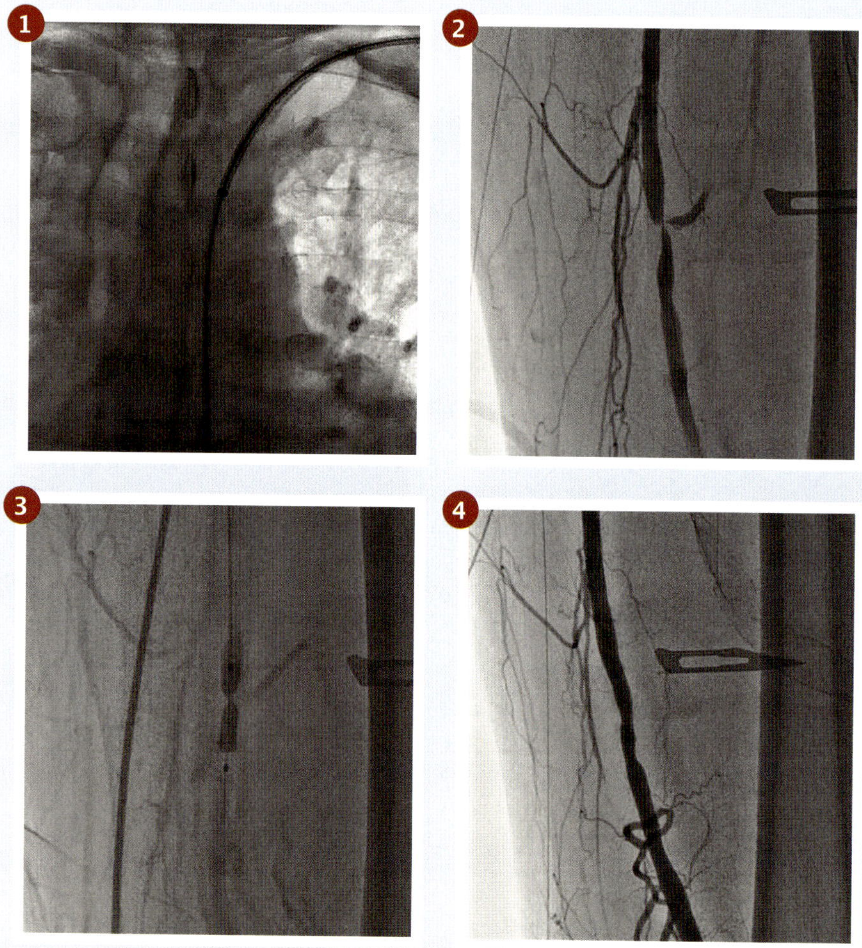

1. A 90 cm long Pinnacle sheath was negotiated into the descending aorta.
2. The lesion was profiled.
3. The PTA was done in the usual fashion using a PTA balloon with a shaft length of 150 cm.
4. The final result is seen.

Example 3

Bilateral iliac and SFA intervention done through the left TRA

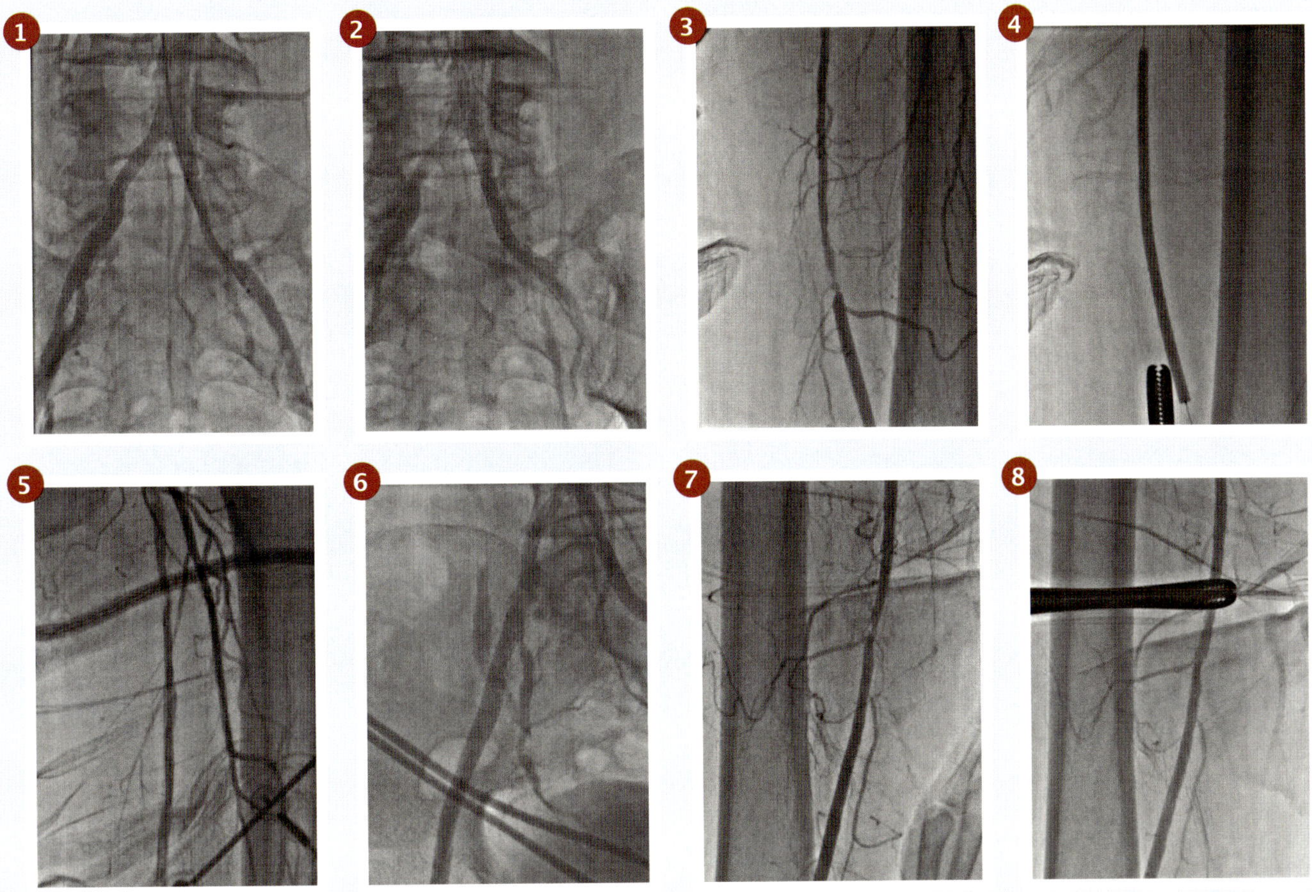

1. Both iliac lesions are profiled.
2. An optimal stent result in the left common iliac stenosis is shown.
3. The left SFA stenosis is profiled.
4. A long PTA balloon is deployed across the lesion.
5. The PTA result is shown.
6. An optimal stent result in the right external iliac stenosis is shown.
7. The right SFA lesion is profiled.
8. An optimal PTA result of the right SFA lesion is seen.

Tips

- The left TRA should be a preferred approach to avoid having to cross the aortic arch. This will allow for 8 cm to 10 cm more working length of the guide catheter.
- The celiac trunk is slightly superior to the renal arteries and can be reached with a normal 100 cm guide catheter from the left radial. The inferior mesenteric arteries may require use of longer guide catheters (125 cm), especially in tall patients.
- Mesenteric arteries arise at a very acute downward angle, especially in very thin patients, leading to easy co-axial cannulation with multipurpose diagnostic or guide catheters through the TRA.
- If the diameter of a mesenteric artery is larger and the stent required does not go through a 6 Fr guide catheter, a long (100 cm or 110 cm) 6 Fr introducer sheath is brought to the descending aorta. A 6 Fr guide catheter is used to selectively cannulate the culprit mesenteric system. After crossing the lesion with a 0.014-inch or a 0.018-inch PTA guidewire, the introducer sheath can be telescoped over the guide close to the ostium of the mesenteric artery. The guide catheter is then carefully removed. A self-expanding, large-diameter stent is negotiated on the same wire and is deployed at the lesion.
- A lateral view is useful for the celiac and mesenteric systems because, most of the time, they arise anteriorly from the aorta.
- For addressing an SFA lesion through the left TRA, a 125 cm long 6 Fr MP or JR guide catheter, a 300 cm long 0.014-inch PTCA guidewire and a long shaft PTA catheter (150 cm) are used. If required, up to a 6 mm self-expanding stent with 150 mm shaft length can be deployed through 6 Fr guides.
- The other approach is to park the distal end of a 110 cm 6 Fr sheath in the Iliac artery in shorter patients. Balloon catheters and self-expanding stents of up to 10 mm diameter can be deployed through 6 Fr sheaths. The longest shaft length of available covered stents in the market is 120 cm, which cannot be deployed in the SFA through the TRA.

Recommended Reading

1. Kelbaek H, Vogt K, Nielsen T, et al. Percutaneous transradial coronary angiography and angioplasty in patients with occlusive atherosclerotic iliofemoral disease. Scand Cardiovasc J. 2000; 34 (1): 84–86.
2. Korabathina R, Yadav S, Coppola J, et al. Transradial approach to lower extremity interventions. Vasc Health Risk Manag. 2010; 9 (6): 503–09.
3. Patel T, Kuladhipati I, Shah S. Successful percutaneous endovascular management of acute post-traumatic superior mesenteric artery dissection using a transradial approach. J Invasive Cardiol. 2010; 22 (4): E61–64.
4. Raghu C, Louvard Y. Transradial approach for percutaneous transluminal angioplasty and stenting in the treatment of chronic mesenteric ischemia. Catheter Cardiovasc Interv. 2004; 61 (4): 450–54.
5. Sanghvi K, Kurian D, Coppola J. Transradial intervention of iliac and superficial femoral artery disease is feasible. J Interv Cardiol. 2008; 21 (5): 385–87.
6. Sharma G, Louvard Y, Morice M, et al. Noncoronary transradial angioplasty with coronary equipment: a less invasive technique. Catheter Cardiovasc Interv. 2002; 55 (2): 197–205.
7. Trani C, Burzotta F, Tommasino A, et al. Transradial approach to treat superficial femoral artery in-stent restenosis. Catheter Cardiovasc Interv. 2009; 1; 74 (3): 494–98.
8. Trani C, Tommasino A, and Burzotta F. Pushing the limits forward: transradial superficial femoral artery stenting. Catheter Cardiovasc Interv. 2010; 76 (7): 1065–71.
9. Yamashita T, Imai S, Tamada T, et al. Transradial approach for noncoronary angiography and interventions. Catheter Cardiovasc Interv. 2007; 70 (2): 303–08.

Rationale for Using the Left Radial Approach

Sanjay Shah, Samir Pancholy and Tejas Patel

19

Most transradial procedures are performed through the right radial artery, but an operator may use the left radial approach just as effectively when the right radial approach is not suitable or not possible.

There is little evidence that there is a significant advantage to using the left radial approach. Some operators prefer it, however, explaining that the anatomical relationship between the left subclavian artery, aortic arch and ascending aorta are more similar to the femoral route and thus make routine catheters (e.g., Judkins) easier to maneuver. (See Chapter 7, "Understanding the Catheter's Course: Radial Versus Femoral.")

Indications for use of the left radial approach

- When the right radial artery pulse is absent.
- For cannulation of a LIMA bypass graft (provided the left radial artery has not been used for the bypass graft). Cannulating and performing interventions on a LIMA bypass graft is very straightforward from the left radial approach because there is no need to cross the aortic arch.
- For diagnostic and interventional procedures in cases of infradiaphragmatic pathology in tall patients (taller than 170 cm) because there is no need to traverse the aortic arch from the left side, thereby saving almost 10 cm of catheter length. Entering the descending aorta is easier and straighter when we approach from the left radial artery. This is an important point given that long catheters and other hardware are still not widely available. Another option in such cases is to go for a high radial puncture, which saves an additional 5 cm to 10 cm of catheter length.
- For left subclavian, left vertebral, LIMA diagnostic and interventional studies, as the approach from the left radial artery is more straightforward.
- For right common and right internal carotid artery interventions; the guide catheter support is much better from the left radial artery because there is no acute bend in the catheter.
- As far as anatomical variations, spasms, or passage challenges go, there is no difference between the right or the left radial artery. Thus, the right is right in most cases.

Recommended Reading

1. Chugh S. Transradial access: right or left? Indian Heart J. 2008; 60 (1 Suppl A): A27-35.
2. Guédès A, Dangoisse V, Gabriel L, et al. Low rate of conversion to transfemoral approach when attempting both radial arteries for coronary angiography and percutaneous coronary intervention: a study of 1,826 consecutive procedures. J Invasive Cardiol. 2010; 22 (9): 391-397.
3. Kanei Y, Nakra N, Liou M, et al. Randomized comparison of transradial coronary angiography via right or left radial artery approaches. Am J Cardiol. 2011; 107 (2): 195-197.
4. Kawashima O, Endoh N, Terashima M, et al. Effectiveness of right or left radial approach for coronary angiography. Catheter Cardiovasc Interv. 2004; 61 (3): 333-337.
5. Mann T, Cubeddu G, Schneider J, et al. Left internal mammary artery intervention: the left radial approach with a new guide catheter. J Invasive Cardiol. 2000; 12 (6): 298-302.
6. Martinez C, Cohen M. Left or right, transradial access for all. J Invasive Cardiol. 2010; 22 (9): 398-399.
7. Santas E, Bodí V, Sanchis J, et al. The left radial approach in daily practice. A randomized study comparing femoral and right and left radial approaches. Rev Esp Cardiol. 2009; 62 (5): 482-490.
8. Sciahbasi A, Romagnoli E, Burzotta F, et al. Transradial approach (left vs right) and procedural times during percutaneous coronary procedures: TALENT study. Am Heart J. 2011; 161 (1): 172-179.

Right Heart Catheterization Through the Radial Approach

20

Ian Gilchrist

Werner Forssmann, MD, reported on and later was awarded a Nobel prize for his early work demonstrating the feasibility of performing a right heart catheterization through a peripheral vein. Over time, the art of peripheral access to the central venous system was increasingly forgotten. But the advent of percutaneous transradial arterial procedures necessitated central venous and right heart access to compliment the eloquent techniques being developed for arterial access. The technique to obtain central venous access from a peripheral arm vein is relatively simple and lets the radialist complete the tool chest for a primarily radial practice.

Venous Anatomy of the Lower Arm

- These veins are highly variable.
- Includes superficial and deep veins.
- The radial (lateral) veins of the forearm feed up either the cephalic or brachial veins.
- Ulnar (medial) veins generally drain up the brachial vein.

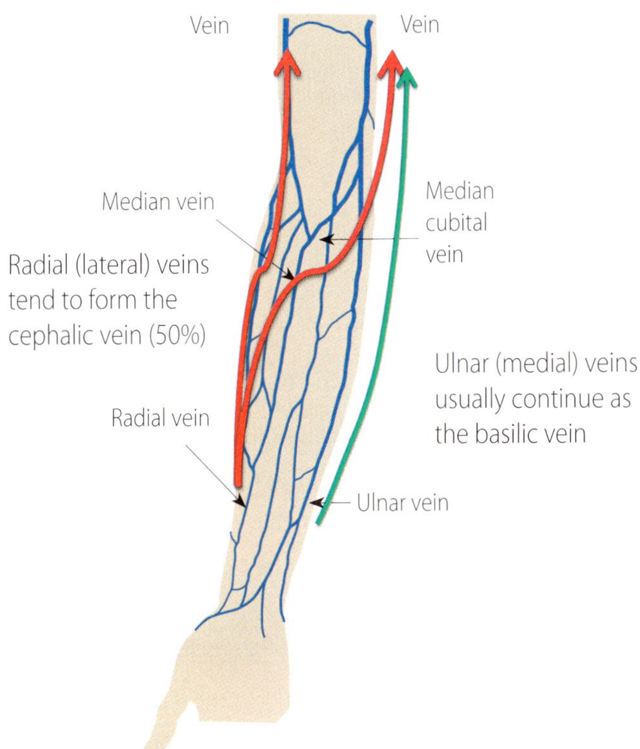

Venous Anatomy of the Upper Arm

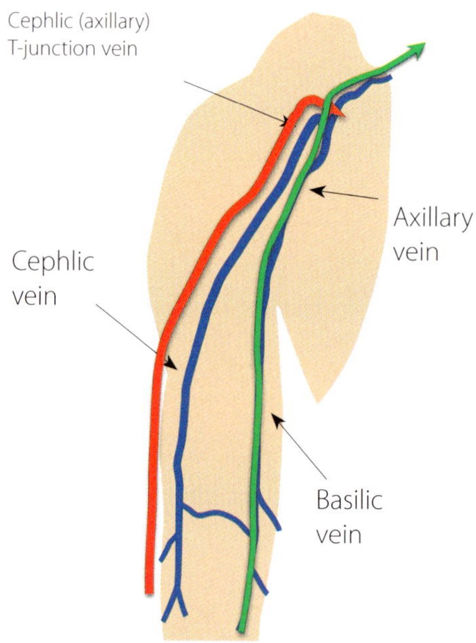

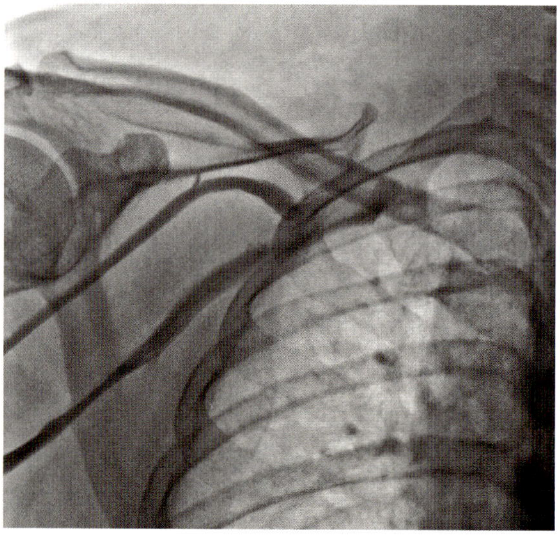

- The axillary and cephalic veins meet to form the subclavian vein.
- The cephalic vein enters the axillary system at a right angle (T-junction) that may misdirect a catheter traversing centrally via the cephalic system.
- Beyond the T-junction is the subclavian vein, which normally passes to the right atrium.

Comparison of Arm Venous and Arterial Systems

- Veins have greater *anatomic variability.*
- Venous collaterals and redundancy are common.
- Veins are *relatively distensible.*
- Venous pressure is much lower than arterial pressure.
- Vasospasm is rare and responds to warmth and nitrates, not Ca^{++} channel blockers.

Obtaining Preliminary Venous Access

- The IV team or nurse establishes IV access *before entering the cath lab* and it is preserved as a heparin cap. This encourages the most efficient use of lab time.
- Staff should use a standard IV angio (e.g., 20 gauge) catheter *in the cath lab* before the start of the procedure.
- The physician should work directly with micropuncture kit +/− tourniquet *in the cath lab.*
- Difficult access may require ultrasound or levophase angiogram techniques.

From Initial Venous Access to Appropriate Vascular Sheath (4 Fr to 8 Fr)

- Lidocaine may be needed at the skin site.
- The vein is often superficial and can be damaged if a blade is used.
- The sheath should be flushed, although low venous pressure may prevent backflow of blood.

Placement of Right Heart Catheter

- Arm passage should be smooth and without resistance.
- Resistance should prompt a limited venogram.
- The fluoroscope should be positioned at shoulder level to confirm the location at the T-junction.

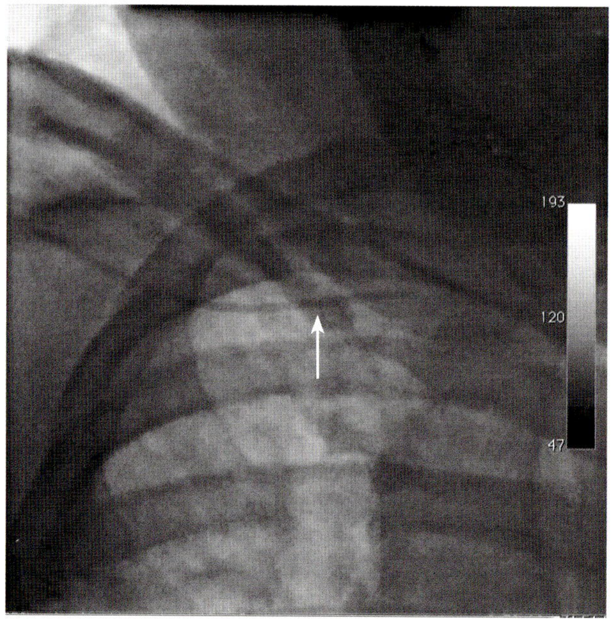

- Passage via the cephalic vein may require an additional wire to help direct the catheter into the subclavian.
- A balloon-tipped catheter should not be inflated until the subclavian vessel has been entered.
- Once into the subclavian region, passage should be similar to the more common subclavian or internal jugular approaches.

Termination of Procedure

- Deflate the balloon. Remove the central venous catheter.
- The sheath can be removed and a simple pressure dressing applied.

Challenges

- Spasm is rare and responds to nitrates and warmth.
- Prior trauma or permanent pacing devices may have thrombosed the central system.
- Lymphedema or previous breast cancer surgery are relative contraindications.
- Commercially available catheters may not allow entry at some patients' wrist levels if the length limited to 110 cm; such peripheral entry may be possible in some patients with shorter arms.
- Similar techniques can be used to place temporary pacemakers and perform right ventricular biopsy.

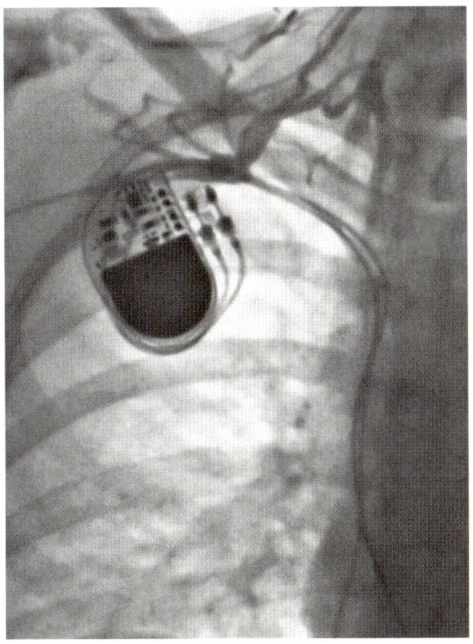

Thrombosis of the subclavian vein has been caused by pacemaker leads. The right heart catheter is seen with contrast in it at the level of the pacemaker can. The right heart catheter was able to negotiate the jugular vein collateral to reach the right heart successfully despite thrombosis.

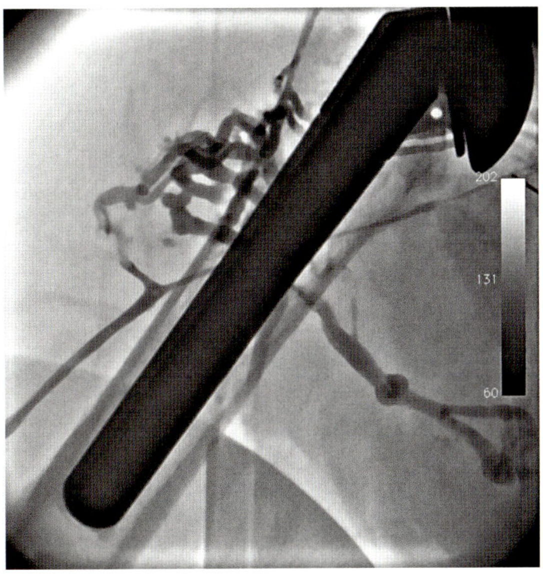

Thrombosis of the brachial/axillary system has been caused by humerus fracture and subsequent repair of the shoulder. A channel to pass the catheter through could not be found.

Recommended Reading

1. Cheng N-J, Ho W-J, Ko Y-S, et al. Percutaneous cardiac catheterization combining direct venipuncture of superficial forearm veins and transradial arterial approach. A feasible approach. Acta Cardiol Sin. 2003; 19: 159-164.
2. Chun HJ, Byun JY, Yoo SS, et al. Tourniquet application to facilitate axillary venous access in percutaneous central venous catheterization. Radiology. 2003; 226: 918-920.
3. Gilchrist IC, Kharabsheh S, Nickolaus MJ, et al. Radial approach to right heart catheterization: early experience with a promising technique. Cathet Cardiovasc Interv. 2002; 55: 20-22.
4. Gilchrist IC, Moyer CD, Gascho JA. Transradial right and left heart catheterizations: a comparison to traditional femoral approach. Catheter Cardiovasc Interv 2006; 67: 585-588.
5. Lo TSN, Buch AN, Hall IR, et al. Percutaneous left and right heart catheterization in fully anticoagulated patients utilizing the radial artery and forearm vein: A two-center experience. J Interven Cardiol. 2006; 19: 258-263.
6. Pancholy SB, Sweeney J. A technique to access difficult to find upper extremity veins for right heart catheterization: The levogram technique. Catheter Cardiovasc Interv. 2010, DOI: 10.1002/ccd.23037
7. Tebet MA, de Andrade PB, de Andrade1 MVA, et al. Safety and efficacy of transradial right and left heart catheterization compared with transfemoral approach: An initial experience. Rev Bras Cardiol Invas. 2008; 16(3): 317-321.
8. Yang C-H, Wu C-J. Percutaneous cardiac catheterization combining direct venipuncture of superficial forearm veins and transradial artery approach. Acta Cardiol Sin. 2003; 19: 166-167.
9. Yang CH, Guo GB, Yip HK, et al. Bilateral cardiac catheterizations: the safety and feasibility of a superficial forearm venous and transradial arterial approach. Int Heart J. 2006; 47(1): 21-27.

Transradial Approach: Present Status and Future Directions

21

Mitchell Krucoff

As evidenced by the growing number of clinical reports, symposia and training programs, and procedural volume, transradial catheterization and intervention (TRI) is rapidly emerging as a widely practiced technique, with progressive advocacy for use as a first-line option rather than for bail-out scenarios. As shown in Tables 1 and 2, which compare and contrast femoral and radial approaches, in the hands of experienced operators, advantages of TRI include

- lower bleeding risk,
- fewer vascular-access complications,
- less post-procedure management,
- increased patient comfort and satisfaction, and
- potentially lower costs.

Despite these perceptions, after more than a decade, uptake of radial technique remains regionally diverse worldwide, with the lowest rates of adoption in some of the world's largest interventional communities such as the United States. Even within single centers, individual practitioners frequently vary in both perspectives and practices.

As a technique rather than a breakthrough technology, since first described for PCI in 1993 by Kiemeneij, TRI has gradually developed acceptance through grass roots evolution, as described by Gilchrist, rather than as a revolution. Femoral arteriotomy, with more than 30 million cases performed over 3 decades, is a mature area of interventional skills, with highly developed equipment, thorough training guidelines, well-defined complication rates, and integration into the logistics and economics of clinical practice. Acceptance and growth of TRI is thus challenged to convincingly show that the disruption of change is outweighed by value — to patients, to practitioners, and to healthcare systems — and to prove this value with robust data. To do this, a broad range of concerns about changes from femoral to TRI need to be directly addressed. These include the following:

- access failure and crossover rates;
- procedural duration, fluoroscopy time and contrast use;
- procedural success rates;
- equipment limitations;
- learning curve metrics and processes for training; and
- clinical outcome benefits.

Dedicated pioneers and investigators, in conjunction with critical advances in state of the art interventional equipment, have led TRI from a niche technique to the tipping point of a new landscape for invasive cardiology — but much work remains to be done. In this chapter, we will review both the current state of these incentives and concerns, as well as look toward key directions for the future with TRI.

Current Technical Influences and TRI Adoption

Negotiating the Learning Curve and Having Confidence That You Can Finish What You Start

As contemporary clinical practice routinely includes ad hoc PCI, confidence that radial access for diagnostic purposes can support successful intervention is critical. With the advent of more flexible, CoCr drug-eluting stents, low-profile RX shaft balloons and 6 Fr guide catheters with inner lumen diameters of > 0.70 inches that will accommodate rotablator burrs up to 1.5 mm or kissing balloon combinations, TRI has become a reliable modality for access in the vast majority of clinical practice cases. In fact, once a guide catheter is well-seated below the sinotubular junction, performing PCI from the wrist is simply identical to that performed from the leg — until the operator goes to pull the sheath.

Reaching this level of confidence requires that the operator conquer the learning curve reaching from the wrist to the aortic root, which has key differences from the femoral approach. Technical obstacles unique to TRI can be divided into six areas:

- access to small-caliber vessel,
- traversing from wrist to aortic root,
- catheters and their manipulation,
- spasm,

- operator attitude; and
- hemostasis, durability and occlusion.

Management of each of these areas is detailed throughout this book. Overall, these technical features are central to both the present status and future direction of TRI. Difficulties with access or with coronary intubation may prolong procedure times. Anomalous branches or loops in the arm or Z-curves and arteria lusoria entering the aortic arch can add to fluoroscopic time and contrast use. Extensive catheter manipulation either traversing these obstacles or intubating coronaries may elicit radial spasm despite the use of vasodilators and sedation. Failure to manage these technical obstacles may lead to access failure, crossover, procedural failure or combinations of all of these.

A study of 1,024 patients randomized to TRI versus a transfemoral approach, in which operator experience level was described as moderate, Brueck and colleagues found that radial access failure was 3.2% versus 0.1% with the transfemoral approach and was related to more frequent procedural failure overall. Average procedural time was about 3 minutes longer, while fluoroscopy time was almost double with TRI. In a meta-analysis of 12 randomized trials of 3,224 patients undergoing diagnostic and interventional procedures, Agostoni reported that odds of procedural failure with TRI were 3.3 times higher (95% confidence interval 1.63 to 6.71), and fluoroscopy time was significantly higher (8.9 versus 7.8 minutes) compared to femoral. Similar observations were also described by Jolly in a more recent report compiling 7,000 patients from 23 studies.

On the encouraging side, these technical concerns improve with experience. In the TALENT study, in which right and left radial approaches were randomized in 1,540 patients, fluoroscopy time from the right for diagnostic procedures was 48 seconds longer for trainees versus 8 seconds longer with experienced operators. Both Spaulding and Jolly have correlated operator volume and experience with lower access failure, shorter procedure times and higher PCI success rates.

Overcoming technical challenges, such as negotiating the TRI learning curve, is the most immediate and most manageable impediment to transradial adoption. Whereas for experienced femoral operators catheter behavior is predictable, easily taught, and identical from either the left or right leg, with TRI, as Patel describes in this book, the operator must get a feel for the catheter. In almost every case, the right and left radial approaches are quite different from one another, and teaching the technique is never by rote. Adoption of gentle technique, heightened awareness of resistance, and education in tips and tricks are fundamental to success. Attention to TRI technique and training are on the rise thanks to established training courses in India, Japan and (recently) by the Society of Coronary Angiography and Intervention in the United States, as well as the development of simulators by industry manufacturers.

Negotiating the TRI learning curve is not only a matter of technical skills, but a state of mind. With due respect to safety and common sense, a problem-solving attitude committed to finishing what you start is as critical as the mechanical techniques. Such a positive state of mind will transform a road of potential frustration and failure into a path of learning that generates experience, success and TRI expertise. This road is quickly reinforced by the happiness of patients. Good mentorship — along with personal patience, commitment, creativity and awareness — breed the confidence to continue, to complete and to grow as a TRI operator, through and beyond the early learning curve.

There must also be awareness of what TRI offers and the conviction to deliver this benefit to patients. In the Brueck study, even with only moderately experienced TRI operators, longer TRI procedures and the use of femoral closure devices in 93% of cases, vascular complications and bleeding were reduced from 3.7% with transfemoral to 0.6% with TRI. In the 3,224 randomized patients collected in the the Agostoni meta-analysis and 5,600 in the Jolly meta-analysis, major hematoma, vascular surgery and arteriovenous fistula were reduced by 80%, and major bleeding by 73%. To traverse the learning curve, TRI operators must develop disciplined attitudes:

- calm, technically creative problem solving;

Example 2

Right common iliac artery stenting using the right TRA.

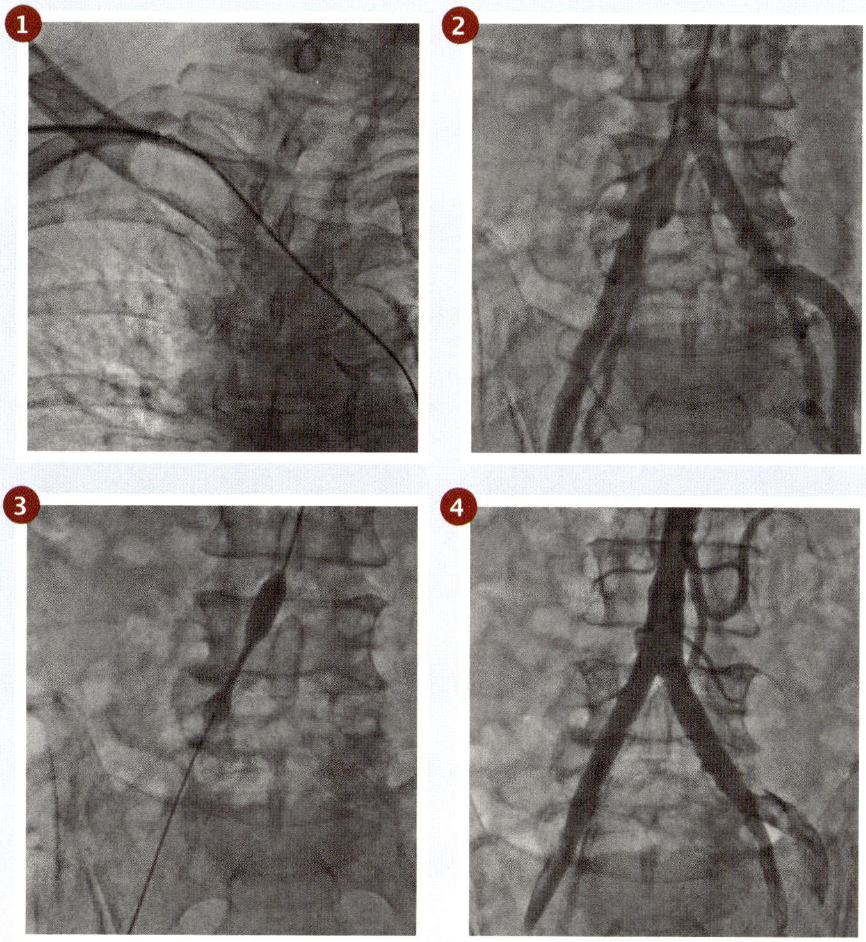

1. A 90 cm long Pinnacle sheath was negotiated from the arch into the descending aorta and kept above the bifurcation.
2. The lesion was profiled.
3. Stenting was done.
4. The final result is shown.

TRA for Addressing Iliac Artery Lesions

Tejas Patel, John Coppola, Kintur Sanghvi and Sanjay Shah

17

Approximately one-third of obstructive lesions in lower-extremity peripheral arterial disease affects the aortoiliac segment. Percutaneous intervention with angioplasty and stenting is less invasive and associated with lower morbidity. PCI is as effective as surgery, with very good long-term outcomes. Although TFA is the most common approach, TRA is evolving as a good alternative approach.

Example 1

Right common Iliac artery stenting using the left TRA

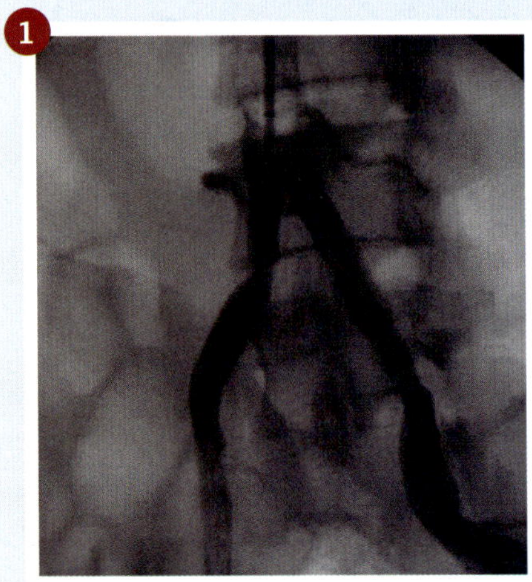

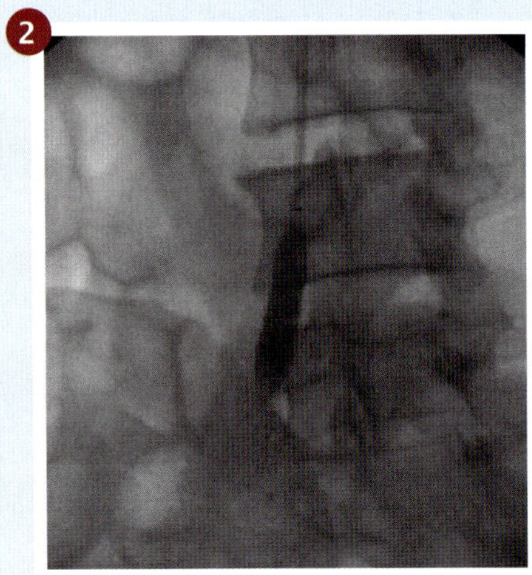

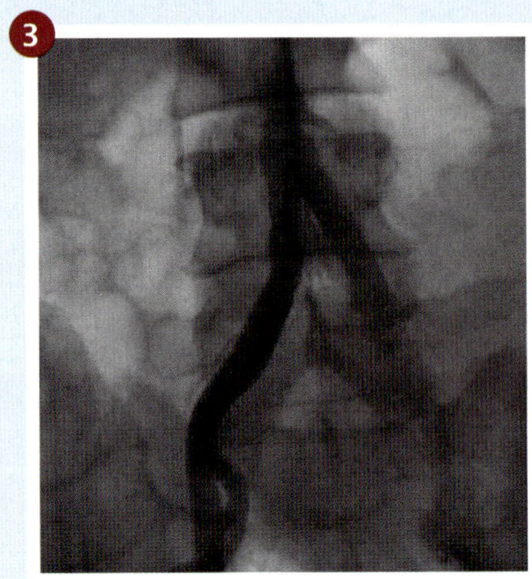

1. A 90 cm long 6 Fr Pinnacle sheath was deployed at the bifurcation, and the lesion was profiled.
2. A balloon-expandable stent was deployed.
3. The final result is shown.

- commitment to completing cases (including common sense and safety awareness); and
- conviction of the benefit to patients.

Understanding and addressing the learning curve is crucial to individual operators and the field itself, as data from outcomes studies may be directly affected by the level of experience of participating operators. High rates of conversion from radial to femoral in randomized trials could offset otherwise-important outcome differences. Procedural delays in access or coronary intubation in time-critical settings such as STEMI could undermine other possible benefits. Reliable results from multicenter trials will emerge only when we have reliable networks of experienced TRI operators.

Finally, in our technical approaches, it must be recognized that patients who undergo catheterization, particularly PCI, may need the procedure repeated. While the superficial anatomy of the radial artery facilitates bleeding reduction, its small-caliber relative to sheaths and catheters makes it more vulnerable to early and late occlusion. Use of anticoagulants and vasodilators is essential. Recently, Pancholy and others have reported randomized use of pulse oximetry-based reverse Allen's testing or mean arterial pressure during compression, or "patent hemostasis," with significant reductions of radial artery occlusion from 12% to under 5% at 24 hours, and from 7% to 1.8% at 30 days. If TRI can be repeated only once or twice in the lifetime of a CAD patient, its adoption will remain limited. While the TRI arteriotomy may be more manageable than femoral with regard to bleeding, operators must pay careful attention to preserving the durability of this much smaller access route.

Clinical Outcomes Data: Where is TRI, and Where Does It Need to Go?

In 26,452 ACS patients from the PURSUIT, PARAGON A, PARAGON B and GUSTO IIb studies, Rao and colleagues reported a greater than fivefold increase in 30-day mortality in patients suffering severe bleeding complications. In patients with specifically procedure-related bleeding, the 30-day mortality was over 15%. In 2,498 ACS patients from the

PREMIER study, Wang and colleagues reported the association of bleeding and early interruption of aspirin, thienopyridine or both during the index hospitalization in around 50% of patients — i.e., interruption of anti-platelet therapy when stent sites are most vulnerable to acute thrombosis.

These and other related data set the conceptual stage for the most profound range of potential benefits associated with TRI's anatomic proclivity for reducing procedural bleeding. Beginning with Ferdinand Kiemeneij's first randomized report of radial, brachial and femoral arteriotomy in 900 patients in the ACCESS study, multiple studies have consistently reported significant reductions in access site complications and bleeding. In the Jolly meta-analysis, the odds ratio of bleeding with TRI was 0.27 (95% 0.16-0.45, $P < .001$). In observational data from more than 500,000 patients undergoing PCI compiled in the National Cardiovascular Data Registry, Rao and colleagues reported even larger reductions in bleeding rates in specific high-risk subgroups, such as ACS patients and women. With a > 70% reduction in bleeding, intuitively the clinical consequences of TRI include the following:

- **potential reductions in death, MI and stent thrombosis;**
- **potential reductions in transfusions, vascular procedures and lengths of stay;**
- **potential cost reductions; and**
- **potential enhancements of post-procedural comfort and satisfaction.**

However, clinical outcomes such as death, MI and stent thrombosis are driven by many factors in the CAD population, and the role of reduced procedural bleeding cannot simply be assumed. Carefully assess caveats for this assumption:

- Non-CABG bleeding is arteriotomy related in 70% of elective PCI patients, but in only 30% of ACS patients.

- Definitions for bleeding and vascular complications vary greatly across studies.
- Bleeding and vascular complication rates vary with body habitus, sex, clinical presentation and adjunctive medical regimens.
- Absolute femoral-access bleeding reports range from less than 2% to more than 5%, averaging 2.3% in the Jolly meta-analysis; non-CABG major bleeding with femoral access was 0.9% in the RIVAL study.
- Bleeding, transfusions and higher mortality have been *correlated*; however mechanistic *causality* that bleeding leads to higher mortality is not established.

Understanding where the field stands in proving the benefits of TRI requires insight into available data in light of these caveats. The risk/benefit profiles are likely to vary with regard to TRI for elective diagnostic patients who do not have coronary disease at all, for elective PCI patients, for ACS and for STEMI intervention compared to femoral access. For the future of TRI, much work needs to be done to define such benefits — and related risks — in each of these cohorts.

Correlation and even causality between reduced bleeding, transfusions and mortality remains another central area of interest. Schiabasi and colleagues reported significant reductions in both in-hospital bleeding (0.7% versus 2.4%, $P < 0.05$) and 1-year mortality (5.5% versus 9.9%, $P < 0.05$) in non-STEMI ACS patients from the PRESTO ACS vascular substudy with TRI versus femoral, respectively. In the British Columbia Cardiac Registry reported by Chase and colleagues in the Mortality benefit Of Reduced Transfusion after intervention via the Arm or Leg (MORTAL) study, which examined 38,872 patients, about 21% of whom had TRI, blood transfusion rates were significantly lower (1.4% versus 2.8%, $P < 0.01$), as were 30-day (1.0% versus 1.7%, $P < 0.01$) and 1-year mortalities (2.8% versus 3.9%, $P < 0.01$). On the other hand, despite significantly reduced access complications, Jolly's meta-analysis showed no mortality

difference between TRI and femoral (1.2 versus 1.8%, OR: 0.74; 95% confidence interval: 0.42–1.30. P = 0.29) with a benefit trend for only combined death, MI and stroke (2.5 versus 3.8%, OR: 0.71; 95% confidence interval 0.49–1.01. P = 0.58).
In the most contemporary and largest randomized trial to date, the RadIal Vs femorAL access for coronary intervention (RIVAL) trial, 7,021 ACS patients were followed for a primary outcome of 30-day composite death, MI, stroke, or non-coronary artery bypass graft (non-CABG) -related major bleeding, with no difference between the groups (3.7% versus 4.0%; hazard ratio [HR] 0.92, 95% CI 0.72–1.17; P = 0.50). Combined death, MI and stroke was also no different (3.2% versus 3.2%, (HR 0.98, 95% CI 0.76–1.28; P = 0.90). Notably, non-CABG-related major bleeding was only 0.9% in the femoral group, not significantly different from the radial group's 0.7% (HR 0.73, 95% CI 0.43–1.23; P = 0.23).

Of equal importance, in a prespecified analysis, benefit for the primary clinical endpoints with radial access interacted significantly with the highest-volume tercile radial centers (HR 0.49, 95% CI 0.28–0.87; P = 0.015). This is illustrated in Figure 1. Another important observation: Improvement in the primary clinical outcome was composite in patients with STEMI randomized to TRI (HR 0.60, 0.38–0.94; P = 0.026), although whether the site experience level had a role (e.g., did only more experienced TRI sites randomize STEMI patients?) in this finding was not described.

Thus the interpretative context for current and future TRI clinical data should include attention to the following:

- the patient population under study,
- the experience of participating operators,
- the application of endpoint definitions, and
- the study design (randomized or observational, single or multicenter).

Economics and Quality-of-Life Data
Another intuitively evident benefit of TRI compared to femoral access is how it reduces patient-management needs, complication rates and lengths of stay — all of which might translate into measurable economic savings and improved

quality-of-life metrics. International differences in charges, hospital costs and reimbursement structures, as well as ongoing changes in these processes over time, make economic data critical and yet complex.
Randomized data from diagnostic catheterization procedures by Cooper et al calculated an average cost savings of \$290 per case based on bed, nursing and pharmacy cost reductions. In a randomized comparison to femoral access with the use of closure devices that allowed faster recovery times, Roussanov et al found costs with TRI still averaged \$184 less per case.

In elective PCI, Amoroso et al reported a 50% reduction in nursing time post-procedure with TRI compared to femoral access. In 142 ACS patients undergoing PCI randomized to femoral or TRI, Roussanov also reported a 1.5-day reduction in length of stay with a cost savings calculated at \$2,913 per procedure. In another elective stenting cohort in which femoral closure devices were routinely used, Mann and colleagues described similar lengths of stay between the groups, with high costs and complication rates in the femoral-closure patients compared to TRI patients.

The TRI literature continues to grow in both volume and quality. Nonetheless, most available reports constitute small, single-center studies — some randomized and others purely observational — whose generalizability is unknown. Recently, much larger reports of outcomes modeled from quality registries have added insight to clinical practice, but do not constitute robust randomized evidence of benefit. Most recently, the RIVAL study further crystallized the critical need for large, multicenter studies to address key questions about the clinical benefits of TRI versus best femoral access.

TRI: Future Needs and Directions

Interventional cardiology includes a broad array of fast-moving technologies applied to an epidemic international patient population. TRI technique, with unequivocal bleeding reduction, enhanced patient comfort and reduced post-procedure management needs, has benefitted from the advent of smaller, more flexible stents and guide catheters, and the dedicated work of investigators willing to perform research and report findings. Together, these efforts have tipped TRI adoption from rare and isolated operators and centers to a progressively expanding and accelerating spread as a standard of care.

To advance TRI from pockets of acceptance to the international standard of care for frontline invasive cardiology, there are five major keys:

1. **Technical needs**
   - dedicated TRI equipment
   - methodological best practices
   - learning curve metrics
   - systematic training and certification program

2. **Clinical data**
   - patient-selection criteria
   - cohort-specific risk and benefit profiles

3. **Economic and quality-of-life (QOL) information**
   - cost-effectiveness models
   - dedicated QOL instruments
   - comparative effectiveness
   - customer satisfaction

4. **New applications**
   - carotid stenting
   - renal intervention
   - peripheral intervention
   - adjunct to structural heart intervention

5. **Vascular access safety training (VAST) and integration**
   - patient-safety orientation
   - TRI competence
   - femoral competence
   - principles of optimal arteriotomy management
   - access techniques
   - use of imaging
   - Compression techniques
   - Risk factors
   - Adjunctive medications
   - Follow-up endpoints and timelines

Technical needs: A major advance that essentially eliminated radial access site granulomas is the advent of dedicated, lubricious radial-access sheaths. Work is ongoing with 7.5 Fr sheathless guide catheters that may facilitate TRI PCI that requires > 6 Fr guide catheters without compromising short- and long-term radial patency. New compression devices have also supported more meticulous approaches to arteriotomy closure and patent hemostatsis to enhance durability of the radial artery for repeated access.

Beyond the arteriotomy site, additional technical innovations are needed to further optimize procedural duration and success. Use of PCI wires and balloons to traverse radial loops is time-consuming and expensive, and more attention to developing wires, sleeves and inserts better suited for wrist arteries is warranted. Dedicated diagnostic and guide catheters for radial procedures should not only accommodate key differences from the femoral approach for coronary intubation and support. It should also be recognized that right and left radial approaches are spatially different from one another, as shown in the TALENT study. Devices suited to special technical challenges, such as patients with both LIMA and RIMA grafts, create opportunities for physicians and engineers to work together. Longer catheters may also have a place in patients for whom the distance to the coronary from the wrist is farther than from the leg.

Continued advances decreasing the size of interventional equipment, including stent-wire technologies and 4 Fr guide catheters represent another area of technological advance ideal for TRI. Such "slim club" constructs in the future could include IVUS, balloon pump and other technologies.

Methodologic best practices for TRI are needed not only for patient care, but to make monitoring and reporting of complication rates more interpretable relative to clinical practice. Risk stratification with the Allen's test, use of sedation, anticoagulation, vasodilators and compression techniques such as patent hemostasis need to be systematized either through expert consensus or data, but not simply relegated to the vicissitudes of individual operator preferences.

Learning curve metrics should be developed based on key areas of concern — access failure, procedure duration and success, fluoroscopic time — then tracked as quality indicators to quantify levels of expertise. More than case volume alone can convey, such metrics are useful for individuals to mark progress, for the field to assess novel training tools that may accelerate the learning curve, and for research efforts in which operator proficiency is clearly a key feature of study design and results.

To pull all of this together, systematic training in TRI and certification standards must be developed. Currently in the United States, the ACC/SCAI Core Cardiology Training Symposium (COCATS) Task Force 3 Training in Interventional and Diagnostic Cardiac Catheterization mentions little more specific than case numbers regarding arteriotomy proficiency, and says almost nothing about radial technique per se. Equally important is the development of training and certification standards for cath lab staff as well as for interventional operators. Converting from femoral access to TRI includes the whole cath lab and recovery team, not just the operator. Developing clear steps to augment this conversion and demonstrate competence at all levels of staffing is mandatory for TRI to emerge as standard of care.

Clinical data: Quantification of clinical benefits and risks associated with TRI will continue to be central to the growth of interest in the technique and growth of the technique itself. Patient selection criteria must be based on the unique risks and benefits associated with specifics of patient age, body habitus, sex and concomitant medications, to name a few. Similarly, risks and benefits specific to clinical presentation and application — diagnostic angiography in patients with no CAD, in patients undergoing elective PCI, in patients presenting with acute coronary syndromes, in patients with STEMI, in patients with shock in conjunction with femoral access for balloon pumps or other assist devices — will vary across these cohorts. Unique settings such as uninterrupted management of patients on warfarin is another area for future exploration. To understand and promote meaningful risk-benefit profiles able to support best practice guidelines will require high-quality, interpretable clinical data.

Economics and QOL: With greater patient comfort, more rapid ambulation and reduced vascular complication rates, TRI has many features that could favorably reduce costs and enhance quality of life. On the other hand, if coronary equipment is used to traverse the wrist, and multiple catheters and more contrast are used for procedures, the balance might be less convincing. Managing vascular complication rates and extended length of stay are significant cost drivers, while the benefits of new paradigms such as same-day discharge for PCI may support lower reimbursement decisions for which hospitals could actually lose money. Other aspects of TRI, such as less nursing-intensive holding areas, which seem favorable, may be balanced against slower overall cath lab throughput, particularly early in the learning curve. Thus the economic impact of TRI is related to many factors beyond reduction of access site complications, and novel models to quantify this impact need to be developed.

TRI's impact on QOL also spans a range of issues that currently available survey instruments may not adequately capture. Some are self-evident — if TRI reduces death, MI and stroke, commensurate impact on QOL is predictable. Other issues may be quite subtle — if a patient who uses the hand professionally, such as a musician, suffers "silent" radial artery occlusion, is it really inconsequential? Short-term index procedure QOL metrics may be easy to gather, but longer-term issues related to repeated use of the radial artery may be more difficult and unique. The development of QOL survey instruments specific to vascular access issues would add greatly to our knowledge.

In the United States, government agencies are showing progressive interest in developing comparative-effectiveness metrics that would quantify the overall benefit of one therapeutic strategy versus other available options. Such metrics are intended to integrate clinical benefit and risk, QOL, cost, and even patient preferences. The development of comparative-effectiveness models for TRI compared to femoral intervention may be an important part of the future.

New applications: Growing confidence in and experience with TRI and the coronaries has spawned bold extensions to other interventional vascular beds, as detailed in several chapters of this book. Carotid stenting, renal intervention and peripheral intervention from the wrist will face many similar challenges to the shift from femoral to TRI in the coronaries, from clinical benefit and risks to technical issues, such as procedure success rates or the need for specially shaped or longer catheters.

Another important area for TRI growth is as an adjunct to structural heart interventions, which require very large sheath sizes or surgically created access in the femoral artery. Ancillary catheters such as a pigtail for aortograms before and after TAVI procedures, or as snares for entrapped tips, portend a hybrid environment where small catheters from the wrist may help with procedural and bleeding safety overall, particularly as these tend to be frail patients.

The Vascular Access Safety Training (VAST) Agenda: Moving TRI From Isolation to Integration

As a relative newcomer to the longstanding femoral access world of PCI, developing from the grassroots efforts of highly motivated and skilled individual operators, for TRI to achieve widespread, first-line, standard-of-care acceptance, it is important to overcome tendencies toward political or emotional advocacy of "femoralists" or "radialists" and restore the focus of the interventional community to the key question at the patient level: the primary issue of vascular access safety. The enthusiasm of pioneers so critical to moving TRI forward must be carefully separated from over-enthusiastic attempts to represent TRI as more beneficial or proven than it is.

While safety has many aspects in this context — including patient and operator safety — the VAST agenda recognizes that interventional cardiologists in the modern era require competence in both TRI and femoral access, not one or the other. Similarly, cath lab staff must be trained, and equipment configurations, recovery facilities and discharge education must be developed for both procedure types. The VAST agenda must be an integrated one. Best practices using TRI and femoral-access options will be delivered to patients only by operators and cath labs who are proficient in both.

Thus the VAST agenda should endeavor to develop core training approaches that highlight similarities and key differences in arteriotomy management of both femoral and radial access — arteriotomy techniques, use of imaging and landmarks, compression techniques, vascular risk factors, adjunctive medications, and appropriate follow-up endpoints and timelines. A balanced and integrated VAST focus is good for the advance of TRI to first-line therapy, even as TRI is good for the vast majority of patients.

Summary: TRI Present and Future

Dedicated pioneers have moved TRI from an isolated niche to a more widely applied technique that potentially benefits clinical outcomes, patient comfort and satisfaction, and healthcare costs and logistics. Building on this progression, bringing TRI to the next level as the accepted front-line approach and standard of care for diagnostic cath and PCI requires the efforts of a dedicated community of practitioners willing to do high-quality, meticulous clinical work and research.

Technical advances and systematic training with key quality metrics remain the core needs for TRI's advance. Metering and mastering the learning curve, both technically and as a state of mind, address both the growth of the TRI community and the growth of TRI's ability to facilitate excellent, randomized multicenter clinical trials that can generate the evidence needed to justify the disruptive nature of change from femoral to radial access on a routine basis.

Making TRI the standard of care also crystallizes how interventional cardiologists must balance the immediate needs of a single patient at the bedside with more national and global questions of public health benefit. Data on outcomes and comparative effectiveness will drive reimbursement decisions and TRI adoption. Toward this end, TRI enthusiasts and experts must recognize the need for randomized trials and the fundamental dilemma of their conduct: If "femoralists" can't randomize because they don't have TRI competence, and "radialists" won't randomize because they consider it unethical, then the studies needed to prove TRI's value will not be done well, if they're done at all. Better to do away with such categories, focus on the central issue of vascular access safety and, in advancing the field of interventional cardiology, advance TRI to first-line standard of care.

Table 1

Advantages and Disadvantages of a Transradial Approach
Advantages
• Reduced bleeding risk • Reduced length of stay costs • Early ambulation • Improved patient comfort • Obviates discontinuation of oral anticoagulant therapy • Same-day discharge possible
Disadvantages
• Learning curve • Not routinely taught in fellowship programs • Limits guide catheter size • Possible greater radiation exposure to the operator* • Long-term consequences to radial (e.g., for re-access or for use as bypass graft) unknown
*May be a function of operator experience.

Adapted from Rao S et al: J Am Coll Cardiol. 2010; 55 (20): 2187-2195.

Table 2

Comparison of Femoral and Radial Access for Cardiac Catheterization		
Feature	**Femoral**	**Radial**
Access-site bleeding	3% to 4%	0% to 0.6%
Artery complications	Pseudoaneurysm, retroperitoneal bleed, AV fistula, painful hematoma	Rare local irritation, pulse loss 3% to 9%
Patient comfort	Acceptable	Great
Ambulation	2-4 hours	Immediate
Extra costs	Closure device	Band
Procedure time*	Perceived shorter	Perceived longer
Estimated radiation exposure*	Perceived shorter	Perceived longer
Access to LIMA	Easy	Hard from RRA
Use of artery for CABG	N/A	Unknown
Learning curve	Short	Longer
> 8 Fr guide catheters	No problem	Maximum 7 Fr (in men)
PVD, obese	Problematic	No problem

*Operator-dependent. Modified from Kern, MJ. Editor's corner: radial artery catheterization: the way to go. Cath Lab Digest. 2009; 9 (7) :4-5.

AV = arterialvenous; CABG = coronary artery bypass grafting; LIMA = left internal mammary artery; N/A = not applicable; PVD = peripheral vascular disease; RRA = right radial artery.

Modified from Kern M, J. Am. Coll. Cardiol. Intv. 2009;2;1055-1056

Recommended Reading

1. Kiemeneij F, Laarman GJ. Percutaneous transradial artery approach for coronary stent implantation. Cathet Cardiovasc Diagn. 1993; 30: 173-178.
2. Lefevre T, Thebault B, Spaulding C, et al. Radial artery patency after percutaneous left radial artery approach for coronary angiography. The role of heparin. Eur Heart J. 1995; 16: 293.
3. Kiemeneij F, Laarman GJ, Odekerken D, et al. A randomized comparison of percutaneous transluminal coronary angioplasty by the radial, brachial and femoral approaches: the access study. J Am Coll Cardiol. 1997; 29(6): 1269-1275
4. Schneider J, Mann T, Cubeddu M, et al. Transradial cforonary stenting: a United States experience. J Invasive Cardiol. 1997; 9 (9): 569-574.
5. Louvard Y, Lefevre T, Morice MC. Radial approach: what about the learning curve? Cathet Cardiovasc Diagn 1997; 42: 467-468.
6. Stella PR, Kiemeneij F, Laarman GJ, et al. Incidence and outcome of radial artery occlusion following transradial artery coronary angioplasty. Cathet Cardiovasc Diagn. 1997; 40: 156-158.
7. Mann T, Cubeddu G, Bowen J, et al. Stenting in acute coronary syndromes: a comparison of radial versus femoral access sites. J Am Coll Cardiol. 1998; 32(3): 572-576
8. Goldberg SL, Renslo R, Sinow R, et al. Learning curve in the use of the radial artery as vascular access in the performance of percutaneous transluminal coronary angioplasty, Cathet Cardiovasc Diagn. 1998; 44: 147-152.
9. Saito S, Ikei H, Hosokawa G, et al. Influence of the ratio between radial artery inner diameter and sheath outer diameter on radial artery flow after transradial coronary intervention. Catheter Cardiovasc Interv. 1999; 46(2): 173-178.
10. Cooper C, El-Shiekh R, Cohen D, et al. Effect of transradial access on quality of life and cost of cardiac catheterization: A randomized comparison. Am Heart J. 1999; 138: 3(1): 430-436.
11. Mann T, Cowper PA, Peterson ED, et al. Transradial coronary stenting: comparison with femoral access closed with an arterial suture device. Catheter Cardiovasc Interv. 2000; 49: 150-156.
12. Beller GA, Bonow RO, Fuster V. ACC revised recommendations for training in adult cardiovascular medicine. Core Cardiology Training II (COCATS 2). (Revision of the 1995 COCATS training statement). J Am Coll Cardiol. 2002; 39: 1242-1246.
13. Hildick-Smith DJ, Walsh JT, Lowe MD, et al. Coronary angiography in the fully anticoagulated patient: the transradial route is successful and safe. Catheter Cardiovasc Interv. 2003; 58: 8-10.
14. Yoo BS, Lee SH, Ko JY, et al. Procedural outcomes of repeated transradial coronary procedure. Catheter Cardiovasc Interv. 2003; 58: 301-304.
15. Agostoni P, Biondi-Zoccai GG, de Benedictis ML, et al. Radial versus femoral approach for percutaneous coronary diagnostic and interventional procedures; Systematic overview and meta-analysis of randomized trials. J Am Coll Cardiol. 2004; 44: 349-356.
16. Lange H, Boetticher H. Randomized comparison of operator radiation exposure during coronary angiography and intervention by radial or femoral approach. Catheter Cardiovasc Interv. 2006; 67(1): 12-16.
17. Kiemeneij F. Cost-effectiveness of transradial coronary access. J Invasive Cardiol. 2007; 19(8): 354.
18. Roussanov O, Wilson SJ, Henley K, et al. Cost-effectiveness of the radial versus femoral artery approach to diagnostic cardiac catheterization. J Invasive Cardiol. 2007; 19: 349-353.
19. Rao SV, Ou FS, Wang TY, et al. Trends in the prevalence and outcomes of radial and

femoral approaches to percutaneous coronary intervention: a report from the national cardiovascular data registry. JACC Cardiovasc Interv. 2008; 1(4): 379-386.

20. Pancholy S, Coppola J, Patel T, et al. Prevention of Radial Artery Occlusion—Patent Hemostasis Evaluation Trial (PROPHET Study): A randomized comparison of traditional versus patency documented hemostasis after transradial catheterization. Catheter Cardiovasc Interv. 2008; 72: 335-340.

21. Doyle B, Ting H, Bell M, et al. Major femoral bleeding complications after percutaneous coronary intervention incidence, predictors, and impact on long-term survival among 17,901 patients treated at the Mayo Clinic from 1994 to 2005. J Am Coll Cardiol Interv. 2008; 1: 202-209

22. Mamas MA, Fath-Ordoubadi F, Fraser DG. Atraumatic complex transradial intervention using large bore sheathless guide catheter. Catheter Cardiovasc Interv 2008; 72: 357-364.

23. Chase A, Fretz E, Warburton W, et al. Association of the arterial access site at angioplasty with transfusion and mortality: the M.O.R.T.A.L study (Mortality benefit Of Reduced Transfusion after percutaneous coronary intervention via the Arm or Leg). Heart. 2008; 94(8): 1019-1025.

24. Jacobs AK , Babb JD et al. Task Force 3: Training in diagnostic and interventional cardiac catheterization endorsed by the Society for Cardiovascular Angiography and Interventions. J Am Coll Cardiol. 2008 22; 51(3): 355-361.

25. Jolly SS, Amlani S, Hamon M, et al. Radial versus femoral access for coronary angiography or intervention and the impact on major bleeding and ischemic events: a systematic review and meta-analysis of randomized trials. Am Heart J. 2009; 157(1): 132-140.

26. Vorobcsuk A, Kónyi A, Aradi D, et al. Transradial versus transfemoral percutaneous coronary intervention in acute myocardial infarction Systematic overview and meta-analysis. Am Heart J. 2009; 158(5): 814-821

27. Brueck M, Bandorski D, Kramer W, et al. A randomized comparison of transradial versus transfemoral approach for coronary angiography and angioplasty. JACC Cardiovasc Interv. 2009; 2(11): 1047-1054.

28. Cubero JM, Lombardo J, Pedrosa C, et al. Radial compression guided by mean artery pressure versus standard compression with a pneumatic device (RACOMAP). Catheter Cardiovasc Interv. 2009; 73: 467-472.

29. Bertrand OF, Larose E, Rodes-Cabau J, et al. Incidence, predictors, and clinical impact of bleeding after transradial coronary stenting and maximal antiplatelet therapy. Am Heart J. 2009; 157(1): 164-169.

30. Dehghani P, Mohammad A, Bajaj R, et al. Mechanism and predictors of failed transradial approach for percutaneous coronary interventions. JACC Cardiovasc Interv. 2009; 2(11): 1057-1064.

31. Sciahbasi A, Pristipino C, Ambrosio G, et al. Arterial access site related outcomes of patients undergoing invasive coronary procedures for acute coronary syndromes (from the ComPaRison of Early Invasive and Conservative Treatment in Patients With Non-ST-ElevatiOn Acute Coronary Syndromes [PRESTO-ACS] Vascular Substudy). Am J Cardiol. 2009; 103: 796-800.

32. Kern M. Cardiac Catheterization on the Road Less Traveled: Navigating the Radial vs. Femoral Debate. JACC Cardiovasc Inter. 2009 (11); 2; 1055-1056

33. Bertrand O, Rao S, Pancholy S, et al. Transradial approach for coronary angiography and interventions: results of the first international transradial practice survey. JACC Cardiovasc Inter. 2010; 3(10): 1032-1034.

34. Gilchrist I. Transradial catheterization's grass

roots epidemic. JACC Cardiovasc Inter. 2010; 3(10): 1032-1034.

35. Cevik C, Izgi C, Nugent K. Radial artery access as an emerging factor for decreasing mortality in cardiovascular interventions. J Interv Cardiol. 2010; 23(1): 95-99.

36. Rao S, Cohen M, Kandzari D, et al. The transradial approach to percutaneous coronary intervention: historical perspective, current concepts, and future directions. J Am Coll Cardiol. 2010; 55(20): 2187-2195.

37. Rathore S, Stables RH, Pauriah M, et al. Impact of length and hydrophilic coating of the introducer sheath on radial artery spasm during transradial coronary intervention: a randomized study. JACC Cardiovasc Interv. 2010; 3(5): 475-483.

38. Sciahbasi A, Romagnoli E, Trani C, et al. Evaluation of the «learning curve» for left and right radial approach during percutaneous coronary procedures. Am J Cardiol. 2011: 15; 108(2): 185-188.

39. Jolly SS, Yusuf S, Cairns J, et al. Radial versus femoral access for coronary angiography and intervention in patients with acute coronary syndromes (RIVAL): a randomised, parallel group, multicentre trial. Lancet. 2011: 3; 377(9775): 1409-1420.

40. Sciahbasi A, Romagnoli E, Burzotta F, et al. Transradial approach (left vs right) and procedural times during percutaneous coronary procedures: TALENT study. Am Heart J. 2011; 161(1): 172-179.

Transradial Approach and Antithrombotic Safety

22

Sunil Rao

Rationale for Antithrombotic Therapy During PCI

Antithrombotic therapy, consisting of anticoagulant and antiplatelet agents, is needed during PCI to minimize the ischemic consequences of iatrogenic plaque rupture that occurs during balloon angioplasty and stenting. The process of crushing the atherosclerotic coronary plaque activates a series of pathways that results in the generation of factor Xa and factor IIa (thrombin). Thrombin, in turn, facilitates the conversion of fibrinogen to fibrin and activates platelets, ultimately resulting in the formation of thrombus. Clinically, this can result in abrupt closure, acute stent thrombosis, thromboembolism to the distal coronary bed, and periprocedural myocardial infarction.

Another rationale for antithrombotic therapy during PCI is the prevention of thrombus formation on angioplasty equipment. Agents that are associated with an increased risk for catheter thrombus, like fondaparinux, have not been accepted for use during PCI without concomitant use of agents, such as unfractionated heparin or bivalirudin, that provide robust anti-thrombin effect.

In the context of TRI, there is one additional consideration for antithrombotic therapy — reducing the risk for radial artery occlusion. This latter point is discussed in detail in previous chapters and will not be covered here.

To summarize, the rationale for antithrombotic therapy during TRI is

- reducing the risk for thrombotic sequelae during PCI;
- reducing the risk for thrombus formation on PCI equipment; and
- reducing the risk for radial artery occlusion.

Risks of Antithrombotic Therapy and Role of Radial Approach

While combination therapy with anticoagulants (directed at thrombin generation) and antiplatelet agents (directed at activated platelets) mitigates these adverse events, it increases the risk for bleeding complications. This risk is compounded by the presence of the arteriotomy in patients undergoing PCI. Indeed, bleeding at the arterial access site accounts for a significant proportion of bleeding complications in PCI patients.

- In patients undergoing elective PCI, access site bleeding accounts for up to 70% of bleeding complications.
- In patients undergoing PCI for non-ST-segment elevation acute coronary syndrome, access site bleeding accounts for up to 30% of bleeding complications.
- In patients undergoing PCI for ST-segment elevation myocardial infarction, access site bleeding accounts for up to 50% of bleeding complications.

The radial approach is associated with a significant reduction in access site bleeding and vascular complications, but does not affect non-access site bleeding. Compared with access site bleeding, non-access site bleeding is more strongly associated with 1-year mortality in patients undergoing PCI. Reducing non-access site bleeding requires judicious use of procedural antithrombotic therapy. The combination of radial approach and appropriate antithrombotic therapy can achieve the lowest bleeding risk for patients undergoing PCI.

To reduce the risk of non-access site bleeding, the following should be considered:

- Dose unfractionated heparin appropriately.
- Dose enoxaparin appropriately with specific attention to the patient's renal function.
- Reserve glycoprotein IIb/IIIa agents (GPI) for "bailout," i.e., procedural complications such as coronary dissection, slow flow, no-reflow, residual or new thrombus, compromised side branches, etc.
- When using GPI, ensure appropriate dosing, especially if using eptifibatide or tirofiban in patients with reduced renal function.
- Use bivalirudin.

Specific Agents

(A) Anticoagulants

(1) Unfractionated heparin

- Has approximately 1:1 anti-Xa and anti-IIa effects.
- Can be administered subcutaneously or intravenously.
- Able to be monitored with aPTT or point-of-care activated clotting time (ACT).
- Reversible with protamine sulfate.
- Dosing for PCI: 70 u/kg bolus to maintain ACT 200–250 seconds if GPI is used; maintain ACT 250–300 seconds if no GPI is used.

(2) Enoxaparin

- Has approximately 12:1 anti-Xa and anti-IIa effects.
- Can be administered subcutaneously or intravenously.
- Cannot be monitored with ACT.
- Partially (50%) reversible with protamine sulfate.
- Dosing for ACS:
    - Normal renal function — 1 mg/kg subcutaneously every 12 hours
    - Creatinine clearance < 30 ml/hr — 1 mg/kg subcutaneously once daily
- Dosing for PCI in patients treated with enoxaparin for ACS:
    - Last subcutaneous dose < 8 hours prior — no additional enoxaparin
    - Last subcutaneous dose ≥ 8 hours prior — 0.8 mg/kg IV before crossing the lesion with the guidewire
- Dosing for elective PCI (no prior treatment with subcutaneous enoxaparin):
    - 0.50–0.75 mg/kg IV before crossing the lesion with the guidewire

(3) Fondaparinux

- Is an indirect factor Xa inhibitor.
- Is administered subcutaneously.

- Cannot be monitored with the ACT.
- Cannot be reversed.
- Must administer additional anti-thrombin agent during PCI:
    - Unfractionated heparin per dosing above
    - Bivalirudin (see below)

(4) **Bivalirudin**

- Direct thrombin (IIa) inhibitor
- Administered intravenously
- Monitorable with an ACT (usually gives high values)
- Cannot be reversed
- Dosing for PCI: 0.75 mg/kg IV bolus followed by 1.75 mg/kg/min infusion during PCI.
    - If creatinine clearance is < 30 ml/min, administer the same bolus dose, decrease infusion dose to 1 ml/kg/hr.

(B) Glycoprotein IIb/IIIa Inhibitors

(1) **Abciximab**

- Made from the Fab fragments of the chimeric human-murine monoclonal antibody directed against the glycoprotein IIb/IIIa receptor.
- Antithrombotic effect reversed by administration of platelets.
- Cleared by the reticuloendothelial system.
- Dosing during PCI: 0.25 mg/kg intravenous bolus administered 10–60 minutes before the start of PCI, followed by a continuous intravenous infusion of 0.125 μg/kg/min (to a maximum of 10 μg/min) for 12 hours.

(2) **Eptifibatide**

- Small-molecule glycoprotein IIb/IIIa inhibitor
- Cleared by the kidney
- Half-life of 2.5 hours

- Dosing for PCI:
  - Normal renal function: 180 mcg/kg bolus followed by infusion at 2.0 mcg/kg/min for 18–24 hours; administer a second bolus of 180 mcg/kg bolus 10 minutes after the first
  - Creatinine clearance < 50 ml/min: administer the same boluses, but reduce the infusion to 1.0 mcg/kg/min
  - Contraindicated in patients on hemodialysis

(3) Tirofiban

- Small-molecule glycoprotein IIb/IIIa inhibitor
- Cleared by the kidney
- Half-life of 2 hours
- Dosing for PCI (high-dose bolus regimen): 25 μg/kg bolus then 0.15 μg/kg/min infusion
- No specific dosage recommendation in patients with renal insufficiency (not recommended for such patients)

Switching Between Anticoagulants

- In general, it is not recommended that you switch from unfractionated heparin to enoxaparin or vice versa.
- The use of fondaparinux for medical therapy before PCI necessitates switching to an agent with greater anti-thrombin (IIa) activity (e.g., unfractionated heparin or bivalirudin).
- Switching from unfractionated heparin or enoxaparin to bivalirudin for PCI is safe based on post-hoc analyses of the REPLACE-2, ACUITY, and HORIZONS-AMI trials as well as the SWITCH randomized trial. The usual dosing of bivalirudin should be used for PCI.

Studies of Agents in the Setting of TRI

Unfractionated heparin

- Most studies comparing radial with femoral PCI have used unfractionated heparin as the background anticoagulant with or without GPI.
  - The radial approach has been consistently associated with a 50% to 70% reduction in major bleeding and/or major access site complications.

Enoxaparin

- The largest study, a post-hoc analysis of the SYNERGY trial, examined the impact of radial approach on outcomes in patients with ACS undergoing PCI.
  - SYNERGY was an open-label randomized trial comparing enoxaparin with unfractionated heparin in 10,027 patients with non-ST-segment elevation acute coronary syndrome.
  - Choice of access site for PCI was left to the discretion of the operator.
  - The radial approach was used in 4.4% of patients.
  - TRI was associated with a significantly lower need for transfusions (0.9% radial versus 4.8% femoral, P = 0.007).
- The ATOLL trial compared intravenous enoxaparin 0.5 mg/kg with weight-adjusted unfractionated heparin in patients with STEMI undergoing primary PCI.
  - The rate of radial approach was very high (67%).
  - The primary endpoints (death, MI-related complications, procedural failure, or major bleeding) did not significantly differ between the enoxaparin and unfractionated heparin groups (unfractionated heparin 33.7% versus enoxaparin 28.0%, P = 0.07).
  - Major bleeding was also not different between the groups (4.9% versus 4.5%, P = NS).
  - This study suggests that the radial approach affects major bleeding in primary PCI bleeding such that the safety advantage of IV enoxaparin is obviated.

Fondaparinux

- There have been no studies specifically examining TRI in the setting of fondaparinux therapy.

Bivalirudin

- A post-hoc analysis of the ACUITY trial examined the role of the radial approach and antithrombotic strategy on ischemic events, major bleeding, and net clinical outcome (a composite of death, (re)myocardial infarction, urgent target vessel revascularization, or major bleeding).
  - The ACUITY trial randomized 13,819 patients with non-ST-segment elevation acute coronary syndrome undergoing early invasive risk stratification to either bivalirudin with provisional GPI, unfractionated heparin with planned GPI, or bivalirudin with planned GPI.
  - The primary endpoint was the 30-day occurrence of death, re-MI, urgent target vessel revascularization, or major bleeding.
  - The bivalirudin with provisional GPI was superior to the other two arms with respect to the primary outcome, primarily driven by a 47% reduction in major bleeding.
  - The choice of access site for PCI was left to the discretion of the operator.
  - Radial approach was used in 6.2% of patients and was associated with a significant 47% reduction in major bleeding compared with the femoral approach (radial 3.0% versus femoral 4.8%, P = 0.02).
  - When the interaction between access site and randomized pharmacotherapy was examined, the use of bivalirudin alone attenuated the difference in bleeding between radial and femoral:

ACUITY Major Bleeding Rates

	Bivalirudin	UFH + GPI	Bivalirudin + GPI
Radial (N = 798)	4.2%	2.2%	2.7%
Femoral (N = 11,988)	3.0%	5.8%	5.4%

Keys to Remember

- The radial approach reduces access site bleeding and complications but does not impact non-access site bleeding.
- When considering procedural pharmacotherapy, appropriate dosing is of paramount importance, especially in patients with reduced renal function.
- The combination of radial approach and judicious antithrombotic therapy results in the best outcomes for the patient.

- This study suggests that TRI is safer overall than the femoral approach, but that the differences in bleeding between the two approaches may be less striking if bivalirudin is used as the procedural anticoagulant. Presumably this is due to bivalirudin's effect in reducing femoral access site bleeding and overall non-access site bleeding.

Summary

Procedural pharmacotherapy is an important aspect of TRI. The combination of anticoagulant therapy and antiplatelet therapy is necessary to reduce the ischemic sequelae of PCI and reduce radial artery occlusion.

Recommended Reading

1. Gibson CM, Ten Y, Murphy SA, et al. Association of prerandomization anticoagulant switching with bleeding in the setting of percutaneous coronary intervention (a REPLACE-2 analysis). Am J Cardiol. 2007; 99(12): 1687-1690.
2. Lincoff AM, Bittl JA, Harrington RA, et al. Bivalirudin and provisional glycoprotein IIb/IIIa blockade compared with heparin and planned glycoprotein IIb/IIIa blockade during percutaneous coronary intervention: REPLACE-2 randomized trial. JAMA. 2003; 289(7): 853-863.
3. Rao SV, Ohman EM. Anticoagulant therapy for percutaneous coronary intervention. Circ Cardiovasc Interv. 2010; 3(1): 80-88.
4. Waksman R, Wolfram RM, Torguson RL, et al. Switching from enoxaparin to bivalirudin in patients with acute coronary syndromes without ST-segment elevation who undergo percutaneous coronary intervention. Results from SWITCH--a multicenter clinical trial. J Invasive Cardiol. 2006; 18(8): 370-375.
5. Winchester DE, Wen X, Brearley WD, et al. Efficacy and safety of glycoprotein IIb/IIIa inhibitors during elective coronary revascularization: a meta-analysis of randomized trials performed in the era of stents and thienopyridines. J Am Coll Cardiol. 2011; 57(10): 1190-1199.

How to Develop a Transradial Program

Jennifer Tremmel and Pinak Shah

23

Starting a transradial (TR) program within a catheterization laboratory can be a challenging undertaking for operators and catheterization laboratories accustomed to performing procedures via the transfemoral (TF) approach. Any change in catheterization laboratory operations that affects a large number of patients will undoubtedly be met with skepticism given the comfort level achieved by staff and operators with the present standard of care. Such a wholesale change in practice will, of course, come with a loss of efficiency within the laboratory as personnel get used to a new protocol for patient preparation and post-procedure care. Therefore, it is paramount that the physicians leading the transition take a methodical and patient approach to making this change. A haphazard attempt at transitioning to TR access may lead to longer procedure times and potentially increased patient discomfort, which will dampen enthusiasm for continuing with attempts at transition. This chapter will outline important steps that should be taken when starting a TR program in order to increase the likelihood of success and make the transition as seamless as possible.

1. Operator Education

Physicians without prior TR-access experience will need to educate themselves regarding the reasons to consider TR access and procedural aspects of TR access. There are several strategies for improving the TR knowledge base.

(A) Transradial Sessions at Cardiovascular Meetings

Given the growing popularity of TR access worldwide, nearly every national and international cardiovascular meeting with some focus on interventional cardiology will have a session devoted to TR access. Such sessions

- are moderated by the world's leaders in TR access.
- provide a broad overview of TR procedures, including key clinical data showing the benefits of TR access, as well as basic procedural steps for gaining TR access and performing catheterization procedures.
- are not always detailed enough to provide the novice operator with sufficient information to independently start a TR program.

(B) Dedicated Transradial Courses

There are a growing number for dedicated one- or two-day TR sessions aimed at educating physicians on every aspect of TR access. Such sessions

- are staffed and moderated by recognized leaders in the field.
- provide a more in-depth discussion of the practical aspects of performing TR procedures.
- discuss specific technical challenges and provide operators with knowledge to deal with difficult issues surrounding TR access, such as maneuvering through tortuous upper extremity anatomy and handling complications unique to the TR approach.
- often include TR access simulators and live case transmissions, but lack in-lab exposure to TR cases.
- are increasingly tailored to operator experience, ranging from the beginning level to master's courses.

(C) Visits to Other Transradial Labs

Most high-volume TR operators are open to hosting visitors for one-day sessions to observe how TR cases are performed in primarily TR laboratories. These visits

- provide invaluable insight into equipment needs for TR cases, strategies for ergonomic TR access site preparation, observation of catheter manipulation for diagnostic and interventional cases, and post-case management.
- vary in format, as different host operators provide more or less structured visits.
- may offer the opportunity for nurses and technicians to also visit and interact with their peers at the host institution.
- demonstrate the technique and protocol of a particular TR laboratory, so visiting several catheterization laboratories may prove valuable.

- are generally observational only, with privileging constraints of the host institution often limiting the ability to physically participate in the procedures.

(D) Visiting Professor Programs

Many physicians are happy to participate in visiting professor programs to present their experience in TR procedures to catheterization laboratory physicians and personnel. Such programs

- present a unique opportunity to facilitate a laboratory's transition to TR with the personal guidance of a TR expert.
- may provide the opportunity to identify and overcome specific transition barriers of a particular laboratory.
- provide personal instruction on all aspects of performing a TR procedure while letting the learners be hands-on.
- train several people (physicians, administration, and staff) simultaneously.
- may be associated with a financial cost of sponsoring the visiting professor.

(E) Transradial Catheterization Proctoring

For many novice TR operators, it will be worthwhile to arrange for a proctor to visit the laboratory for the performance of the first TR cases performed in a catheterization laboratory in transition. These proctor visits

- ideally give the proctor can temporary privileges so that she/he can participate in the cases with the novice operator.
- should select several cases to be performed with the proctor.
- should discuss with the selected patients that they will be the first TR patients in your laboratory's experience and that an expert proctor will be guiding the cases.

2. Catheterization Laboratory Personnel Education

Converting a cardiac catheterization laboratory from TF to TR is a multidisciplinary effort that will not succeed unless the entire laboratory team is educated on the TR procedure and motivated about the change. The catheterization laboratory needs to be educated on the data surrounding TR access, reasons for the laboratory conversion to TR access, as well as the TR procedure itself. In addition, the technical staff responsible for patient preparation will need to be educated on the differences between TR and TF access. It will be important to arrange for staff to participate in TR courses, many of which now have dedicated sessions for catheterization laboratory technologists and nurses. When making visits to other TR laboratories, include nurses, technical staff, physician colleagues and trainees when possible.

To facilitate conversion to TR access, it is advisable to identify "champions" among the nursing and technical staff to help promote the transition. Staff members with strong leadership skills and an interest in novel treatment strategies in the catheterization laboratory are ideal candidates. Additionally, depending on the size of the laboratory and the number of physicians, it is important to partner with several colleagues to help start the program. A collegial approach to learning TR access will enhance learning and education. Even more importantly, the more physicians involved, the more frequently the technical and nursing staff will be exposed to the procedure, making the cases less likely to be considered novelties each time they are performed.

Unique aspects of TR access with which the staff will need to become familiar include the following:

(A) Procedural Placement of the IV, BP Cuff, and Pulse Oximeter

- For patients undergoing TF catheterization, the procedural IV is generally placed in the easiest place to access a vein and the blood pressure cuff is placed on the upper arm contralateral to the IV site. More careful consideration will be needed prior to placing the procedural IV and blood pressure cuff for TR procedures, as well as the pulse oximeter.

Avoid placing the IV in the same arm that access will be obtained.

- IVs placed at the access site may be compressed by the post-procedure hemostatic device, rendering the IV non-functional and causing the patient discomfort if the hub of the IV is compressed into the soft tissue.
- IVs placed distal to the access site in the hand may not be functional after the hemostasis device is placed due to venous compression.
- IVs placed proximal to the access site may be in the way if more proximal access is desired, if right heart venous access is planned, or if there are unexpected complications in the arm requiring external compression.

1. Ideally, the IV should be placed proximally in the contralateral arm from which access will be obtained. A more proximal location of the IV will still allow the radial artery ipsilateral to the IV to be used for access, if necessary.
2. Because there will be arterial access in one arm and venous access in the other arm, and because a blood pressure cuff on the upper arm would intermittently disrupt flow of either the arterial or venous system, the blood pressure cuff is generally placed on the leg. Blood pressures from this location, however, may be less accurate.
3. The pulse oximeter should be placed on the ipsilateral hand for ongoing monitoring.

(B) Pre-Procedure Assessment of the Radial and Ulnar Arteries

It is good practice to educate the nursing staff on assessing collateral ulnar flow prior to catheterization. While some experienced operators suggest this may not be necessary given the very low risk of ischemic complications to the hand, novice operators should continue to assess ulnar flow until they are fully comfortable with TR access and complications associated with TR procedures. This should be documented in the catheterization laboratory record.

Modified Allen's Test

- Compress both the radial and ulnar arteries while the patient opens and closes the hand several times.
- Have the patient hold the blanched hand open while the ulnar artery is released.
- Count the number of seconds it takes for reperfusion of the hand (normal is ≤ 7 seconds, abnormal is ≥ 15 seconds).

Alternative (objective) Allen's Test

- Same as the modified Allen's Test, but with plethysmography on the thumb to access collateral flow, rather than using return of palm color.

Barbeau Test

- More sensitive than the modified Allen's Test (excludes only 1.5% of patients).
- Compress the radial artery for 2 minutes.
- The presence of an arterial waveform (even if delayed or reduced in amplitude) and a hemoglobin oxygen saturation > 90% confirms the adequacy of collaterals to the hand.
- TR should be avoided with a type D Barbeau Test.

Inverse Allen's Test

- Used to determine patency of the radial artery.
- Useful for repeat procedure from the same radial artery. If the inverse Allen's Test is negative (abnormal), the radial artery may not be suitable for a repeat procedure.

(C) Femoral Preparation

- Operator preference will dictate whether the femoral region should be prepped in the event that TF access is necessary.
- When first starting a TR program, it is recommended that the femoral region be prepped and ready for use.

- Over time, as crossover to the femoral artery becomes rare, concurrent preparation of the femoral region is no longer necessary and the practice can be abandoned for low-risk procedures.
- Even in experienced labs, at least one femoral artery should be prepped for high-risk cases in the event that an emergent cardiac support device becomes necessary.

(D) Radial Artery Access Site Preparation

There are several ways to prep the radial artery access site. When starting a program, it will be important to learn at least three of these preparations so physicians and laboratory staff can determine which will work best for the laboratory. Although a variety of specialized drapes are available, some operators continue to use standard femoral drapes shifted to one side so one access site on the drape can be placed on the radial access site and the other access site can be placed on the ipsilateral femoral access site in the event that TF access is required.

(E) Transradial Catheterization Equipment

Different equipment is required for TR catheterization compared to TF catheterization and the technical staff will need to be educated on these differences (see "TR Catheterization Equipment List").

(F) Post-Procedure Managment

The recovery staff needs to be educated about management of the post TR-catheterization patient. A variety of radial hemostasis devices are available.

- Regardless of the hemostatic device used, education on how to properly use the device is necessary for both the physicians and the staff.
- The goal is non-occlusive hemostasis to reduce the risk of radial artery occlusion.

- Nursing staff will need to know what complications to monitor during recovery, including venous congestion from the hand secondary to the hemostatic device, lack of collateral flow to the hand during radial hemostasis, and local hematoma formation.

3. Transradial Catheterization Equipment List

Prior to starting a TR program, the catheterization laboratory will need to be stocked with appropriate equipment. In addition, laboratories performing only diagnostic cases may want to keep equipment typically used for interventional procedures. Specifically required equipment before consideration of starting a TR program includes the following:

(A) Arm Boards and Drapes

Depending on how the access site will be prepped, specialized arm boards that allow for abduction of the arm may be necessary to gain access before positioning the arm close to the body for performance of the procedure. Specialized drapes can also be used, but are not absolutely necessary.

(B) Access Needles

There are two standard ways of gaining radial access, and which is used depends solely on operator preference.

- Anterior wall stick with a micro-puncture needle (21 gauge).
- Through-and-through puncture with an angiogath needle (21 gauge or 22 gauge).
- Needles can be purchased separately or as part of a pre-packaged radial access kit.

(C) Access Wires

- Once access is gained in the radial artery, a 0.021-inch or 0.025-inch hydrophilic wire is advanced into the radial artery for sheath placement.

- Due to its hydrophilicity, care must be taken to avoid perforation or dissection of the radial artery and its small branches.
- These wires can be purchased separately or part of a pre-packaged radial access kit.

(D) Sheaths

- A hydrophilic-coated sheath, rather than a traditional TF sheath, is optimal for easy placement and removal of the sheath from the smaller caliber radial artery.
- The hydrophilic coating also helps reduce the likelihood of radial artery spasm.
- 5 Fr and 6 Fr sheaths should be available, but there is no specific reason to stock sheaths longer than 11 cm when first starting a TR program.

(E) Arterial Guidewires

There are multiple guidewires that can be used for advancing catheters through the upper extremity vasculature.

- The standard 3 mm J-tipped 0.035-inch guidewire is commonly used, although smaller radial arteries may not be large enough to accommodate the 3 mm J tip.
- The floppy straight-tipped 0.035-inch wire is another option.
- A straight or angled 0.035-inch hydrophilic wire may be helpful, particularly for tortuous arterial anatomy, although caution should be used to avoid perforation or dissection.
- When starting a TR program, it will be helpful to have 0.035-inch wires that are 300 cm in length to facilitate catheter exchanges without having to relinquish ascending aortic access, which may be difficult to achieve in some patients.

(F) Interventional Wires

- For diagnostic-only catheterization laboratories, a stock of 0.014-inch and 0.018-inch interventional wires (hydrophilic-coated, preferably) will be helpful for navigating tortuous radial anatomy. An example is a radial artery loop, which cannot easily be traversed with standard 0.035-inch guidewires.

(G) Diagnostic and Guiding Catheters

Diagnostic and guiding catheters in 5 Fr and 6 Fr are necessary when starting a TR program. Minimizing French size is felt to reduce the risk of radial artery occlusion, so most diagnostic cases will be performed with a 5 Fr catheter, as will many coronary interventions. In addition, catheter manipulation is slightly different from the radial artery compared with the femoral artery; however, operator familiarity with the catheter shape and response will enhance learning the TR approach.

Femoral catheters

- Standard Judkins catheters are excellent for radial access and should be considered by new radial operators if they are already familiar with their use.
- A recent international survey of transradial practice showed that most radial operators use standard Judkins catheters rather than specialized radial catheters.
- The disadvantage of the Judkins shapes is that the catheter has to be exchanged for performance of left and right coronary angiography.

Radial-specific (Universal) catheters

- Have the advantage of allowing one catheter to engage the right and left coronary arteries.
- Have a learning curve that needs to be overcome before operators become facile with these catheters.

Guiding catheters

- The majority of TR coronary interventions can be successfully completed using standard TF-guiding catheter shapes.

- When first starting TR coronary intervention, it is recommended that the operator choose guide catheters they are familiar with before trying specialized guiding catheters.
- Many of the radial specific guide catheters offer improved seating and support because they are designed to fit the aorta from the arm. Therefore, operators should aim to increase their experience with radial specific catheters over time.
- Once the operator is comfortable with 6Fr coronary interventions, they should consider increasing their experience with 5 Fr coronary interventions.

(H) Hemostasis Devices

A variety of hemostatic devices are available for compression of the radial artery after sheath removal. New operators should try several models to find out what they will be most comfortable using.

- Arterial monitoring should be performed following placement of the hemostatic device to ensure non-occlusive hemostasis.
- Every effort should be made to remove the sheath as early as possible after the procedure while the patient is still in the catheterization laboratory.
- Proper in-servicing by the device manufacturer is important so physicians, recovery room nurses, and nurses on the inpatient floors will be comfortable with managing the device post-procedure.

(G) In-Lab Vascular Ultrasound

While not an absolute requirement, in-lab vascular ultrasound can be an invaluable tool for TR procedures.

- In patients with small radial arteries or with difficult access, ultrasound can be used to identify the radial artery and allow for direct puncture with visualization.

- Ultrasound can be used to identify sites of bleeding from a forearm branch vessel perforation in patients who develop forearm hematoma during or after TR catheterization procedures, allowing for a more clear delineation of where to apply pressure to achieve hemostasis.

4. The First Transradial Cases

Once physicians and technical/nursing staff have been educated and appropriate equipment is available, consideration can be given to performing the first cases. There are several points to consider when performing the first cases in the catheterization laboratory.

(A) Patient Selection

Appropriate patient selection is key in ensuring success for the first cases. Care must be taken to ensure that the first cases will provide the greatest likelihood for success so physician and staff confidence will be built quickly. Difficulties with TR catheterization in the early phase of a program will lengthen procedure times and may reduce the enthusiasm to maintain the program. Ideal first patients are:

Diagnostic-only cases

- Avoid cases in which ad hoc coronary intervention is a high likelihood.
- The operator and laboratory should feel comfortable with the management of diagnostic patients prior to proceeding with TR coronary intervention.

Elective cases

- Do not attempt the TR approach for urgent cases where time delays in treatment may be deleterious to the patient.

Patients in whom access is likely to be straightforward

- Patients with a very palpable radial pulse and a good test of collateral ulnar flow

- Larger patients, who tend to have larger arteries
- Male patients, who have a lower rate of crossover to TF than female patients.
- Taller patients (patients shorter than 165 cm have shorter ascending aortas and less room to manipulate catheters entering the ascending aorta from the upper extremity, making catheter engagement more difficult)
- Younger patients (as patients age, there is a greater likelihood of radial, brachial, and innonimate/ subclavian tortuosity that may make catheter manipulation difficult)
- Patients without prior coronary artery bypass grafting (CABG) surgery
- Non-anxious patients (patients who appear to be overly anxious may not be ideal early cases because significant anxiety may lead to radial artery spasm, making the case more difficult and uncomfortable than necessary)

Patients in whom TR access should be avoided

- Dialysis patients with AV fistula or shunt potential
- Patients with a failed Allen's test
- Patients with Raynaud's phenomenon
- Planned large-bore (8 Fr or more) procedures
- Known pathology in proximal arteries (stenosis, tortuosity, abarrent right subclavian [arteria lusoria])

(B) Patient Education and Consent

- It is important to discuss the reasons for using a particular access site with patients.
- Explain that TR access is being used because it is considered safer (reduced bleeding and vascular complications) and more comfortable.
- Also discuss the potential downsides of TR access, including radial artery spasm and radial artery occlusion.

- Discuss the operator's lack of experience with TR access and that this may lead to a longer procedure time or crossover to the femoral artery.

(C) Gradual Increase in Transradial Volume

It should be expected that the first cases will be longer for a catheterization laboratory that is new to TR catheterization. The technical staff will take longer to prepare the patient for the procedure, and the operator will take longer to gain access and engage the coronary arteries. Having a systematic approach to increasing TR volume, such as the one described below, may be helpful, particularly in very busy catheterization laboratories.

- Aim to perform at least one TR case per day, while completing the remainder of the cases transfemorally.
- The operator/laboratory should complete approximately 20 cases in this fashion over a short period of time to minimize long gaps in the experience of doing TR cases.
- Once these cases have been completed, the operator can gradually increase the daily volume.
- Similarly, as confidence grows, the operator can loosen selection criteria to include more potentially difficult cases.
- Performing TR procedures from the left radial artery rather than the right radial artery may offer a shorter learning curve.
- Success with TR interventions depends on the operator's experience, with a case volume of $\geq$ 50 cases needed to achieve outcomes comparable to experienced operators.

5. Maintaining Commitment and Reaffirming Benefits

Every operator who has transitioned their practice from TF to TR has had difficult cases early in their experience that may have shaken their confidence with TR catheterization. Many find having to convert to TF access to complete a procedure frustrating. It is important to keep in mind that this is going to be part of the early experience, but with maintained commitment to TR catheterization, the difficult cases and the TF conversions will decrease dramatically. Many high-volume operators no longer prep the femoral arteries and will attempt the contralateral radial artery for access before considering TF access. With continued commitment, TR access will become the default strategy, and more patients at higher risk of bleeding and vascular access site complications (small women, STEMIs) will benefit from the paradigm shift. The drive to maintain commitment to transitioning to TR access can be bolstered by reaffirming the benefits of TR access.

(A) Discuss Experience With Patients

- The majority of patients find TR access to be very comfortable, and the maintenance of mobility post-procedure is a major benefit, particularly for patients with orthopedic/spine problems.
- Patients who have had prior TF procedures and are now undergoing their first TR will nearly uniformly want future procedures performed via TR access.
- Patients often relay their positive experiences to the physicians who referred them, increasing the likelihood of subsequent referrals.

(B) Discuss Experience With Referring Physicians

- Referring physicians who are not familiar with catheterization procedures are generally amazed that cardiac catheterization and coronary intervention can be performed via the radial artery.
- Referring physicians are generally pleased to know that their patients' procedures can be done in a safer and more comfortable manner, and they often refer patients to operators specifically for this approach.

(C) Discuss Experience With Catheterization Laboratory Staff

Once the catheterization laboratory staff has become comfortable with the procedure, they will likely prefer radial access as a default strategy as well.

- Recovery room nurses will generally report that patient monitoring is simpler for TR patients compared with patients who have undergone TF access.
- Nurses also appreciate that patients are more comfortable and independent when they are not required to be on bed rest.
- Concern for insidious life-threatening bleeding is virtually eliminated.
- Local complications, if they occur, are easily seen and managed.

SUMMARY

Starting a transradial program is a methodical process that involves a multidisciplinary approach involving physicians, technical staff, and nursing. Education of the entire health care team is required to gain familiarity with TR procedures. Much can be learned by observing seasoned radial operators and inviting recognized experts in TR access to proctor cases. With continued commitment, a successful TR program is achievable for all catheterization laboratories.

Keys to Remember

- There are multiple formats in which to build a cognitive and technical knowledge base about TR procedures, and taking advantage of more than one may be helpful.
- Identify a technician and nurse to help champion the laboratory's transition to TR.
- Ensure proper stocking of the catheterization laboratory with equipment necessary for the performance of TR cases before starting a program.
- Initially select cases that have a high likelihood of success. Gradually introduce more complicated patient subsets.
- All operators will have difficult cases and high TF conversion rates during their early experience. With maintained commitment and reaffirmation of the benefits of TR access, cases will become easier and TF conversion rates will be very low.

Recommended Reading

1. Bertrand OB, Rao SV, Pancholy S, et al. Transradial approach for coronary angiography an interventions: results of the first international transradial practice survey. J Am Coll Cardiol Intv. 2010; 3: 1022–1031.
2. Barbeau GR, Arsenault F, Dugas L, Simard S, Lariviere MM. Evaluation of the ulnopalmar arterial arches with pulse oximetry and plethysmography: comparison with the Allen's test in 1010 patients. Am Heart. J 2004; 147: 489–493.
3. Pristipino C, Pelliccia F, Granatelli A, Pasceri V, Roncella A, Speciale G, Hassan T, Richichi G. Comparison of access-related bleeding complications in women versus men undergoing percutaneous coronary catheterization using the radial versus femoral artery. Am J Cardiol. 2007; 99: 1216–1221.
4. Dehghani P, Mohammad A, Bajaj R, Hong T, Suen CM, Sharieff W, Chisholm RJ, Kutryk MJB, Fam NP, Cheema AN. Mechanism and predictors of failed transradial approach for percutaneous coronary interventions. J Am Coll Cardiol Intv. 2009; 2: 1057–1064.
5. Sciahbasi A, Romagnoli E, Trani C, Burzotta F, Pendenza G, Tommasino A, Leone AM, Niccoli G, Porto I,, Penco M, Lioy E. Evaluation of the "learning curve" for left and right radial approach during percutaneous coronary procedures. Am J Cardiol. 2011; 108: 185–188.
6. Ball WT, Sharieff W, Jolly SS, Hong T, Kutryk MJB, Graham JJ, Fam NP, Chisholm RJ, Cheema AN. Characterization of operator learning curve for transradial coronary interventions. Circ Cardiovasc Interv. 2011; 4: 336–341.
7. Jolly SS, Yusuf S, Cairns J, et al. Radial versus femoral access for coronary angiography and intervention in patients with acute coronary syndromes (RIVAL): a randomized, parallel group, multicenter trial. Lancet. 2011; 377: 1409–1420.
8. Tremmel JA. Launching a successful transradial program. J Invasive Cardiol. 2009; 21(Suppl A): 5A–10A.
9. Caputo RP, Tremmel JA, Rao S, et al. Transradial arterial access for coronary and peripheral procedures: Executive summary by the transradial committee of the SCAI. Catheter Cardiovasc Interv. 2011; 78: 823–839.

Transulnar Approach: Pros and Cons

Sasko Kedev

24

Background

The transulnar approach for diagnostic and percutaneous coronary interventions is a safe and effective alternative to the transradial approach, as both techniques share a high success rate and an extremely low incidence of entry site complications, and reduce costs and length of hospital stay. Additionally, it provides greater comfort for patients and allows early ambulation, as compared with femoral and brachial approaches.

The transulnar approach is not inferior to the transradial approach when performed by operators well experienced in radial cannulation. For institutions that routinely use the radial approach with transulnar experienced operators, this technique is of particular benefit when the radial artery access site is not available or at high risk of failure or complications, mostly after repeat radial artery puncture.

The transulnar approach is used in cases of radial access failure due to small-caliber or thin radial pulse, severe spasms and most challenging variations in radial artery anatomy. It also has the potential to spare injury to the radial artery (RA) in anticipation of its use as a coronary-bypass conduit.

Anatomy of the Ulnar Artery

The ulnar artery (UA) is the larger of the two branches (ulnar and radial artery) of the brachial artery. The UA/RA ratio is 1.35. The UA begins below the bend of the elbow, and, passing obliquely downward, reaches the ulnar side of the forearm at a point about midway between the elbow and the wrist. Then it runs along the ulnar border to the wrist, crosses the transverse carpal ligament on the radial side of the pisiform bone, and immediately beyond this bone divides into two branches that enter into the formation of the superficial and deep volar arches. At the wrist, the ulnar artery terminates in the superficial palmar arch, which provides most of the blood supply to the fingers. Just above the middle of the forearm, the ulnar nerve joins the artery (lying to its ulnar side) and accompanies it down into the hand.

Interosseous branch:

About 1 inch below the origin of the UA, the common interosseous artery arises and divides into the anterior (volar) branch and the posterior (dorsal) branch.

- In the forearm, the UA is deeper than the radial artery; as it passes down the forearm, it is lying just lateral (deep) to the ulnar nerve.

Note: In the instance of a high takeoff of the ulnar artery, the interosseous branch in the majority of cases arises from the radial artery or from the brachial artery.

Ulnar artery in hand:

- The radial and ulnar arteries terminate by dividing into superficial and deep branches.
- A line drawn across the palm at the level of distal border of a fully abducted thumb marks the approximate location of the superficial arch.
- Immediately distal to this point, the artery divides into its larger branch, which forms most of the superficial arch, and its smaller branch, which forms the lesser part of deep the palmar.
- The superficial arch is much larger and more important than the deep arch.
- Just proximal to pisiform bone, the UA gives off volar and dorsal carpal branches, which unite with the volar and dorsal branches of the RA to form an arterial wristlet about the carpal bones.

Abnormal Course of the Ulnar Artery

The UA was found to deviate from its usual mode of origin nearly in proportion of one in 13 (~7.7%), similar to the 7% incidence of high bifurcating radial artery take-off.

- The lower part of the brachial artery was the source from which the UA sprang more frequently than the axillary or the upper part of the brachial artery (BA).

- The ulnar artery can have a high axillary origin, where the vessel was connected with the BA opposite the elbow joint by means of a transverse branch.
- The superficial UA is a rare variation of the upper limb arterial system that arises from the BA or axillary artery and runs superficial to the muscles arising from the medial epicondyle. The variable incidence is about 0.7 to 7%.

Reverse Allen's Test, Doppler, Plethysmography and Pulse Oximetry

A reverse Allen's test is done on the right or left wrist and its purpose is to determine radial artery patency and adequate radial-ulnar collaterals to the hand. A reverse Allen's test is performed by compressing both the radial and ulnar arteries and having the patient clench the fist several times. In contrast to the Allen's test — in which pressure on the ulnar artery is released — the Reverse Allen's test maintains occlusion of the ulnar artery while pressure on the radial artery is released. If blush returns to the palm within 10 seconds, the test is considered positive and indicates adequate collateral supply to the hand.

For the Doppler plethysmography test, the radial and ulnar arteries are compressed sequentially while confirming normal audible signal intensity in the palmar arch.

The pulse oximetry test is performed with occlusion of the ulnar artery, and a normal waveform and percentage oxygenation is confirmed.

Doppler plethysmography and pulse oximetry are of particular importance for providing patent hemostasis after sheath removal.

Technique:

- The skin is prepared with local anesthesia (1 ml lidocaine, 2%).

- The ideal puncture site is around 3 cm proximal to the flexor crease along the axis with the most powerful pulsation of ulnar artery.
- Puncture angle should be 45° along the axis of vessel.
- The ulnar artery is punctured with a 20-G plastic cannula, and a 0.025-inch Glidewire is inserted in the vessel. Then a hydrophilic sheath is introduced.
- To prevent ulnar artery spasm, inject blood mixed with verapamil 5 mg through the cannula or through the sidearm of the sheath.

Note: Procedure failure is almost always related to puncture, which can be more difficult than radial artery puncture, due to the deeper UA course and lower intensity of pulsations.

High puncture of the UA: Although the ideal site for puncture is 3 cm proximal to the os pisiforme, the ulnar artery can be punctured up to the mid-forearm as long as the pulsations can be felt. This approach may be useful for an experienced operator performing coronary or endovascular interventions requiring larger-bore devices. However, the ulnar nerve is very close to the artery in that region, so the puncture has to be very acurate and the operator has to be very cautious avoiding accidental nerve damage.

Retrograde ulnar arteriography

Retrograde ulnar arteriography is performed after administration of the arterial vasodilatator to define the ulnar artery anatomy from mid forearm to ulnar-brachial anastomosis and to delineate radial artery anatomy as well. A solution of 3 ml of contrast mixed with 7 ml of blood (to dilute the contrast) is injected briskly through the cannula or through the side arm of the sheath under fluoroscopy in AP position. If anomalous anatomy is identified, the operator can plan the procedure on that basis. Retrograde arteriography is of particular importance when there is some resistance in guidewire advancement and in patients after several previous transradial interventions.

Post-Procedure Management

The sheath is removed immediately after the procedure, regardless of the level of anticoagulation, and a compressive dressing or closure device is applied. To decrease the rate of UA occlusion, it is important to provide patent hemostasis. In our practice, we use the TR band and confirm the distal pulse with Doppler

plethysmography after hemostasis is achieved.
Compressive dressing is mandatory with higher puncture, because of the deeper artery position and greater risk of hematoma.

Complications

Rare minor complications:

- Ulnar artery spasm (less frequent than radial artery spasm)
- Asymptomatic ulnar artery occlusion (3% of cases in our series, and strongly associated with larger sheath size)
- Ulnar artery dissection/perforation
- Branch perforation/forearm hematoma

Very uncommon complications:

The following very uncommon complications are described in the literature, but we have not seen any of these after performing over 500 transulnar procedures:

- Ulnar nerve damage
- A-V fistula
- Pseudoaneurysm
- Compartment syndrome
- Hand ischemia (where there is coexistent radial artery flow compromise)
- Granuloma formation at the access site (has been associated with specific hydrophilic sheath use)

Pros:	Cons:
• All the associated benefit of transradial access: comfort, earlier ambulation, less complications • Larger diameter than the radial artery • Straighter course than the radial artery • Loops and curvatures are very rare • Less prone to spasm than the radial artery • Procedure after puncture is the same as transradial	• Ulnar artery puncture more difficult than radial artery puncture • Deeper position of the ulnar artery • Ulnar artery runs closely to the ulnar nerve • High-origin ulnar artery more prone to spasm, thus making the procedure more challenging at times

Indications for Transulnar Access

- Failed radial artery puncture (only puncture without sheath insertion)
- Confirmed, complex, challenging loops and curvatures of the radial artery
- Previous multiple transradial interventions — but the patient must have a positive Reverse Allen's Test (< 10 seconds)
- After previous large-bore (7 Fr/8 Fr sheath) transradial interventions with confirmed radial artery patency
- Stronger pulsation of the ulnar artery
- The radial artery has to be used for a bypass graft in multi-vessel disease

Examples

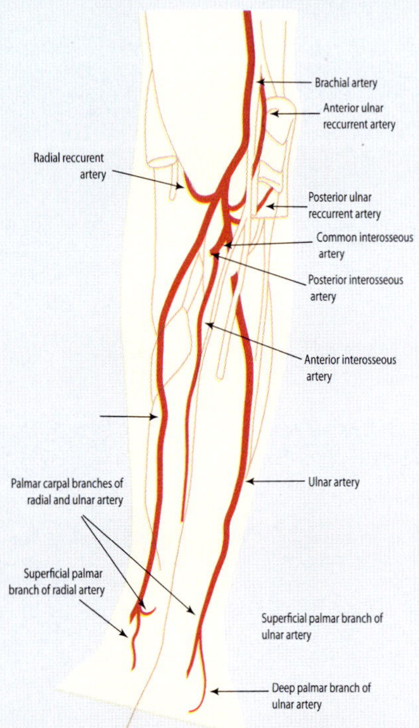

Normal anatomy of the forearm

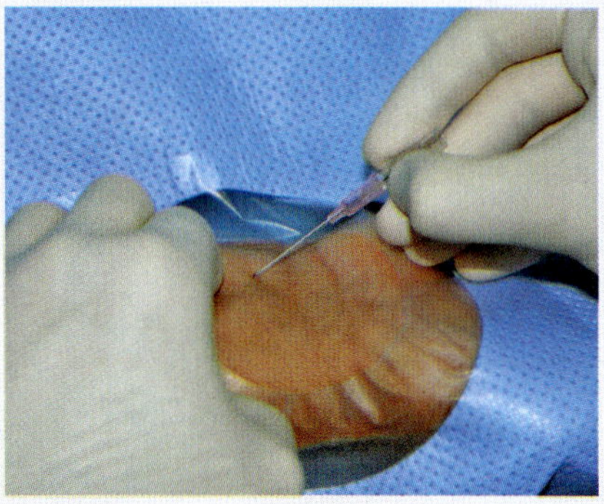

Ulnar artery puncture

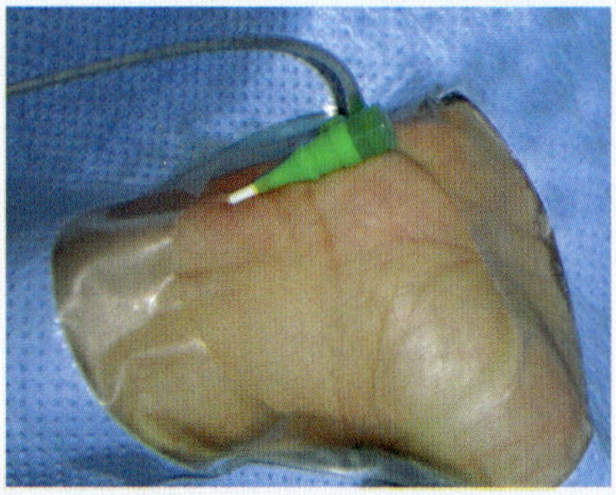

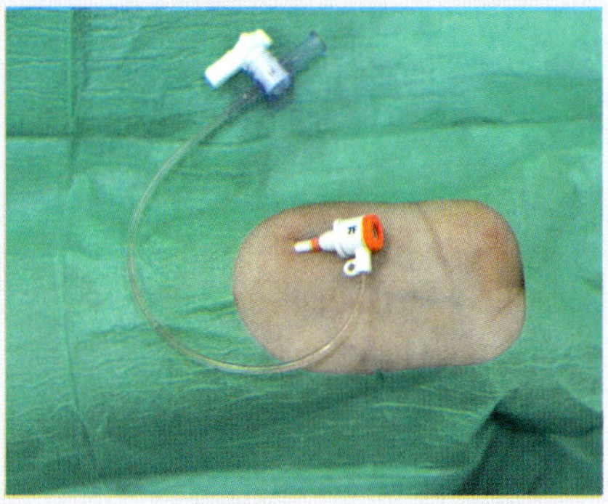

Ulnar artery cannulation with a 6 Fr and 7 Fr sheath

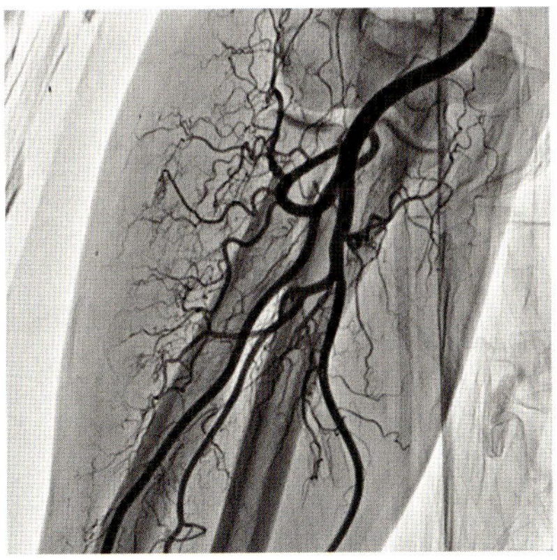

Retrograde ulnar artery arteriography

High origin of the ulnar artery

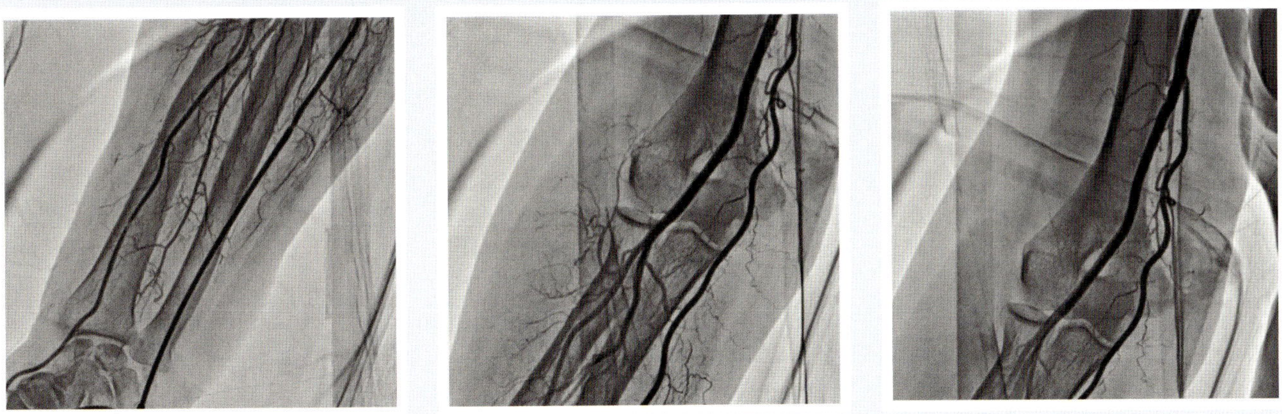

Ulnar artery arising high from the brachial artery in the region of the mid-humerus

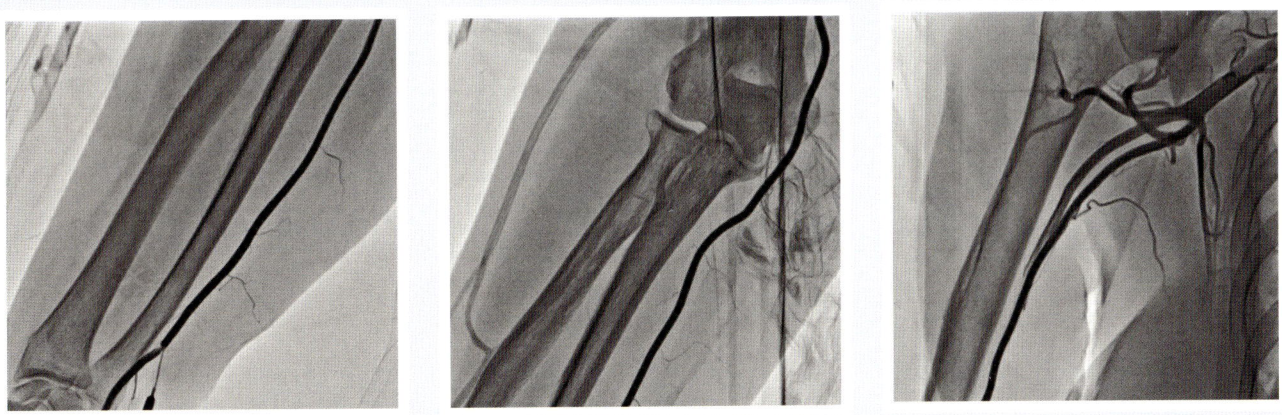

Ulnar artery high take-off from the axillary artery

- Superficial ulnar artery — the patient had easily felt pulsations all the way up the ulnar artery, until the cubital fossa.

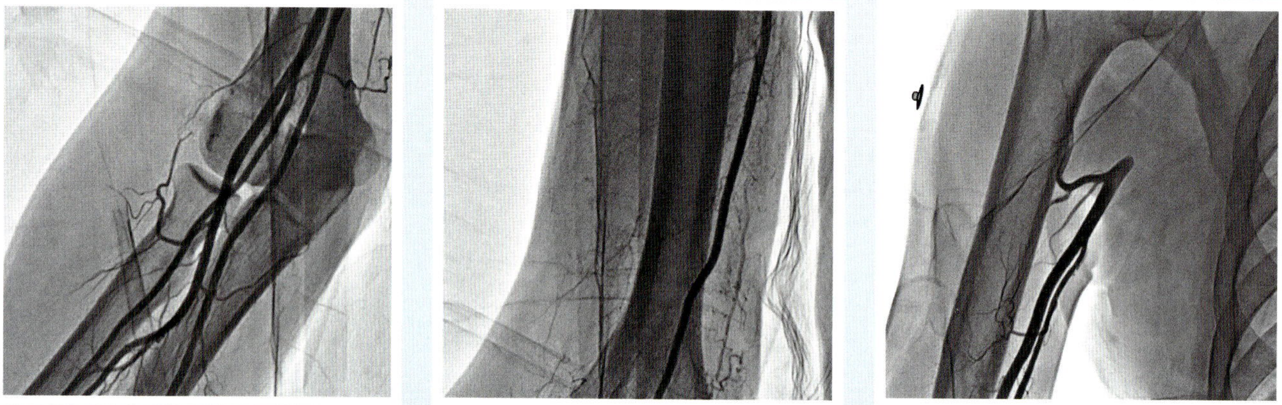

Angiographic images of the superficial ulnar artery

Note: As we can see from the images, the superficial ulnar artery has a high take-off from the axillary artery. The radial artery also has a high take-off from the lower part of the brachial artery. The brachial artery terminates with the interosseous arteries 5 cm distally from the cubital fossa.

- Failed TRA — on the picture, you can see the failed puncture on the radial artery (left arrow) and successful puncture and sheath placed in the ulnar artery. There is a spasm of the ulnar artery at the end of the sheath (right arrow).

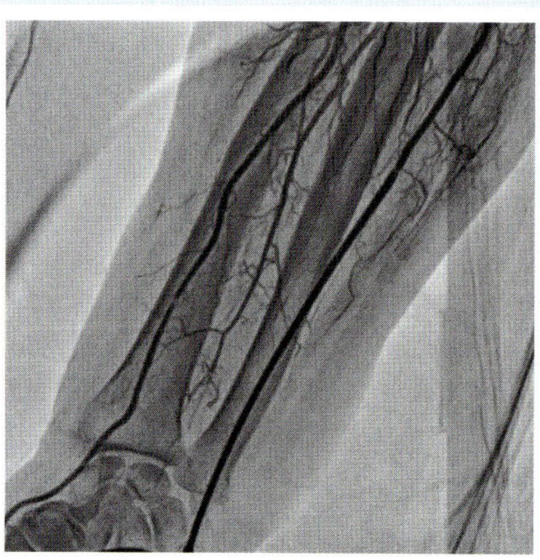

High puncture of the ulnar artery

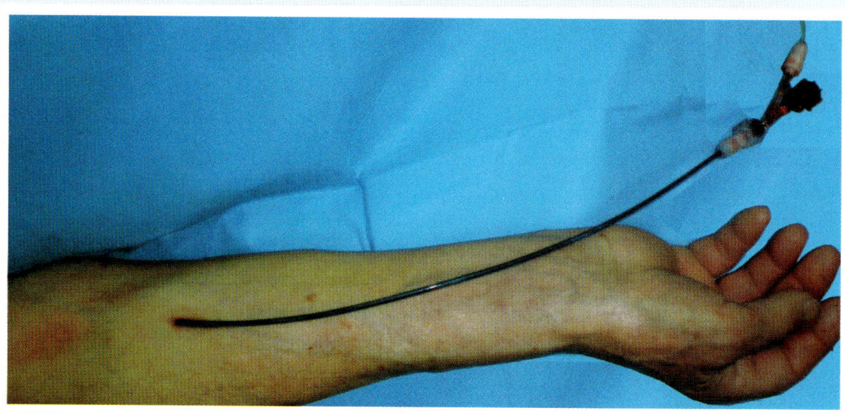

Puncture site in high puncture of ulnar artery, and a catheter placed in the artery

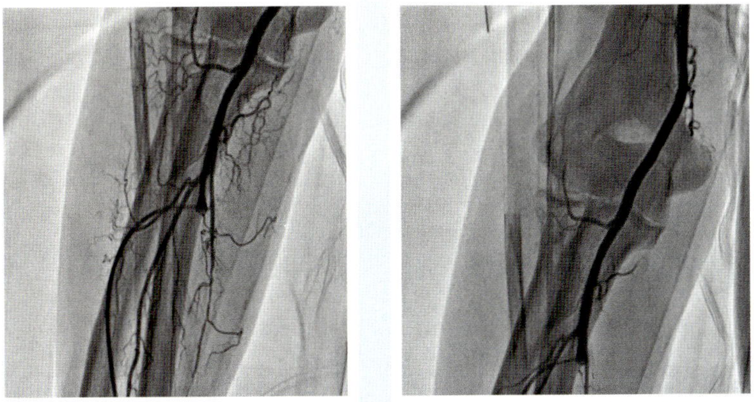

Angiographic image of the high puncture of the ulnar artery in the same patient with high take-off of the radial artery

- We can see that the lower part of the ulnar artery has atherosclerotic changes.
- Complications

Note: Always check the radial artery before placing the sheath. It is easy and doesn't take a lot of time. After puncture, inject contrast into the needle cannula. If the radial artery is small, or there is difficult anatomy, loops or tortuosities, the operator can switch to the ulnar approach and simultaneously avoid damaging the radial artery with the placement of the sheath.

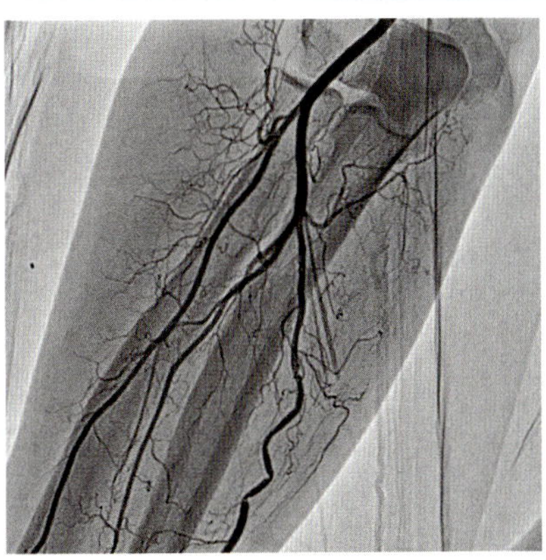

Left ulnar artery canulation with spasm of the ulnar artery

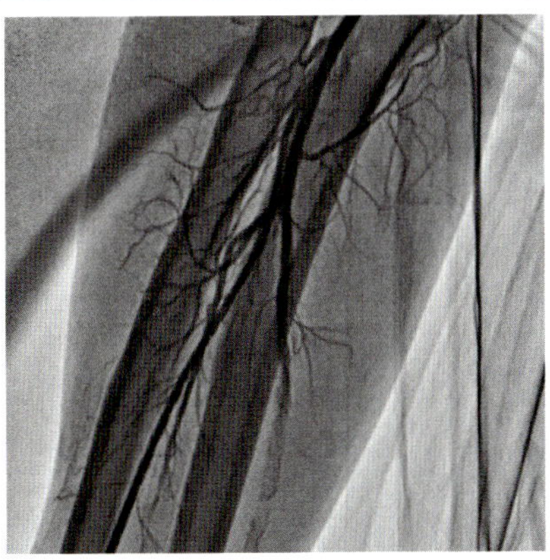

Calcified and atheromatous ulnar artery

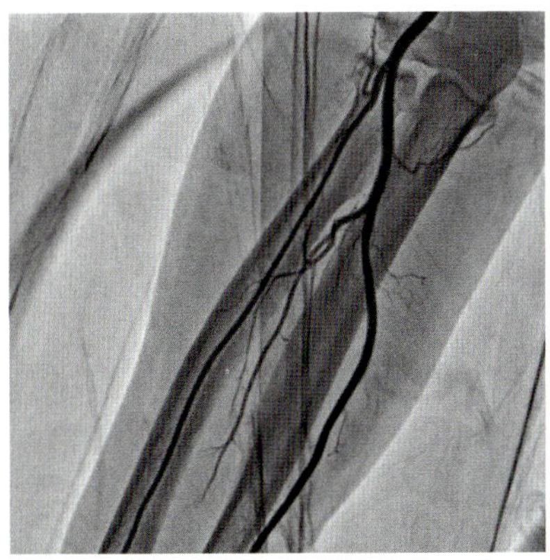

Case with hypoplastic radial artery and regular-sized ulnar artery

- Case reports: the transulnar approach after repetitive transradial interventions

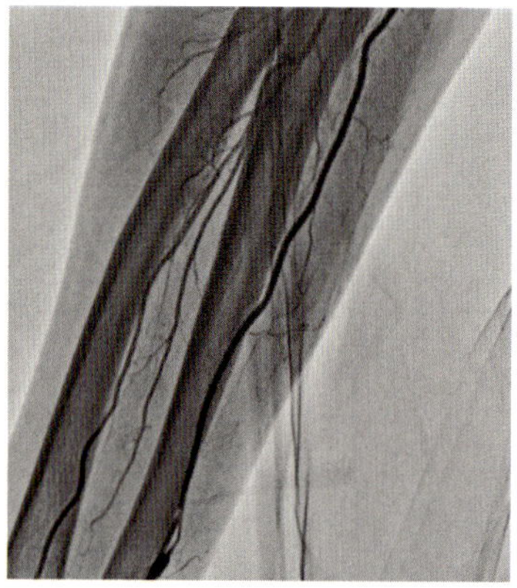

Step 1: After puncture, we check with contrast through the cannula to see if the radial artery is patent, as we can see in this picture.

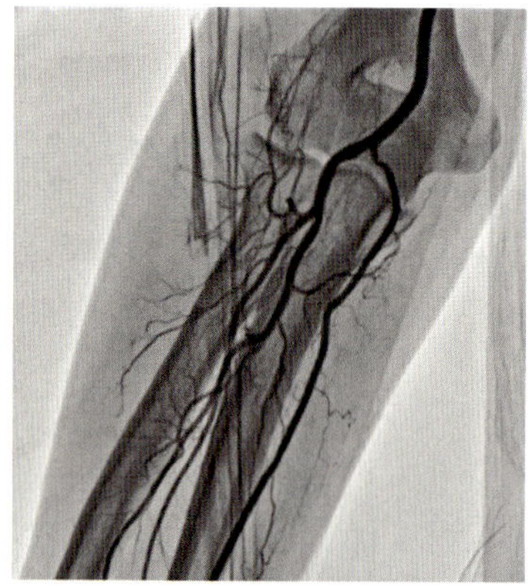

Step 2: We puncture the ulnar artery and insert the sheath.

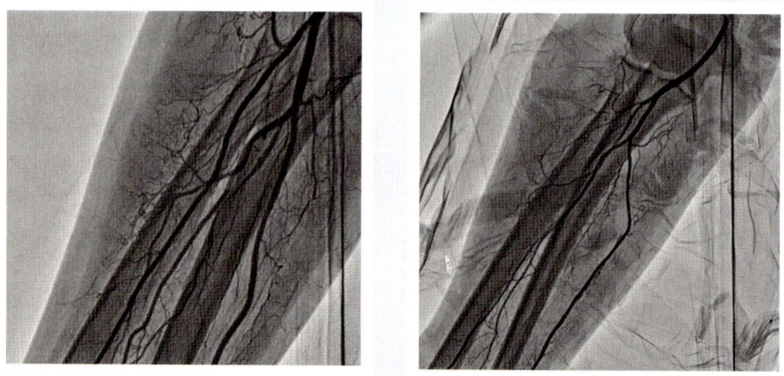

Other cases of a transulnar approach after previous TR interventions are shown.

In these cases, a 5 Fr/90 cm guiding sheath was used.

Note: Each of these procedures resulted in successful carotid artery stenting through the transulnar approach after previous transradial interventions.

- Patient with two interventions, 20 days apart. The first intervention is through the transradial approach, and the second is the transulnar approach.

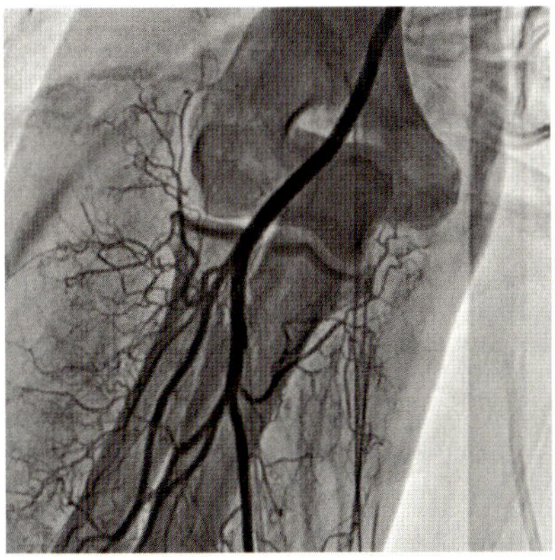

Transradial intervention

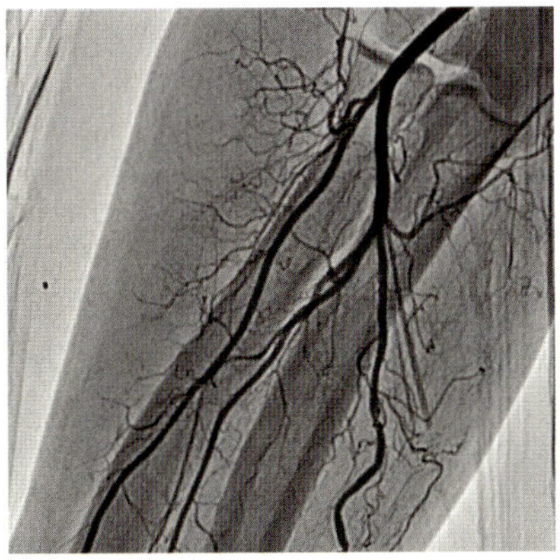

Transulnar intervention

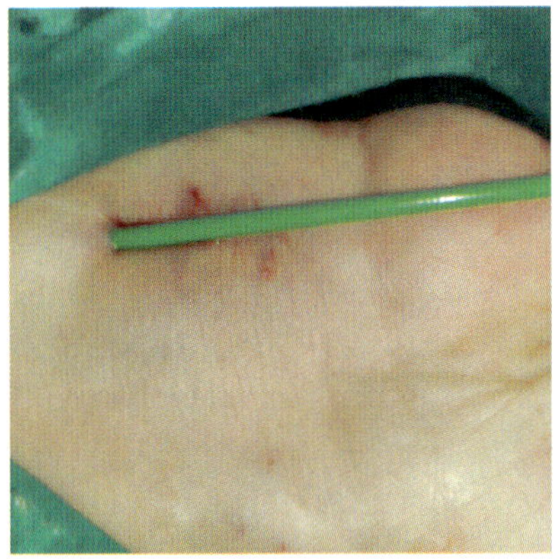

Patient with a 6 Fr guiding sheath in the ulnar artery

Note: At that time, intervention was done on the right internal carotid artery. One month prior, the same patient had had a successful carotid artery stenting of the left internal carotid artery.

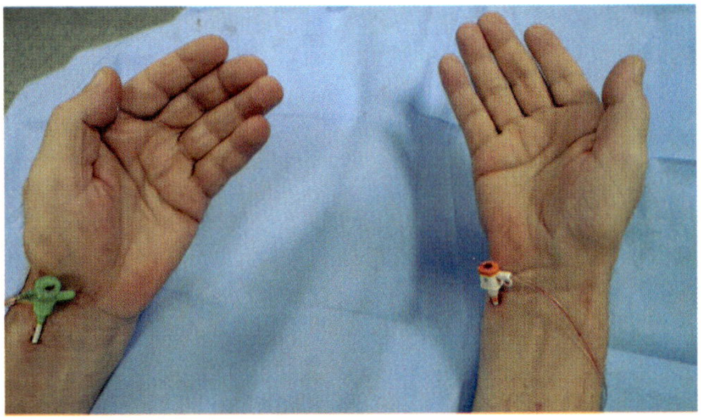

A complex double-vessel PCI CTO procedure was done through the right ulnar access with a 7 Fr guiding catheter and with contralateral injection through a 6 Fr left radial access.

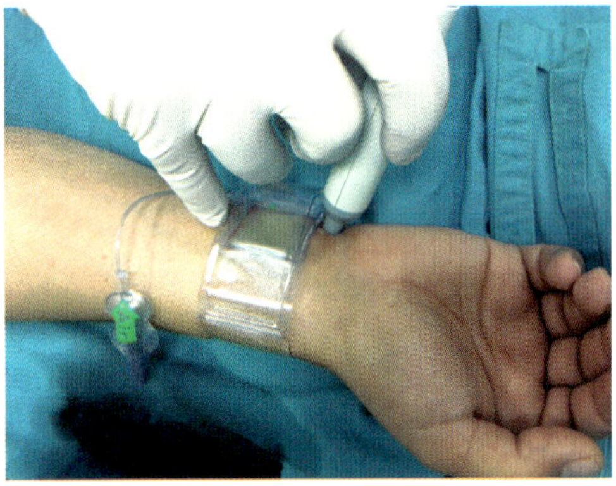

Doppler evaluation of the signal intensity of the ulnar artery after procedure is shown.

Recommended Reading

1. Andrade P, Tebet M, Andrade M, et al. Primary percutaneous coronary intervention through transulnar approach: safety and effectiveness. Arq Bras Cardiol. 2008; 91 (4): e49-52, e41-44.
2. Aptecar E, Dupouy P, Chabane-Chaouch M, et al. Percutaneous transulnar artery approach for diagnostic and therapeutic coronary intervention. J Invasive Cardiol. 2005; 17 (6): 312-317.
3. Aptecar E, Pernes J, Chabane-Chaouch M, et al. Transulnar versus transradial artery approach for coronary angioplasty: the PCVI-CUBA study. Catheter Cardiovasc Interv. 2006; 67 (5): 711-720.
4. Chiam P, Lim V. Transulnar artery approach for percutaneous coronary intervention: an alternative route in a patient with challenging transfemoral access and hypoplastic radial artery. Singapore Med J. 2010; 51 (5): e81-84.
5. Dashkoff N, Dashkoff P, Zizzi J Sr, et al. Ulnar artery cannulation for coronary angiography and percutaneous coronary intervention: case reports and anatomic considerations. Catheter Cardiovasc Interv. 2002; 55 (1): 93-96.
6. Knebel AV, Cardoso CO; Safety and feasibility of transulnar cardiac catheterization. Tex Heart Inst J. 2008;35(3):268-272.
7. Lanspa T, Reyes A, Oldemeyer J, et al. Ulnar artery catheterization with occlusion of corresponding radial artery. Catheter Cardiovasc Interv. 2004; 61 (2): 211-213.
8. Lanspa T, Williams M, Heirigs R. Effectiveness of ulnar artery catheterization after failed attempt to cannulate a radial artery. Am J Cardiol. 2005; 95 (12): 1529-1530.
9. Layton K.F.; Kallmes D.F.; Kaufmann T.J.; Use of the ulnar artery as an alternative access site for cerebral angiography. Am J Neuroradiol. 27:2073-2074.
10. Li Y, Zhou Y, Zhao Y, et al. Safety and efficacy of transulnar approach for coronary angiography and intervention. Chin Med J. 2010; 123 (13): 1774-1779.
11. Limbruno U, Rossini R, De Carlo M, et al. Percutaneous ulnar artery approach for primary coronary angioplasty: safety and feasibility. Catheter Cardiovasc Interv. 2004; 61 (1): 56-59.
12. Lo TS, Nolan J, Fountzopoulos E, Behan M, Butler R, Hetherington SL et al. Radial artery anomaly and its influence on transradial coronary procedural outcome. Heart. 2009;95:410-415.
13. Mc Cormack LJ, Caldwell EW, Anson BJ Brachial and antebrachial patterns. Surg Gynecol Obst. 1953; 96: 43-54.
14. Pancholy S, Coppola J, Patel T, Roke-Thomas M. Prevention of radial artery occlusion-patent hemostasis evaluation trial (PROPHET study): a randomized comparison of traditional versus patency documented hemostasis after transradial catheterization. Catheter Cardiovasc Interv. 2008;72:335- 340.
15. Terashima M, Meguro T, Takeda H, et al. Percutaneous ulnar artery approach for coronary angiography: A preliminary report in nine patients. Catheter Cardiovasc Interv. 2001; 53 (3): 410-414.
16. Vassilev D, Smilkova D, Gil R. Ulnar artery as access site for cardiac catheterization: anatomical considerations. J Interv Cardiol. 2008; 21 (1): 56-60.
17. Vogelzang RL. Arteriography of the hand and wrist. Hand Clin. 1991;7:63-86.
18. Fu X-H, Ma N, Liu J, et al; Feasibility of percutaneous coronary intervention via transulnar artery approach in selected patients with coronary heart disease. Chinese Journal of Cardiology. 2003-05-006.

Same-Day, Outpatient Practice Using the Transradial Approach

25

Olivier F. Bertrand

Introduction

Each year, more than 3 million percutaneous coronary interventions (PCI) are performed worldwide, with almost 50% done in the United States. The current outlook estimates that the largest increases in the future will occur in emerging countries such as Brazil, China and India. While the percentages of patients diagnosed with chronic angina have remained stable, catheterization laboratories have been busier, primarily because more patients are being referred for acute coronary syndromes (ACS). This is because fast-track PCI improves ACS outcomes, compared with medical management, as shown in several multicentre international trials. This increased activity in PCI laboratories creates a significant burden for hospital bed turnover and management.

With the advent of coronary stents and antithrombotic regimens, PCI have also become much safer than a decade ago. Several other medical disciplines have witnessed the development of outpatient programs, a direct consequence of improved care with planned surgical procedures. Laparoscopic cholecystectomy, eye surgery and selected vascular surgeries under general anesthesia are now performed with same-day discharge. Percutaneous procedures in interventional radiology for renal, peripheral arteries or carotid arteries are also often performed as outpatient practice.

Risks Associated With PCI

The two risks related to PCI have evolved since the early days of percutaneous transluminal coronary angioplasty (PTCA). The first can be ascribed as the ischemic risk. After PTCA, sub-acute vessel occlusions occurred in ~5% of the cases within 24 to 48 hours, bringing significant morbidity and mortality risks. In the early days, the ischemic risk was tightly linked to the clinical presentation and to the angiographic appearance of coronary lesions before interventions. Today, the risks of sub-acute vessel occlusion after uncomplicated coronary stenting are negligible whatever the clinical presentation or lesion complexity.

The second risk can be described as the bleeding risk. This risk can be further sub-categorized into access site and non-access site bleeding. With standard femoral access, there is also a ~5% risk of vascular complications, which include large hematoma, retroperitoneal hemorrhage, pseudoaneurysm and A/V fistulas. Vascular complications and bleeding associated with the femoral approach are also closely linked with the use of ≥ 7 Fr sheaths and catheters. Femoral access imposes a period of strict bed rest, which needs to be accounted for in the context of same-day discharge. There is debate regarding the exact benefit of closure devices to reduce the risks of post-PCI vascular complications. The transradial approach has been associated with ~70% reduction in access site bleeding and vascular complications, compared to the standard femoral approach. Therefore, transradial appears an optimal technique to limit the bleeding risk. It is also associated with faster hemostasis, which does not require the patient's lying in bed until hemostasis completion.

In order to establish a safe, effective same-day discharge program, it is vital to be able to reduce and control the risks of post-PCI ischemia and bleeding. In this chapter, we will discuss current experience with same-day discharge PCI and review persisting challenges to wider adoption of a same-day strategy after uncomplicated PCI.

Economic Impact of Same-day Discharge Programs

Modern medicine faces increasing pressure to reduce cost-escalation in patient care and maintain adequate access to state-of-the art technologies for an aging population. Indeed, as patients age, healthcare policy-makers and managers struggle to cope with increasing demand for a limited number of beds, which cannot grow. As acute PCI results have dramatically improved, shorter hospital stays could have a major effect on maximizing limited resources. At least theoretically, resources freed by an outpatient strategy for a selected group of patients could be reallocated to more valuable and cost-effective purposes. In the United States, where ~1 million PCIs are performed annually, related health costs have been estimated around $10 billion. A cost analysis of the EASY trial, which enrolled elective PCI patients and those presenting with ACS, suggested that for every 1,000 PCI patients treated with same-day discharge, cost savings could yield over $1 million in the Canadian system. The same analysis applied in the U.S. system: Elective PCI as outpatient procedures or with moderate risk ACS could produce cost savings between $200 and $500 million per year. This analysis critically depends on the type of reimbursement. In the United States, reimbursement for elective PCI has shifted to Ambulatory Payment Classification billing for outpatient procedures, as opposed to the better-reimbursed Diagnosis Related Group (DRG) system for inpatient procedures. Simply said, this means that U.S. hospitals could actually lose money by transferring PCI activity to outpatient practice instead of the current inpatient routine. Therefore, it is critical that proper selection criteria be validated and that the different players — physician groups, medical societies, taxpayers, hospital managers and insurance providers — interact closely. However, as outpatient practice has expanded in surgical procedures, and even includes those performed under general anesthesia, there is no reason to oppose adoption of an outpatient post-PCI practice in appropriate patients.

Previous Experience

In carefully selected patients and simple coronary lesions, a few investigators reported their experiences with same-day discharge and PTCA in the early 1990s. As discussed previously, expanding this strategy was limited by the inherent risks of sub-acute vessel occlusion after balloon angioplasty without stent implantation. Interestingly, soon after describing the first transradial PCI, Dr. Kiemeneij and his group in The Netherlands described their initial experience with patients pre-treated with Coumadin derivatives before stent implantation. Another group in Europe established that a 4- to 6-hour observation period after uncomplicated PCI was safe before re-transferring patients to their referring centers. Over the next decade, several groups using either radial approach or femoral approach ± closure devices reported their single-center experiences with a few thousand patients. Progressively, these studies included not only patients with stable angina and simple lesions but also patients with unstable angina undergoing multi-lesion procedures. With proper guidance and early follow-up, the majority (~90%) of same-day discharge patients expressed satisfaction and preference for this simplified strategy. Using clinical judgment and a few angiographic criteria, patients at higher risk of ischemic complications can be identified and hospitalized for observation. Furthermore, to include higher-risk patients, some observational studies with bolus-only or abbreviated treatment with platelet glycoprotein IIb/IIIa inhibitors were reported — and did not show higher rates of bleeding or ischemic complications.

At a time when a growing number of ACS patients are being referred to catheterization laboratories, my colleagues and I (in Quebec, Canada) conducted the EASY randomized trial. At that time, we were facing two issues. First, same-day home discharge was occurring very infrequently, and was limited to patients living nearby and presenting for elective PCI. Second, referring centers were reluctant to retransfer post-PCI patients the same day with an ongoing intravenous drip of glycoprotein IIb/IIIa inhibitors.

From 2003 to 2005, we enrolled 1,348 patients representing all who presented to a busy catheterization laboratory (> 3,000 PCIs per year). After transradial diagnostic angiogram, most patients underwent ad hoc coronary stenting and received abciximab bolus. Before the procedures, a few exclusion criteria precluded participation in the trial: STEMI ≤ 72 hours, a history of LV ejection fraction < 30%, intolerance to ASA or thienopyridines, and co-morbidities precluding same-day discharge or contraindication to abciximab. After stent implantation, unsuccessful PCI defined as persisting ≥ grade B dissection, < 3 final TIMI flow, compromised side-branch, or angiographic evidence of thrombus prevented randomization. Patients undergoing uncomplicated transradial coronary stenting were randomized either to same-day home discharge and did not receive additional abciximab or to overnight hospitalization and received the standard 12-hour abciximab infusion. As described previously, patients with periprocedural complications remained in a registry and received the 12-hour abciximab infusion. All lesions had to be stented unless there were daughter branches in bifurcation lesions or in case of re-dilatation for in-stent restenosis. During the study period, 1005 patients were randomized and 343 entered the registry. Thus from this experience, 25% of patients presented some sort of clinical or angiographic complications precluding safe same-day discharge. From the 504 patients randomized patients to home discharge, 88% ultimately left the hospital 4 to 6 hours after PCI completion, as planned. Of note, only one randomized patient presented with vessel occlusion within 2 hours of uneventful PCI and underwent emergency repeat PCI. In a lower-risk population of patients undergoing elective PCI by the femoral approach, another group of investigators in Europe performed a randomized trial. From 2000 to 2003, they randomized 800 patients from 1,453 patients deemed eligible for same-day discharge before PCI. Patients were randomized after a 4-hour observation period; approximately 20% were considered ineligible for same-day discharge at that time, but 77% were effectively discharged the same day.

In both trials, ischemic and bleeding events were similar in the same-day and overnight hospitalization groups. As expected, in the EASY trial, patients excluded from randomization showed significant increases in ischemic and bleeding complications compared to randomized patients during early and late follow-up.

How to Select Patients

At the present, there are no definite criteria for selecting patients eligible for same-day discharge. As discussed, the most important parameter is that patients be undergoing uncomplicated PCI, rather than basing selection strictly on clinical presentation (e.g., stable versus unstable angina, or lesion type or complexity). The U.S. Society of Cardiac Angiography and Intervention published a white paper defining the length of stay after PCI. The authors were extremely conservative, as they proposed limiting outpatient practice to patients with stable angina or silent ischemia presenting with single-vessel disease and normal ejection fraction. The society's procedural criteria include single-vessel PCI with a single stent (< 28 mm) by radial, brachial or femoral access. It says the patient should live within 20 miles of the PCI center with adequate home or emergency medical support. However,

Gilchrist et al have reported that only 15% of patients from their center who were effectively discharged home the day of the PCI would have met this criterion. There is an urgent need for a political and proactive effort from interventional cardiology societies to promote outpatient practice.

From several reports originating from different parts of the world with various health systems, it appears safe to propose same-day discharge to a much larger group of patients. If the logistics can be managed (see below), patients with stable angina or moderate-risk ACS (unstable angina or troponins) can be considered for same-day discharge before diagnostic angiography and possible ad hoc PCI. Initial angiographic appearance or lesion complexity should not preclude eligibility, although the risks of peri-procedural complications can be higher with those types of lesions. In several cases, left ejection fraction is not known before PCI, so this could theoretically be a problem if a patient presents with ischemic event, arrhythmia or ischemia-related complications after uncomplicated PCI. It should be recognized that although many institutions routinely place patients under telemetry surveillance post-PCI, the incidence of severe arrhythmia occurring after uncomplicated PCI is extremely low. Moreover, patients with < 30% ejection fraction are usually equipped with pacemaker defibrillators, which protect them from life-threatening ventricular arrhythmia post-PCI. The use of glycoproteins IIb/IIIa, bolus-only or with abbreviated infusion, has been shown to be non-inferior to the standard bolus followed by several-hour infusion. Although their up-front use has dramatically decreased in recent years, they should not preclude same-day discharge. It should also be emphasized that asymptomatic cardiac biomarkers bumps after uncomplicated PCI should not prevent same-day discharge, as these rises do not predict PCI complications 24 to 48 hours post-PCI.

Choice of Access Site

Same-day discharge has been described after percutenous brachial, femoral and radial access. With femoral access, delayed hemostasis or local complications may prevent early discharge and lead to crossover to overnight hospitalization. Still, if hemostasis has been completed (with or without closure devices), patients can safely be discharged home after uncomplicated PCI. With radial access and current techniques, hemostasis is usually achieved within 2 hours. It is prudent to observe the patient for an additional 2 hours to ensure the patient does not have rebleeding. A minimal observation period of 4 hours after uncomplicated PCI is also recommended to detect any ischemic complications before discharge.

Logistic Aspects

Of course, to propose same-day discharge to patients coming from home is relatively easy. The logistics for hospitalized patients or transferred patients, however, is more complex. Most patients undergo diagnostic angiography and PCI in the same setting sothat immediate results should be shared with referring physician and/or center before discharging patients home directly. In some instances, it might be preferable to simply transfer the patients back to their referring hospitals, where they can be discharged after short medical contact with medical staff to plan the next outpatient visit.

In our facility, we have instituted the positions of liaison-nurse and liaison-pharmacist to assist physicians with logistics. The liaison-nurse meets with the patient in the recovery room immediately after PCI, once informed by the operator that the patient is eligible for same-day discharge. During the observation period, the nurse meets again with the patient and his or her relatives on the ward to explain the results (using a graphic made by the operator) and to make recommendations for radial bandage management for the next 24 to 48 hours. The nurse also provides information regarding secondary prevention and, eventually, provides relevant information regarding rehabilitation, especially after ACS.

If the patient was referred from a different hospital, the nurse phones the referring cardiologist to detail the results and to plan a first follow-up visit 4 to 6 weeks later. For patients coming from far away, she might also find nearby hosting families or book a room in a hostel situated just outside the hospital. For safety, the nurse will do a follow-up phone call the next day, and a direct phone line to the ward opened 24 hours a day is provided to the patient in case of emergency or medical concern. In our experience, the direct line has been very rarely used.

The liaison-pharmacist is devoted to medication management. For outpatients, the pharmacist emphasizes the role of antiplatelet therapies and ensures the patient leaves the hospital with prescriptions for all required medications, including aspirin and clopidogrel or a newer antiplatelet agent. If the patient was referred from another hospital, the pharmacist may contact the patient's pharmacy, the referring center and the operator to ensure that all cardiology medications are updated and that optimal dosages are prescribed before hospital discharge.

Radial Lounges

Dr. Kiemeniej introduced the concept of a radial lounge based on an airport lounge. In this area, pre- and post-PCI patients have relaxing seats, can watch TV, use the Internet, and remain ambulatory before and after PCI. A few years ago, a new 150 m^2 space was built without any beds. This concept ultimately benefits patient management after transradial interventions. In the Czech Republic, Dr. Bernat has developed a smaller sized radial lounge that can accommodate four patients per day. In this institution, they have produced several educational brochures so when patients are scheduled for exams, they can choose in-hospital admission or be managed as outpatients using the lounge. For safety, it is mandatory that a member of the family be able to pick up the patient by late afternoon. In

Radial Lounge at OLVG Amsterdam, The Netherlands (Dr. Kiemeneij)

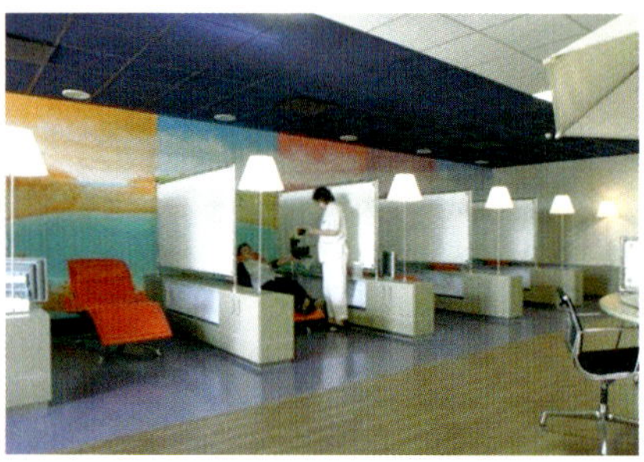

- In this 150 m^2 space, beds have been replaced by comfortable chairs.

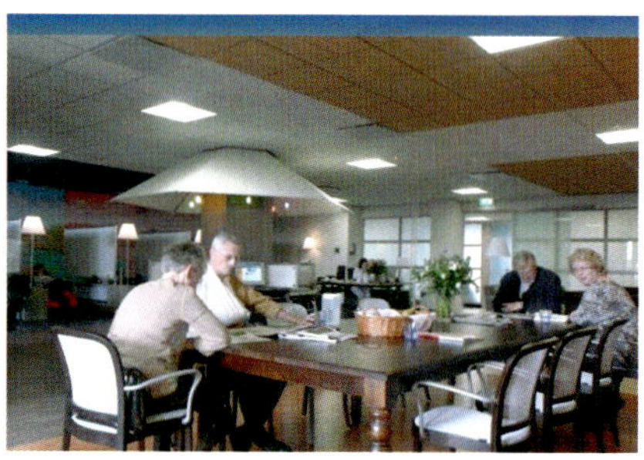

- Patients and families can sit at a table or take advantage of Internet access.

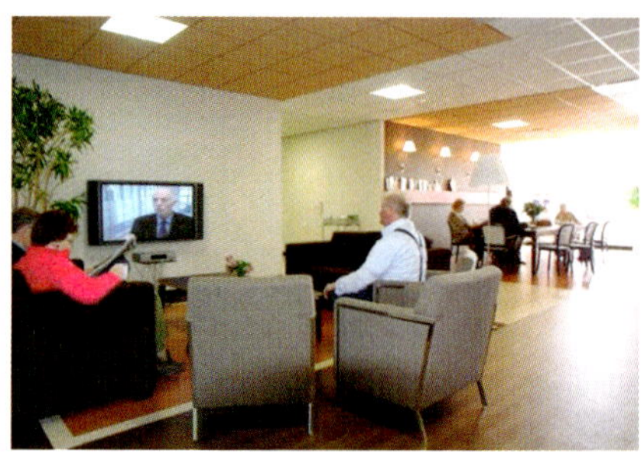

- Patients and families have also access to TV in a relaxed environment.

Radial Lounge at Pilsen Hospital, Czech Republic (Dr I Bernat)

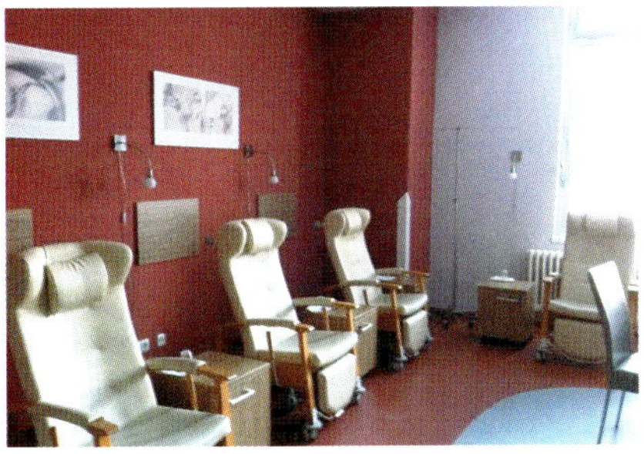

- In this 50 m^2 space, four confortable chairs are available each day.

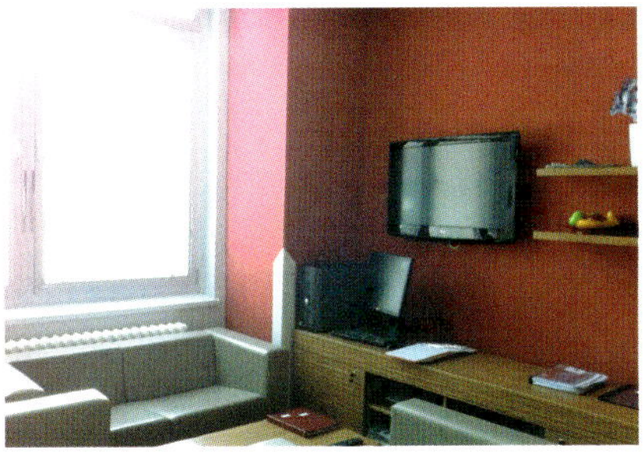

- Patients and families have access to TV and the Internet.

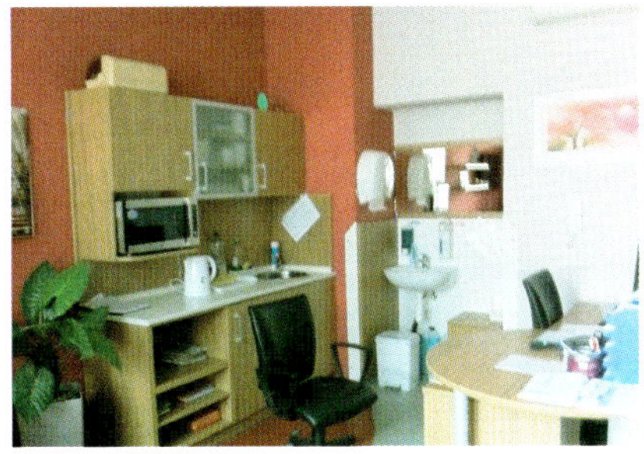

- One nurse is in charge of the four patients and monitors radial access before and after procedures.

the United States, the first radial lounge was recently installed in Saint Joseph's Hospital (Atlanta, GA).

Future and Conclusion

Although same-day discharge after uncomplicated PCI has been described for more than a decade, its practice remains limited around the world. A recent survey among radial operators

Radial Lounge at St Joseph's Hospital, Atlanta, USA (Dr. J.P. Chen)

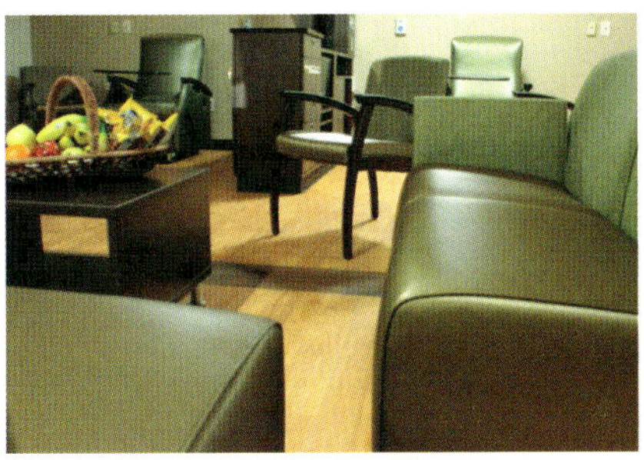

showed that < 50% of radial operators discharge post-PCI patients home the same day, and 45% never transferred patients to their referring hospitals the day of the procedures. In the United States, a recent analysis of a large registry showed that 1.25% of post-PCI patients older than 65 were discharged home the same day. Beyond medical reasons, there are several financial and logistic burdens that need to be removed before the practice could be extended. As with radial adoption, once patients are properly educated and reassured, they simply love to be discharged from the hospital a few hours after PCI — and spend their first night in their regular beds instead of being hospitalized until the next morning.

Recommended Reading

1. Bertrand OF, De Larochelliere R, Rodes-Cabau J, et al. A randomized study comparing same-day home discharge and abciximab bolus only to overnight hospitalization and abciximab bolus and infusion after transradial coronary stent implantation. Circulation. 2006; 114(24): 2636-3643.
2. Bertrand OF, Larose E, De Larochelliere R, et al. Outpatient percutaneous coronary intervention: Ready for prime time? Can J Cardiol. 2007; 23 Suppl B:58B-66B.
3. Chambers CE, Dehmer GJ, Cox DA, et al. Defining the length of stay following percutaneous coronary intervention: an expert consensus document from the Society for Cardiovascular Angiography and Interventions. Endorsed by the American College of Cardiology Foundation. Catheter Cardiovasc Interv. 2009; 73(7):847-858.
4. Gilchrist IC, Nickolaus MJ, Momplaisir T. Same-day transradial outpatient stenting witha 6-hr course of glycoprotein IIb/IIIa receptor blockade: A feasibility study. Cathet Cardiovasc Interv. 2002; 56: 10-13.
5. Gilchrist IC, Rhodes DA, Zimmerman HE. A single center experience with same-day transradial-PCI patients: A contrast with published guidelines. Catheter Cardiovasc Interv. 2011 May 3. [Epub ahead of print]
6. Heyde GS, Koch KT, de Winter RJ, et al. Randomized trial comparing same-day discharge with overnight hospital stay after percutaneous coronary intervention: results of the Elective PCI in Outpatient Study (EPOS). Circulation. 2007; 115(17): 2299-2306.
7. Jabara R, Gadesam R, Pendyala L, et al. Ambulatory discharge after transradial coronary intervention: Preliminary US single-center experience (Same-day TransRadial Intervention and Discharge Evaluation, the STRIDE Study). Am Heart J. 2008; 156(6): 1141-1146.
8. Kiemeneij F, Laarman GJ, Slagboom T, et al. Outpatient Coronary Stent implantation. J Am Coll Cardiol. 1997; 29: 323-327.
9. Rao SV, Kaltenbach LA, Weintraub WS, et al. Prevalence and outcomes of same-day discharge after elective percutaneous coronary intervention among older patients. JAMA. 2011; 306(13):1461-1467.
10. Ziakas A, Kllinke P, Fretz E, et al. Same-day discharge percutaneous coronary interventions: Why do patients prefer it? (Abstract). Am J Cardiol. 2002; 90: 152H.
11. Ziakas AA, Klinke BP, Mildenberger CR, et al. Safety of same-day-discharge radial percutaneous coronary intervention: a retrospective study. Am Heart J. 2003; 146(4): 699-704.